Valvular Heart Disease: Comprehensive Evaluation and Treatment

Second Edition

Books Available in Cardiovascular Clinics Series

Valvular Heart Disease: Comprehensive Evaluation and Treatment

William S. Frankl, M.D. / Editor

Professor of Medicine
Regional Director of Cardiovascular Programs
Medical College Hospitals
The Medical College of Pennsylvania
Philadelphia, Pennsylvania

Albert N. Brest, M.D. / Editor

James C. Wilson Professor of Medicine
Jefferson Medical College
Philadelphia, Pennsylvania

CARDIOVASCULAR CLINICS
Albert N. Brest, M.D. / Editor-in-Chief

 F. A. DAVIS COMPANY • Philadelphia

Printed in the United States of America

Last digit indicates print number: 10 9 8 7 6 5 4 3 2 1

acquisitions editor: Robert H. Craven
production editor: Gail Shapiro

As new scientific information becomes available through basic and clinical research, recommended treatments and drug therapies undergo changes. The author(s) and publisher have done everything possible to make this book accurate, up to date, and in accord with accepted standards at the time of publication. The authors, editors, and publisher are not responsible for errors or omissions or for consequences from application of the book, and make no warranty, expressed or implied, in regard to the contents of the book. Any practice described in this book should be applied by the reader in accordance with professional standards of care used in regard to the unique circumstances that may apply in each situation. The reader is advised always to check product information (package inserts) for changes and new information regarding dose and contraindications before administering any drug. Caution is especially urged when using new or infrequently ordered drugs.

Library of Congress Cataloging in Publication Data

Cardiovascular clinics.
   Philadelphia, F. A. Davis, 1969–
      v. ill. 27 cm.
      Editor: v. 1- A. N. Brest.
      Key title: Cardiovascular clinics, ISSN 0069-0384
      1. Cardiovascular system—Diseases—Collected works   I. Brest,
Albert N., ed.
      [DNLM: w1 CA77N]
   RC681.A1C27   6.6.1   70-6558
   ISBN 0-8036-3792 6   MARC-S

Preface

The success of our previous volume entitled *Valvular Heart Disease: Comprehensive Evaluation and Management* prompted us to assess the need for an update of the material given the many conceptual and technological advances since 1986.

In the past several years, we have seen a resurgence of rheumatic fever and the likelihood that rheumatic valvulitis will be encountered in increasing numbers in the future. The early management of rheumatic fever will need to be reassessed in light of this resurgence as well as the early evaluation of valvular disease when it appears.

Color-flow Doppler evaluation of cardiac valves and the entirely new procedure, transesophageal echocardiography, have in many ways revolutionized the diagnostic approach to valvular heart disease. Indeed, some workers in the field have even suggested that cardiac catheterization might not be required in many cases because of the high degree of accuracy of these techniques (although the editors would dispute that concept). The new technique of cardiac magnetic resonance imaging, although largely investigational, appears to hold out another sophisticated and noninvasive method for assessing valvular disease.

The high incidence of complications surrounding mitral valve and tricuspid valve replacement has led to the concept of valvular reconstruction, which appears to maintain the integrity of the supporting valvular apparatus that could not be attained with the use of a prosthesis.

Balloon valvuloplasty has provided a new and exciting technique in the management of aortic stenosis and mitral stenosis. Although aortic balloon valvuloplasty has been a disappointment as a long-term method of management, it has been a great help as a "bridge" to aortic valve replacement especially in the elderly who present in congestive heart failure or who are deemed to be at high risk until medically stabilized. On the other hand, mitral valve balloon valvuloplasty has been quite successful in the management of mitral stenosis, especially in those without heavily calcified valves.

The approach to valvular replacement in the elderly has become increasingly complicated and challenging given the advanced age and relatively good physiologic state of our patients who require evaluation and often replacement of severely stenosed aortic valves. Special care in the preoperative evaluation, intraoperative techniques and postoperative management of these patients is clearly required and has become a specialized activity for many cardiologists and cardiac surgeons.

At a time when new diagnostic and surgical procedures have become available, so have new pharmacologic agents that have made the medical management of valvular disease more feasible as well. Thus, surgery can often be delayed and the patient managed medically, postponing the eventual time that one disease (the native diseased valve) is replaced by a new disease (the prosthetic valve). Finally, with the appearance of resistant organisms, new and highly potent antibiotics, and an increasing threat of prosthetic valve endocarditis, the entire subject of infective endocarditis requires careful reconsideration.

We are still faced with the dilemma that was cited in the 1986 volume. Even with these very sophisticated diagnostic, pharmacologic, interventional, and surgical techniques have we really affected the long-term prognosis of patients with valvular heart disease? Have we changed the natural history of valvular heart disease in a fashion that has improved the quality of life for our patients?

In producing this update, we have once again called on a distinguished group of physicians and surgeons who have written "state-of-the-art" chapters covering a wide and complex field. As in our previous volume, there is some overlap in subject matter among the various authors but we believe that this was necessary so that each chapter could stand on its own, providing a truly comprehensive overview to the reader. We are, as always, grateful to the contributing authors and we hope that you, the reader, will find this volume both useful and stimulating.

William S. Frankl, M.D.
Albert N. Brest, M.D.

Editor's Commentary

The first issue of CARDIOVASCULAR CLINICS appeared in 1969. This book, the 67th in the series, will be the finale.

Over the years, CARDIOVASCULAR CLINICS has examined virtually all aspects of cardiovascular diseases—not only the various heart conditions but essentially all of the clinical vascular disorders as well.

In such a long series, there are an almost endless number of individuals who have contributed to its success. About one thousand individual physicians and scientists, the bulk of whom are acknowledged academic and clinical leaders, have written superb individual chapters, and guest editors have generously guided the formulation of various books. I am forever indebted to all of them because it is their efforts in particular that have made this series successful. Of course, only the publisher can take the material we provide and, in turn, produce the books we read. More people than I know have labored long and hard at F. A. Davis Company and the finished product has been exemplary. I extend my deepest and sincerest gratitude to all of those who have toiled in the publication of these books. Additionally, one person stands out beyond all others with regard to the founding and nurturing of CARDIOVASCULAR CLINICS, namely Robert Craven, Sr. Bob Craven and I conceived the idea of this book series and he made it possible. He deserves full recognition for whatever success has been achieved.

As for myself, the countless hours spent on organization, editing of all the manuscripts, galleys, and proofs have been rewarded by the intellectual stimulation provided by the superb content of each and every chapter. In this regard, I received far more than I gave.

Finally, I am grateful to those who subscribed to this series. Hopefully the contents had a positive impact on their medical lives.

Albert N. Brest, M.D.
Editor-in-Chief

Contributors

Stanley K. Brockman, M.D.
Professor and Chairman
Department of Cardiothoracic Surgery
Hahnemann University Hospital
Philadelphia, Pennsylvania

Bruce M. Brown, M.D.
Director of Cardiology
Tobey Hospital
Wareham, Massachusetts

Daniel J. Burge, M.D.
Clinical Instructor in Medicine
Division of Clinical Immunology/Rheumatology
Hahnemann University
Philadelphia, Pennsylvania

Krishnaswamy Chandrasekaran, M.D.
Associate Professor of Medicine
Director, Cardiac Ultrasound Laboratory
Likoff Cardiovascular Institute
Hahnemann University Hospital
Philadelphia, Pennsylvania

Adnan Cobanoglu, M.D.
Professor of Surgery
Chief, Division of Cardiopulmonary Surgery
Director, Heart and Lung Transplantation Programs
The Oregon Health Sciences University
Portland, Oregon

Lawrence S. Cohen, M.D.
The Ebenezer K. Hunt Professor of Medicine
Deputy Dean
Yale University School of Medicine
New Haven, Connecticut

Raphael J. DeHoratius, M.D.
Professor of Medicine
Associate Director for Clinical Services
Division of Rheumatology
Jefferson Medical College
Philadelphia, Pennsylvania

Leonard S. Dreifus, M.D.
Professor of Medicine
Director, Division of Cardiovascular Diseases
Hahnemann University
Philadelphia, Pennsylvania

Mark A. Goldstein, M.D.
Division of Cardiovascular Diseases
Hahnemann University
Philadelphia, Pennsylvania

Richard J. Gray. M.D.
Director, Surgical Cardiology
Professor of Medicine
UCLA School of Medicine
Los Angeles, California

Richard H. Helfant, M.D., F.A.C.C.
Professor of Medicine
UCLA School of Medicine
Los Angeles, California

Irving M. Herling, M.D.
Associate Professor of Medicine
University of Pennsylvania School of Medicine
Consultant Cardiologist
University of Pennsylvania Medical Center
Philadelphia, Pennsylvania

Alfred Ioli
Chief Research Technician
Albert Einstein Medical Center
Philadelphia, Pennsylvania

Larry E. Jacobs, M.D.
Director, Echo-Doppler Laboratory
Albert Einstein Medical Center
Assistant Professor of Medicine
Temple University School of Medicine
Philadephia, Pennsylvania

Dean G. Karalis, M.D., F.A.C.C.
Assistant Professor of Medicine
Likoff Cardiovascular Institute
Hahnemann University Hospital
Philadelphia, Pennsylvania

Robert B. Karp, M.D.
Chief of Cardiac Surgery
Professor of Surgery
The University of Chicago Medical Center
Chicago, Illinois

Daniel M. Kolansky, M.D.
Assistant Professor of Medicine
University of Pennsylvania School of Medicine
Philadelphia, Pennsylvania

Morris N. Kotler, M.D.
Chief of Cardiology
Albert Einstein Medical Center
Professor of Medicine
Temple University School of Medicine
Philadelphia, Pennsylvania

Robert M. MacMillan, M.D.
Director, Cardiac Magnetic Resonance Imaging
Hahnemann University
Philadelphia, Pennsylvania

Kevin P. Marzo, M.D.
Assistant Professor of Medicine
State University of New York at Stony Brook
School of Medicine
Interventional Cardiologist
Winthrop University Hospital
Mineola, New York

Colin B. Meyerowitz, M.D.
Cardiology Division
Albert Einstein Medical Center
Philadelphia, Pennsylvania

Eric L. Michelson, M.D.
Professor of Medicine
Hahnemann University
Philadelphia, Pennsylvania

Abdolghader Molavi, M.D.
Associate Professor of Medicine
Director, Division of Infectious Diseases
Hahnemann University School of Medicine
Philadelphia, Pennsylvania

Gary Y. Ott, M.D.
Assistant Professor of Surgery
The Oregon Health Sciences University
Portland, Oregon

Leo A. Podolsky, M.D.
Cardiology Division
Albert Einstein Medical Center
Philadelphia, Pennsylvania

William C. Roberts, M.D.
Chief, Pathology Branch
National Heart, Lung and Blood Institute
National Institutes of Health
Bethesda, Maryland

Clinical Professor of Pathology
and Medicine
Georgetown University
Washington, DC

John J. Ross, Jr., R.C.P.T.
Administrative Director
Cardiac Ultrasound Laboratory
Likoff Cardiovascular Institute
Hahnemann University Hospital
Philadelphia, Pennsylvania

Mark E. Sand, M.D.
Assistant Professor of Surgery
University of Chicago Medical Center
Chicago, Illinois

Michael D. Strong, III, M.D.
Associate Professor
Department of Cardiothoracic Surgery
Hahnemann University Hospital
Philadelphia, Pennsylvania

Zoltan G. Turi, M.D.
Associate Professor of Medicine
Wayne State University School of Medicine
Director, Cardiac Catheterization Laboratory
Harper Hospital
Detroit, Michigan

Contents

PART 1

Etiologic Considerations

CHAPTER 1

Acute Rheumatic Fever

Daniel J. Burge, M.D.
Raphael J. DeHoratius, M.D.

During recent years, rheumatic fever has received much attention in the scientific community as demonstrated by multiple reviews.[1-9] This renewed interest was sparked by reports of the resurgence of rheumatic fever across the country in the mid-1980s.[10-16] Clinicians in the first half of this century were all too familiar with the devastating outcome of rheumatic carditis. Younger clinicians, though unfamiliar with rheumatic fever, still encounter the long-term effects of rheumatic heart disease. Approximately 15 million to 20 million new cases of rheumatic fever occur each year in Third World countries where rheumatic heart disease is currently the leading cause of heart disease.[17]

Although the etiologic agent for acute rheumatic fever is known to be the group A β-hemolytic streptococcus, researchers still do not have a clear understanding of the precise pathogenesis of this disease. The pathogenesis is obscured by the fact that streptococci have a multitude of cellular and extracellular proteins, structures, and toxins. With many of these producing ill effects in humans, discerning which are involved is difficult. Making our understanding additionally difficult is the latency period of several weeks between infection and development of acute rheumatic fever. This delay denies the opportunity to investigate the early processes involved with this disease. Prospective studies would not only be unethical but would also require enormous numbers of volunteers because of the low incidence of rheumatic fever following group A β-hemolytic streptococcal infection. The predisposing factors allowing one patient to develop rheumatic fever while another does not have been both puzzling and intriguing to clinicians. Uncovering these mechanisms is the interest of many investigators and will hopefully yield a treatment that will benefit many. Unfortunately, without an animal model for this disease, the study has been slow and tedious.

HISTORIC AND EPIDEMIOLOGIC PERSPECTIVE

HISTORIC PERSPECTIVE

In the late nineteenth century, the reports of acute rheumatic fever worldwide were numerous.[8] In the United States, Philadelphia, New York, and Boston hos-

3

pitals reported thousands of cases during 15- to 25-year periods. Convalescent hospitals were set up solely for recovering victims of the disease. In the early 1900s, incidence reports in the United States were sparse and were not duplicated to note trends. However, Denmark had set up a registry in the late 1800s and these data seem to illustrate what was occurring in most of the industrialized world.[9,18] At the turn of the century, Denmark had an annual incidence of rheumatic fever that was as high as 250 per 100,000 people.[18] By 1930, the incidence had decreased to approximately 100 cases per 100,000. This decline continued until World War II at which time there was a brief rise in incidence. The increase at this time was largely due to involvement of the military recruits. The decline was more precipitous after the war. In 1962, the annual incidence of rheumatic fever had diminished to 12 per 100,000,[18] and by 1983, the incidence was reported at 0.3 cases per 100,000 inhabitants.[19] In Turkey,[20] the incidence of rheumatic heart disease was halved in a 10-year period from 1976 to 1986. The prevalence fell from 1% to 0.56%.

The United States had problems similar to Denmark during World War II. From 1943 to 1945, the incidence of rheumatic fever in army personnel in the northeastern United States was 388/100,000.[8] However, like Denmark, the postwar era was more favorable in the United States. In San Francisco, 116 cases were reported in 1946. By 1955, the number had dropped to 29.[21] A 20-year study in Chicago[22] confirmed 200 to 400 cases a year from 1961 to 1971, which subsequently declined steadily to the end of the surveillance period in 1977 when less than 20 cases were reported. Gordis[23] reported rates of disease involving school-age children in an inner city community in the 1960s to be 21/100,000.[23] Many reports from the late 1970s and 1980s revealed very low incidences of rheumatic fever, ranging from 0.23 to 1.14 per 100,000 school-age children.[11,24-27]

By the mid-1980s, many clinicians were feeling optimistic that rheumatic fever would soon be a thing of the past. However, the observations of "epidemics" of rheumatic fever in multiple sites around the country stifled these hopes for at least a while longer. Study of the epidemiology of rheumatic fever, the reasons for its decline, and the features of the recent epidemics may aid our understanding of the disease, its pathogenetic processes, and its status in the current medical community.

EPIDEMIOLOGY

In the past, researchers believed that the epidemiology of acute rheumatic fever was simply that of the group A β-hemolytic streptococcus. However, the persistent high frequency of streptococcal pharyngitis[1] and the considerably lower incidence of rheumatic fever today indicate that this is obviously an oversimplification. Environmental factors, which are generally believed to be risk factors for streptococcal pharyngitis and still of importance in the epidemiology of rheumatic fever, may play less of a role than previously imagined. The virulence and strain of the organism and the role of the host are important but unclear ingredients.

Environmental Factors

Environmental factors have long been credited for the high incidence of rheumatic fever. The majority of affected people were of lower socioeconomic backgrounds and primarily minorities.[6,23] Reasons proposed have been overcrowding, poor nutrition, and poor hygiene. Streptococcal infections, which are spread by droplets of secretions, can be transmitted more easily in this kind of environment. Furthermore, this environment may promote a more virulent organism. Virulence of the organism may be enhanced when spread rapidly from host to host.[28]

Demographics can be illustrated by work done in Turkey.[20] Two schools were studied in 1976. A history of rheumatic fever was found in 5.7% of the students at the school serving the lower socioeconomic group whereas only 2.2% of the economically more advantaged group had a history of the disease. The prevalence of rheumatic heart disease was 1% and 0.2%, respectively.

Military populations are another example of increased risk in an overcrowded situation. Quinn[8] compiled data on the incidence of rheumatic fever and rheumatic heart disease. The military has been afflicted with high rates of disease for more than a century. Reports of British troops in the early 1900s state an annual incidence of up to 1%. Of the American soldiers in the Civil War, 0.65% of the Union troops and 0.9% of the Confederate troops were affected annually.

Rheumatic fever most commonly strikes the school-aged child in whom social contact is high, but involvement of adults is not rare. Rheumatic fever also tends to occur more in winter and spring.[8]

The Role of the Group A β-hemolytic Streptococcus

Although the group A β-hemolytic streptococcus has been shown to be the etiologic agent, the pathogenesis remains a mystery. The epidemiologic data have thus become a riddle that each investigator hopes to solve, unveiling the truths that have so long eluded us. Each hypothesis is scrutinized and challenged to fit the lessons of history.

The military was a common place for rheumatic fever epidemics in the past.[8] Rammelkamp[29] described epidemics in the military population during World War II. These epidemics provide the most dependable statistics on the natural evolution of rheumatic fever following untreated streptococcal pharyngitis. During these epidemics, these men developed rheumatic fever at a rate of approximately 3% following exudative streptococcal pharyngitis. Siegel and coworkers[30] reported a much lower rate in the sporadic cases in a pediatric population. The difference in the attack rates raised the question of a qualitative difference in the organism.

Virulence of the organism was initially thought to be the important factor involved in producing acute rheumatic fever. Although at least two distinct parts of the streptococcus have been implicated in the virulence of the organism, many feel that the hyaluronic capsule may play the more important role. The hyaluronic capsule has been shown to help resist phagocytosis and has been known to be doing so for nearly half a century.[31] The virulent richly encapsulated organism appears as a mucoid colony on culture plate. These mucoid colonies have been involved in a high percentage of epidemics.[32] The M protein is also most certainly involved in virulence. Whitnack and Beachey[33] demonstrated that the M protein was involved in opsonization. However, virulence alone cannot be the determining factor for rheumatic fever. Highly virulent strains resulting in severe pharyngitis have been noted for the absence of sequelae. Very mild strains have been observed to cause severe complications.

A major consideration leading to the idea of rheumatogenic strains of group A streptococci is the fact that the two nonsuppurative sequelae, acute rheumatic fever and poststreptococcal glomerulonephritis, rarely, if ever, occur together.[34] Also, rheumatic fever occurs only following an upper respiratory infection of group

A streptococci whereas glomerulonephritis can occur following either a skin infection or a pharyngeal infection. Studies in the preantibiotic era reveal epidemics of group A streptococci that failed to cause rheumatic fever even in high-risk patients.[35] Majeed and associates[36] studied populations with each nonsuppurative sequela and noted that the serotypes were different. Studies of the particular M serotypes using monoclonal antibodies and rheumatic fever sera have shown that the strains associated with rheumatic fever epidemiologically also share antigenic epitopes with human end-organ tissue. Bessen and colleagues[37] described a common domain on the M protein that is shared by most of the serotypes associated with rheumatic fever. Each of these pieces of information points to the conclusion that some types are more likely to cause rheumatic sequelae whereas others are more likely to produce renal effects. M types that have been associated with epidemics include types 5, 18, 24, 3, 14, 19, 6, 27, and 29.[3] The most prevalent endemic serotypes are 12, 2, and 4. With these missing from the "rheumatogenic" list, one is led to believe that these very common strains are not often, if ever, involved in acute rheumatic fever.

Bisno,[4] in an editorial, cites several case reports of rheumatic fever with concomitant glomerulonephritis, both overt and subclinical. This has aided the concept that a few of these strains may have the potential to produce rheumatic and renal disease. The work of Kraus and coworkers[38] on the M protein of one such strain has demonstrated common antigenic determinants with kidney and heart tissue.

The Host

Several observations have been made concerning the host and rheumatic fever. First, the degree of immune response has been positively associated with risk of rheumatic fever. Second, genetic factors have long been considered to be involved in susceptibility to rheumatic fever.

HOST ANTIBODY RESPONSE. Following an acute streptococcal infection, certain patients tend to mount much higher antibody responses than others. Those with greater immunologic responses, as typically measured with antistreptolysin, anti-DNAase B, and antihyaluronidase, are statistically more likely to develop acute rheumatic fever when compared with those who mount a lesser response. Researchers postulate that this hyperresponive state is necessary for the initiation of the pathologic mechanisms.

GENETICS. Genetic factors have been suspected since the late 1800s because of apparent clustering within families. A considerable amount of investigation has evaluated the genetic contribution to the risk of disease. Twin studies have shown a low level of concordance among monozygotic twins.[39] Studies on the Maoris in New Zealand, a group with an inordinately high incidence of rheumatic fever, revealed no HLA-A or HLA-B antigen association.[40] In 1979, Patarroyo and colleagues[41] discovered an antibody (labeled 883) in a patient that marked cells in 71% to 75% of rheumatic fever patients both in New York and Bogotá, Colombia. This sparked excitement about a universal marker. This antibody marked lymphocytes in only 20% of controls and was not HLA-associated.

In 1986, Ayoub and associates[42] searched for different associations with different ethnic groups. They demonstrated an association of HLA-DR2 in blacks and HLA-DR4 in whites with acute rheumatic fever.[42] About that same time, Zabriskie and associates[43] developed a monoclonal antibody that had similar characteristics to Patarroyo's 883. It detected an alloantigen in 59% to 76% of 84 rheumatic patients, including all but one of the 883-positive patients. This antibody also was tested on cells from other parts of the world, and 77% of 39 acute rheumatic fever patients from New Mexico and 60% of 22 patients from India were tested positive. Controls were positive at a rate of 16% to 18%. A second monoclonal antibody detected an alloantigen in five of the seven 883-negative patients cells from the previous studies. Combined, 92% of all rheumatic fever patients tested positive with one of the two antibodies. This suggested diallelic genetic markers for susceptibility.

Khanna and coworkers[44] used another monoclonal antibody, D8/17, that seemed to recognize rheumatic fever patients who were either 883-positive or 883-negative. Nearly 99% of patients were positive for an antigen that bound this antibody. About 14% of controls were positive. The test seemed to have quantitative importance as well. A third of the B cells were positively labeled in rheumatic fever patients whereas their siblings and parents had only about 12% to 15% of their cells marked. Control cells had only 5% to 7% labeled. Taneja and colleagues[45] used D8/17 in India where only 63% of the patients were positive for this marker. Interestingly, these D8/17-positive patients had an assciation with HLA-DQ2.

The role of genetics in the pathogenesis of rheumatic fever is still not clear. Rich and associates,[46] using complex segregation analysis, rejected the null hypothesis of no gene involved. Undoubtedly, a marker will be found that clearly enables us to know who is at high risk for this disease.

THE DECLINE OF RHEUMATIC FEVER

As the decline of rheumatic fever began before the advent of antibiotics, the decrease in disease was generally attributed to improvement in social circumstances. Less crowding and better sanitation were major reasons for this early decline. A second factor that undoubtedly has played a role in the decline of the morbidity and mortality of this disease is penicillin.

In military recruiting centers, many young men are brought together in crowded living conditions with a high turnover of personnel, giving ample opportunity for rapid spread of infection from individual to individual. Because rheumatic fever in this population was a serious problem in the 1950s, administration of intramuscular benzathine penicillin G was given to incoming recruits. This prophylaxis was widely used in armed forces training centers by the end of the next decade,[47] and the incidence of rheumatic fever among recruits decreased to <1/100,000.

Massell and others[48] demonstrate that although the decline in disease began before the discovery of penicillin, this drug had an impact on the rate of decline. The institution of routine antibiotics to prevent recurrence of rheumatic fever began shortly after World War II.[1] Although secondary prevention was relatively quickly received, it took 20 years of public and professional education to increase the awareness that sore throats could lead to heart disease.[1] This leads us to a third important factor in the decline in rheumatic fever, the availability of medical care.

Inasmuch as most of the people affected by rheumatic fever were of low socioeconomic background, access to medical care was likely a major roadblock to prevention in a large percentage of cases. With few resources available, the poor were not likely to seek medical care for a sore throat, which itself was self-limited. Gordis[23,27,49] addressed this problem with a series of studies in an inner-city region

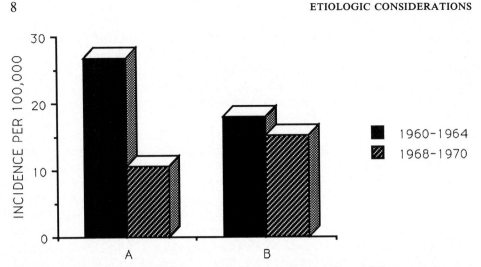

Figure 1-1. Effect of available medical care on incidence of rheumatic fever. (*A*) Represents the population located in the region that was served by the public health care system. This system was initiated in 1965. (*B*) Represents the population of a nearby community that was not eligible for the public health care.

of Baltimore. From 1960 to 1964, he studied several populations in the inner city. In the mid-1960s, a public health center was set up in one of the poor communities. With more available care, Gordis re-evaluated the populations from 1968 to 1970. The area served by the public health center had a decline in incidence in 5- to 14-year-old children from 26.8/100,000 to 10.6/100,000. A nearby community without access to the public health center had an incidence of 18.1/100,000 in the earlier survey and an incidence of 15.3/100,000 in the latter period (Fig. 1-1). An

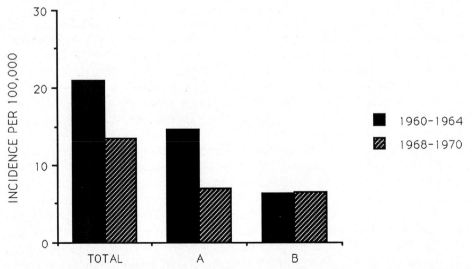

Figure 1-2. Symptomatic vs. asymptomatic pharyngitis preceding acute rheumatic fever. Incidence of rheumatic fever declined in Baltimore with the institution of a public health care system (TOTAL). (*A*) As expected, the cases that presented after clinically evident pharyngitis declined dramatically with readily available health care, whereas (*B*) the incidence of rheumatic fever after an asymptomatic infection was unchanged. In 1968 to 1970, a much higher percentage of cases followed asymptomatic infections.

Table 1–1. Reported Cases
of Rheumatic Fever*

Dates	Cases
1956–1959†	26,163
1960–1964	42,491
1965–1969	20,154
1970–1974	13,625
1975–1979	7,937
1980–1984	1,038
1985–1989	681

*Data from the Centers for Disease Control. Rheumatic fever is not a reportable disease and the number of actual cases is likely highly underrepresented. Additionally, the reporting habits likely have varied and therefore trends may be skewed accordingly.
†This period includes only 4 years.

interesting observation was that the incidence of rheumatic fever following clinically evident pharyngitis was cut in half (14.6/100,000 to 7.0/100,000) whereas the incidence of disease without an apparent antecedent infection was unaffected (6.3/100,000 to 6.5/100,000) (Fig. 1–2). This indicates that the decrease in incidence was due to intervention of clinical infections in the population with newly available medical care. Budetti and colleagues[50] showed that with the institution of the Medicaid system, the average number of visits to the doctor per year increased in the poor populations almost to the level of the nonpoor. This further supports the idea that better medical care has contributed to the decline of disease.

A third report by Gordis[27] in Baltimore from 1977 to 1882 showed the incidence of rheumatic fever to be 0.5/100,000. Obviously, inasmuch as asymptomatic pharyngeal infections were resulting in more than six cases per 100,000 in the late 1960s, other factors must have been in force to decrease the rate of attack to this very low number. Changes in the virulence or rheumatogenicity of the organism were suspected.

The cases reported to the Centers for Disease Control are shown in Table 1–1. Rheumatic fever has not been a reportable disease, and the figures cannot be deemed as reliable total counts. However, several conclusions may be made. Great strides have been made in the prevention of this disease, however, with more than 100 cases reported yearly, the disease has not been eradicated and should be considered a diagnostic possibility in the appropriate setting.

RECENT OUTBREAKS

Several regions of the United States, including Utah,[11] Ohio,[14,15] Pennsylvania,[16] and West Virginia,[10] reported an increased number of cases of acute rheumatic fever in the mid-1980s. In many of these regions, more cases were reported during a relatively brief period than had been previously reported during an entire decade.[1] The patients in these areas seemed to have a different epidemiology, had severe disease, and demonstrated a trend toward certain strains of streptococci known to be associated with rheumatic fever.

In contrast to the accepted epidemiology of rheumatic fever, these patients were almost all white, the majority lived in rural or suburban communities, they had above-average incomes (reported in only two of the studies), and had adequate access to medical care. The incidence of clinically apparent antecedent infection also was surprising. In several studies,[11,16] less than one third of cases had evidence of pharyngitis. In the Utah study,[11] an attempt was made to determine if adequate treatment was given to those with clinically apparent infections. Of the eight patients who were informed that they had positive cultures, appropriate therapy was apparently issued in all cases. Unfortunately, compliance was thought to have been less than adequate.

In the Utah study, mucoid M-18 and M-3 were obtained from siblings and classmates of patients.[51] In Ohio, an increase in mucoid strains was also encountered. All of these were M-18 type.[52] The peak incidence of this mucoid strain was in the spring of the year and coincided with the outbreak of rheumatic fever. The group in Utah also had a high incidence of cardiac involvement. Seventy-two percent had cardiac involvement clinically, and echocardiography detected an additional 19%. Congestive heart failure was noted in 19%, and two patients even required mitral valve replacement. Only three of the involved patients had a prior history of rheumatic fever.

There were several reports that involved a significant number of adults. Two of these reports were from military bases.[12,13] In West Virginia, two thirds of the patients were adults.[11] In San Diego, the Naval Training Center had ten definite cases of rheumatic fever. This rate of attack was 80/100,000 recruits for the 6-month period involved and compares with a normal rate of 0.75/100,000 from 1982 to 1986. The Naval Training Center had discontinued routine prophylaxis of its incoming recruits in 1980. Durng the same period, the Marine Corps Recruit Department, which is adjacent to the naval center, had no cases of rheumatic fever. The marine corp center had continued its prophylactic program. The report from Fort Leonard Wood in Missouri, an army training center, describes an increase in highly mucoid colonies from throat cultures at the base concomitant with the 13 cases of rheumatic fever that occurred. Although, again, no cultures were available from the patients, the base had a high percentage of mucoid M-18 (74%) and M-3 (20%). Reinstitution of prophylaxis at both bases resulted in a dramatic decrease in occurrence.

In West Virginia, two thirds of the cases (23 total) involved adults. Unique to this report is that 10 of the 23 cases were patients with a history of rheumatic fever. Nine of the recurrences were among adults. Only one of these nine patients had been receiving prophylaxis (intramuscular benzathine penicillin G), and this patient missed the injection in the month prior to infection. The period from the most recent bout of rheumatic fever in these adult patients ranged from 8 to 35 years with six of the cases having a disease-free interval of more than 20 years. Five of these nine adults had clinical carditis and an additional patient was found to have mitral regurgitation by echocardiography (a 28 year old). One had a normal echocardiogram and two without clinical evidence of carditis did not have an ultrasound.

Collectively, these recent reports cause us to re-think our current understanding of disease. High-risk patients may not be as easily defined by standard of living as once thought. We are once again presented with evidence that the organism itself, by way of the present prevalent serotype, is playing a major role in determining outcome of streptococcal pharyngitis. With the low incidence of clinically apparent pharyngitis observed in several of these studies and evidence that compliance with treatment for pharyngitis is suboptimal, further evaluation of primary prevention is warranted. Additionally, secondary prevention for high-risk groups such as military recruits and those with previous rheumatic fever (especially those with previous heart disease) deserves continued thought.

PATHOGENESIS

As previuosly discussed, a variety of factors undoubtedly contribute to the pathogenesis of acute rheumatic fever. Most important is the requirement of a group A streptococcal infection of the upper respiratory tract that persists long enough to initiate a significant antibody response in the host. Conditions that promote rapid transfer of a virulent strain will likely result in a higher incidence of poststreptococcal sequelae. Evidence that there are rheumatogenic strains has already been presented. Their role in the immune mechanism will be discussed in this section.

SITE OF INFECTION

The site of the infection required to result in rheumatic fever has been established to be the upper respiratory tract. The reasons behind this are obscure but there are several ideas that may play a part. First, it may be necessary for the infection to involve the mucous membranes of the upper respiratory tract because the skin, via lipids, is capable of blunting the immune response.[53] A second possibility is suggested by Hafez and associates.[54] They studied the ability of the streptococci to adhere to pharyngeal cells. They compared adherence of many different strains to the cells of rheumatic fever patients, their family members, and controls (no family member had a history of rheumatic fever). When using strains not associated with rheumatic fever, no difference was seen in any group. When using strains of streptococci associated with rheumatic fever, patients with a rheumatic history had an increased avidity for adherence when compared with uninvolved siblings and controls. No significant difference was seen between uninvolved siblings and controls. Is this increased ability of rheumatogenic strains to adhere to lymphoid tissue in diseased patients a risk factor for the patient or a result of infection? The answer is unclear at the present time. A final observation is that T cells labeled with monoclonal antibodies against rheumatic antigens, seem to be compartmentalized. Gray and coworkers[55] analyzed T cells from tonsillar tissue and peripheral blood in rheumatic fever patients and controls. The tonsillar tissue from the rheumatic fever patients had no cells labeled by the antibody whereas the cells from peripheral blood in these same patients were labeled 71% of the time. T cells from tonsils and blood were labeled in controls 50% and 17% of the time, respectively. Perhaps this lack of T-cell antigens at the infection site promotes risk for disease. The mechanism by which each of these observations may play a part requires further investigation.

IMMUNOLOGIC ASPECTS

T-Cell and Lymphokine Dysregulation

Several studies have investigated the changes in lymphocytes in rheumatic fever patients. Studies examining the changes of T-cell subsets during the disease often gave conflicting results.[56-58] Alarcon-Riquelme and associates[56] found that the

CD4+ T cells increased in the acute phase of rheumatic fever whereas the CD8+ cells remained at a normal absolute level. Interleukin-2 (IL-2) production fell at this stage. Three months later, these patients were restudied and the CD4+ cells had decreased to normal levels and the CD8+ cells had increased more than 60% from the acute phase levels. Interestingly, the study demonstrated decreased suppressor activity during that time. At the recovery phase, IL-2 production was decreased further. T cells, predominantly CD4+, have been demonstrated in heart valve tissue in rheumatic heart disease patients.[59]

Other studies, including those by Cairns,[58] have demonstrated increased production of IL-2 during the acute phase of rheumatic fever. The interesting aspect of his study is that he used a monoclonal antibody to measure a receptor on T cells for IL-2 (TAC). The TAC receptor was present in levels two to three times higher in rheumatic fever patients when compared with controls. This was quantitatively more significant in patients with carditis. This IL-2 receptor increase persisted long after acute phase reactants had returned to normal and was most marked on CD4+ T cells. Cytokine production has been shown also by others to be dysregulated.[60] Whether these changes are the result of rheumatic fever and rheumatic heart disease or a susceptibility factor is unclear. What role the dysregulation of lymphocytes and cytokine production plays in the pathogenesis of the disease is unknown.

Complement and Immune Complexes

Another immunologic aspect of rheumatic fever deals with alterations of complement and the production of circulating immune complexes. Circulating immune complexes may play a part in pathogenesis. Van de Rijn and colleagues[61] demonstrated that almost 100% of patients with rheumatic fever had measurable circulating immune complexes during early stages of the disease. They noted no significance in the absolute levels and suggested that the components of the complexes themselves may play an important role. Gupta and coworkers[62] determined that the circulating immune complexes in their patients consisted of polypeptides of streptolysin O, antibodies to streptolysin O, and C-reactive protein. Svartman and associates[63] studied synovial fluid in children and young adults with acute rheumatic fever. Complement levels were significantly reduced, suggesting immune complexes are involved. Again, further study is necessary to determine the significance of these findings.

Complement has been difficult to study because some of the components are acute phase reactants. Kaplan and coworkers,[64] however, demonstrated in the 1960s that C3 was deposited in the myocardium of patients who had died of rheumatic carditis. Complement levels have been low in some patients' sera.[65] The role of complement in the pathogenesis has continued to be a curiosity.

Molecular Mimicry and Autoantibodies

The best-studied aspect of the immunology of rheumatic fever and how it relates to pathogenesis has been the idea of antibody production against streptococcal antigens that also react with host tissue. Kaplan and colleagues[64] were among the first to recognize heart-reactive antibodies. Antibodies to group A β-hemolytic streptococci have been identified that cross-react with many tissues, including the heart[66,67] and brain.[68–70] Many questions remained unanswered. Their importance in pathogenesis is not known. Which of the many detected antibodies contributes to disease and which are merely epiphenomena? This section will look at the current level of understanding of autoimmunity induced by streptococci.

M PROTEIN. The M protein has received the most attention in recent investigation into the molecular mimicry of streptococci with human tissues. Structurally, it is a coiled-coil and has portions that are closely homologous to myosin, tropomyosin, keratin, and neural fibers.[67-74] An antiphagocytic component is responsible for much of its virulence.[75] More than 80 different M proteins have been identified.

In the early 1960s, Kaplan[76] was involved in identifying the type of antibodies produced after exposure to streptococci. Using immunized rabbits, he found that antibodies that cross-reacted with cardiac tissue could be absorbed with specific M-type proteins. Using acute rheumatic fever patients' sera, a sarcolemmal protein was identified that was of similar molecular weight as a protein identified to cross-react with a particular M-protein epitope.[77] Additionally, a protein on the streptococcal membrane that absorbed all of the heart reactive antibody was recognized.[78]

Cunningham and associates[67,73] have used murine monoclonal antibodies and noted cross-reactivity with the heavy chain of myosin. Dale, Beachey,[72] and others[72,79] have continued to identiy epitopes that are cross-reactive with cardiac tissue. They have shown that some streptococcal epitopes are involved in opsonization, others are involved in cross-reactivity, and others have both capabilities.[80-82] Further localization of these epitopes has used synthetic peptides and pepsin-cleaved proteins.[38,83] Localization of potentially cross-reactive epitopes and opsonic epitopes will be of the utmost importance when considering a vaccine.

Although most of the work done by Dale and Beachey has been looking at the NH_2 terminal end of M protein, the portion that protrudes away from the microorganism, work also has been focused on other portions of this protein. Bessen and Fischetti[84] identified a constant region on the M protein proximal to the pepsin cleavage site. Mice that were immunized intranasally with this section were protected from an intranasal challenge of similar organisms. In a later study by the same group,[37] they noted that the majority of M proteins with rheumatogenic potential had an amino-acid sequence with dramatic homology to this previously noted constant region. This homology between two sample serotypes, M-6 and M-12, was <27% on the more distal part of the protein. However, when this constant region was reached, the homology was 97%. Other serotypes, without rheumatic fever potential, did not share these sequences. They proposed that streptococci could be classified into one of two categories depending on the presence or absence of this domain, thus identifying organisms with high risk of producing rheumatic fever.

GROUP A CARBOHYDRATE. Antigenic similarity of human and bovine heart valve glycoprotein and group A streptococcal carbohydrate was demonstrated by Goldstein and colleagues[85] in 1967. Dudding and Ayoub[86] measured antibodies to group A carbohydrate in patients with rheumatic fever both with and without rheumatic heart disease. Although both started with high titers of antibody in their sera, the patients with heart disease had prolonged elevation. The role these antibodies play in valvular disease remains obscure.

MEMBRANE PROTEINS. The number and complexity of proteins that are contained in the membrane of the streptococcus has led to investigation of their possible roles in the pathogenesis of acute rheumatic fever. The structure consists of 72% proteins, 26% lipids, and 2% sugars.[87] In addition to the many unique proteins in the cell membrane, studies using cell membrane very likely include some M-protein pieces as the M protein extends down to this level. Early studies using immunized rabbits demonstrated that cell membranes can induce antibodies that are reactive with muscle tissue, including cardiac, skeletal, and vascular smooth muscle.[88] Other researchers studied the interaction of antibodies to cell-membrane proteins and brain tissue. Kingston and Glynn[70,74] demonstrated antibodies, present in group A streptococcal antisera, that reacted to astrocytes. Husby and coworkers[69] showed preferential binding of antibodies in rheumatic fever sera to caudate and subthalamic nuclei of the human brain. The incidence of this reaction was considerably higher in patients with chorea when compared with those with carditis and no chorea (46% vs. 14%). These antibodies were completely absorbed with group A cell membrane, only partially absorbable with cell-wall preparations (which were known to be contaminated with membrane), and not absorbed by group A carbohydrate. Additionally, these antibodies were absorbed more completely by membranes of rheumatogenic strains when compared with skin strains.

The Streptococcus as an Immune Modifier

Not only does the streptococcus have these cross-reactive epitopes, but it also has the capability of modifying the host's immunologic reaction. The hyaluronic capsule has been shown to activate neutrophils. Muramyl peptides and cell peptidoglycan aid in stimulating immune response.[58] Lipoteichoic acid can bind to platelets and leukocytes and induce the production of tumor necrosis factor. O'Conner and Cleary[89] located a protein, C5a peptidase, bound to the bacterial cell surface that specifically cleaves C5a to an inactive compound, eliminating a potent chemoattractant. The organism modifies the response of the host as it induces autoantibodies through its mimetic structural features.

CLINICAL ASPECTS

PRESENTATION

Acute rheumatic fever follows streptococcal pharyngitis after a 2- to 3-week latency period. The pharyngitis may be asymptomatic in a considerable number of patients. The onset can be very acute, usually presenting with arthritis. It can occur more insidiously when the presenting manifestation is carditis or chorea. The symptoms usually last for several weeks if untreated and gradually resolve without residua. The important exception is carditis and when rheumatic heart disease occurs, its sequelae can be very serious. The incidence of the major manifestations are listed in Table 1–2.

Arthritis

Arthritis occurs in most patients with rheumatic fever. The incidence varies with age; virtually all adult patients and about two thirds of children develop arthritis. Classically, large joints, particularly of the lower extremities, are involved in rapid succession. Maximal pain does not last more than several days in any one joint. Usually the pain is more dramatic than the physical findings. If untreated, an average of six joints are affected and the entire course subsides after a 2- or 3-week period. Permanent joint damage rarely, if ever, occurs. The arthritis responds to aspirin in a dramatic fashion.

A patient with arthritis as the only major manifestation can be difficult diag-

Table 1–2. Clinical
Manifestations of Acute
Rheumatic Fever

	1920–1950	1980s
Number of patients	1000	154
Arthritis*	81%	63%
Carditis	65%	58%†
Chorea	52%	23%
Erythema marginatum	7%	6%
Nodules	9%	4%

*Arthritis and arthralgia grouped together in early records.
†By clinical examination and not including those detected by echocardiogram.
Sources: 1920–1950 data from Bland, EF and Jones, TJ: Rheumatic fever and rheumatic heart disease: A 20-year report on 1000 patients followed since childhood. 1980s data compiled from references 10–14.

nostically. Arthritis should be carefully distinguished from arthralgia, a much less specific symptom. At least two joints must be involved, and this should be associated with at least two minor criteria and high titers of an antistreptococcal antibody.

Carditis

Carditis is the most concerning aspect of rheumatic fever. Not only can it lead to long-term sequelae, but it can also cause acute heart failure and death. Although carditis has serious acute and chronic implications, it most commonly causes no symptoms of its own. It is usually detected on physical examination by the presence of murmurs. The addition of echocardiography will undoubtedly yield a higher incidence of carditis, and this may be important when one considers prophylaxis. Carditis may occasionally be the only manifestation of disease, and if the carditis does not cause symptoms, the disease may not be diagnosed until years later when the patient is found to have rheumatic heart disease.

Rheumatic carditis may occur as a pancarditis. The valvular disease is probably the most familiar, but a myocarditis may be associated with cardiac dilation that can accentuate the murmurs. Pericarditis is also a frequent manifestation. A previous book in the *Cardiovascular Clinic Series* discussed at length the valvular disease that results from rheumatic fever.[90] Most commonly, the mitral valve is involved, followed by the aortic and mitral valves in combination, and lastly the aortic valve alone. Rheumatic heart disease is the most common etiology of mitral stenosis.

Chorea

Chorea is typically a late manifestation of rheumatic fever, occurring as late as 1 to 6 months after streptococcal pharyngitis. It is never encountered simultaneously with arthritis but may occur either in combination with carditis or alone. When chorea occurs alone, all other criteria may be absent (pure chorea).[91] It is characterized by rapid, purposeless, involuntary movements and also may be associated with muscular weakness and emotional lability. The movements are abrupt and erratic rather than fluid as occurs in athetosis. Regardless of the severity, all movements disappear during sleep. After puberty, this manifestation occurs in women almost exclusively. It rarely occurs in adults. The clinical course of chorea can last from several weeks to several years, but it is more typically 8 to 15 weeks.

Erythema Marginatum

Erythema marginatum is an evanescent, nonpruritic rash that is typically observed on the trunk but occasionally may involve the proximal limbs. It appears as a bright pink ring that spreads serpiginously. It blanches and is not painful or indurated. The lesions spread centrifugally, with gradual fading of the center, whereas the outer edge remains sharply defined.[92] The lesions may appear and remit in a matter of hours and may change shape before one's eyes. A hot bath may make them more prominent. Erythema marginatum is rare in adults and is associated with carditis.[93]

Subcutaneous Nodules

Subcutaneous nodules are a relatively infrequent manifestation of rheumatic fever. They occur over bony prominences and tendons, particularly of the hands and feet. They may be as small as several millimeters or as large as 2 centimeters. They may last several weeks but rarely last longer than 1 month. Nodules are rarely encountered in adults and occur almost exclusively in patients with carditis. They may be confused with nodules of rheumatoid arthritis and systemic lupus erythematosus.

Other Manifestations

Fever occurs in almost all attacks of acute rheumatic fever. Exceptions include isolated chorea and occasionally isolated carditis. Fever usually ranges from 38.4°C to 40°C. It does not have the huge swings that are characteristic of fever associated with juvenile rheumatoid arthritis. Typically, the fever becomes low grade after a week even without antipyretic therapy. Low-grade fever may then persist for several more weeks.

Abdominal pain, anorexia, nausea, and vomiting also may occur with rheumatic fever and occasionally cause diagnostic confusion.

Laboratory Findings

There are no diagnostic tests for rheumatic fever. Nonspecific findings such as an increased erythrocyte sedimentation rate (ESR) or C-reactive protein (CRP), a mild leukocytosis, or anemia are often present. Mild elevations of liver enzymes also occur. Synovial fluid, obtained to exclude septic arthritis, has a leukocyte count ranging from several hundred to almost 100,000. polymorphonuclear cells (PMNs) account for 50% to 100% of the white blood cells.

Evidence of a recent streptococcal infection is present in almost all cases. Stollerman and associates[94] demonstrated antibodies to streptolysin O in 78% of patients. When antihyaluronidase and antistreptokinase antibodies are additionally sought, 95% of patients have one or more positive test results. Anti-DNAase B also has proved to be a useful test. Rapid tests for streptococcal antigens have been proven to be specific but have less than desirable sensitivity.[95]

Table 1–3. Jones Criteria (Modified 1984)

Major Manifestations	Minor Manifestations
Carditis	Fever
Polyarthritis	Arthralgia
Chorea	History of rheumatic fever or rheumatic heart disease
Subcutaneous nodules	Elevated ESR, CRP or white blood cells
Erythema marginatum	Prolonged PR interval

Two major or one major and two minor manifestations, with supporting evidence of a recent streptococcal infection, indicate the probable presence of rheumatic fever.

DIAGNOSIS

In 1944, Jones[96] established criteria for the diagnosis of acute rheumatic fever. These criteria were chosen, not because they were necessarily the most common manifestations, but because they were most likely to differentiate rheumatic fever from other diseases. The Jones Criteria have been modified several times and were most recently reviewed in 1984 (Table 1–3). The presence of two major manifestations or one major and two minor manifestations, in conjunction with evidence of a recent streptococcal infection, indicate the probable presence of rheumatic fever. Two situations that are exceptions are isolated chorea and insidious carditis. In these situations, the evidence of recent streptococcal infection may no longer be present and other manifestations may have resolved.

Evidence of a previous streptococcal infection has included scarlet fever, a positive culture for streptococcal pharyngitis, or an elevated antistreptococcal antibody. Several concerns exist regarding this aspect of the criteria. First, a positive throat culture in a patient with pharyngitis does not distinguish between pharyngitis secondary to streptococcal infection and that of a viral etiology in a streptococcal carrier.

Second, a single elevated titer for antistreptococcal antibody does not establish the timing of the streptococcal infection. Antibody titers may remain elevated for variable lengths of time after streptococcal infection. If several antibodies are tested (such as antistreptolysin O, antihyaluronidase, and antistreptokinase) and all are negative, this is more useful in ruling out rheumatic fever as a diagnosis.[97] Serial tests that demonstrate a rising titer are more useful, but if both sets reveal high titer antibodies, this is also nonspecific.

Kaplan,[95] in a discussion of rapid tests for evidence of streptococcal infection, states that a positive test result is ample evidence for streptococcal pharyngitis and to treat as such, but a negative test result must be followed by a throat culture because the sensitivity of these tests are less than desirable.

MANAGEMENT

Treatment of Acute Disease

Patients with rheumatic fever should be examined daily for the first several weeks of disease to look specifically for evidence of carditis. If heart failure ensues, prompt treatment is necessary. In general, rest is advised during the acute phase but the prolonged bedrest advocated in the past is unnecessary.

After the diagnosis is made, salicylates in anti-inflammatory doses are appropriate for the treatment of arthritis. This therapy usually results in prompt resolution of arthritis symptoms. Management of carditis can be a challenge. If carditis is present but there is no evidence of heart failure, salicylates alone are appropriate. If fever, discomfort, or tachycardia persist, some advocate the use of corticosteroids but there are no controlled studies that prove efficacy of this treatment. If carditis is severe and heart failure is present, most clinicians use corticosteroids (40–60 mg/day of prednisone or equivalent as initial dose). Again, no controlled studies provide evidence of efficacy but since adrenocorticotropin hormone (ACTH) was first used in 1950,[98] steroids have been employed in cases of severe disease.

Prevention[34]

PRIMARY PREVENTION. Primary prevention requires the elimination of group A β-hemolytic streptococci from the throat. Treatment of streptococcal pharyngitis, though not significantly altering the course of pharyngitis, has been shown to prevent primary attacks of rheumatic fever even if started several days after onset of pharyngitis. Therapy with penicillin should be given to all except those with penicillin allergies. Injectable benzathine penicillin G has been shown to be the best method of administration, but oral penicillin V can be used. A full 10 days of treatment is necessary and compliance must be stressed. If the patient is allergic to penicillin, erythromycin is the best alternative (Table 1–4).

SECONDARY PREVENTION. Patients with a history of rheumatic fever are at much higher risk of recurrent infection. Recurrences are typically wrought with the same features as the initial attack.[99] The incidence of recurrence declines with length of time since the previous attack.[100] In the study by Bland and Jones,[100] 19% had recurrences in the first 5 years, 11% in the second 5 years, 6% in the next 5 years, and 1.4% in the 16- to 20-year range. Because of the high risk, secondary prevention was initiated in the 1950s. Because the risk is once again relatively low after 10 or 15 years, some discontinue prophylaxis after that time if the patient has reached adulthood. Increased concern about the duration of prophylaxis has occurred, especially in light of the West Virginia report[10] previously noted. Perhaps this secondary prevention should continue indefinitely in patients with increased exposure to group A streptococcus, including parents of small children, health-care workers, military recruits, teachers, day-care workers, and others. Additionally, patients with a history of carditis also should consider more highly the idea of indefinite prophylaxis. Prophylaxis should continue even after valve replacement as they continue to be at increased risk.[101] Conversely, patients without evidence of carditis may consider discontinuing prophylaxis earlier. Risks and benefits should be discussed prior to discontinuation.

Table 1–4. Primary Prevention of Rheumatic Fever:
Treatment of Streptococcal Pharyngitis

Benzathine penicillin G IM 1,200,000 units (600,000 units if patient is <60 lb)
or
Penicillin V 250 mg orally tid for 10 days

If penicillin allergic:
Erythromycin orally 1 g/d for 10 days (20–40 mg/kg per day divided in 2–4 doses)

Table 1–5. Secondary Prevention of Rheumatic Fever
(Recurrences)

Benzathine penicillin G, 1,200,000 units IM ever 4 weeks

or

Penicillin V, 250 mg orally twice daily

or

Sulfadiazine, 1 g orally once daily (500 mg for patients <60 lb)

If allergic to penicillin and sulfadiazine:
Erythromycin, 250 mg orally twice daily

Secondary prevention recommendations include parenteral penicillin or oral penicillin, sulfadiazine, or erythromycin. Intramuscular penicillin is the most effective regimen and is given every 4 weeks. Some countries have had breakthrough with this schedule and recommend every 3 weeks. Oral medications have been slightly less effective and probably should not be recommended to those at high risk. Some have switched their patients to oral agents after 5 or more years when they are at a lower risk. Erythromycin should only be given to allergic patients. In Japan, routine use of erythromycin resulted in mass resistance of the streptococci to this drug. When penicillin replaced the erythromycin, the resistance subsided. Doses are given in Table 1–5.

IMPORTANT: Secondary prophylaxis does not replace the necessity to use subacute bacterial endocarditis prophylaxis prior to procedures in patients with valvular disease.

VACCINE. With the incidence of asymptomatic pharyngitis and the difficulty of making primary prophylaxis available to the masses worldwide, a vaccine is very desirable. However, there are several major concerns regarding a vaccine. First, many streptococcal products have been very toxic. Primitive vaccines used in the 1960s were highly toxic. Second, one must ensure that the vaccine antigens include opsonic antigens of many of the different serotypes of streptococci while being devoid of any cross-reactive antigens. Identification of the rheumatogenic strains and their respective rheumatogenic epitopes would obviously short cut this difficulty. The work of Bessen and coworkers,[84] indicating a common sequence on most of the rheumatogenic strains, also may prove very useful for creating a vaccine.

Poirer and colleagues[102] produced a vaccine using attenuated *Salmonella typhimurium* and a cloned streptococcal M-5 protein. This hybrid, when given orally to mice, protected the mice from *S. typhimurium* and M-5 streptococci. This method avoided the potentially serious toxic reactions encountered with streptococcal products while delivering the required antigenic stimulus. Certainly, a solution to the vaccine for rheumatic fever is near.

CONCLUSION

Rheumatic fever remains a serious health concern in the United States. Although the number of patients has decreased dramatically, a low-level incidence persists with sporadic clustered outbreaks. Treatment of streptococcal pharyngitis should proceed with continued diligence. This obviously will not eliminate the cases of rheumatic fever that occur after asymptomatic pharyngitis and inasmuch as rheumatic heart disease occurs in the majority of patients, secondary prophylaxis also will continue to be important. We are hopeful that, through the efforts of the many individuals studying rheumatic fever and the mechanisms and epidemiology of the disease, high-risk individuals will be identified and a safe and effective vaccine will be available for administration.

SUMMARY

During the first half of this century rheumatic fever was a common disease with significant morbidity and mortality in the United States. In the 1980s, when many clinicians were hoping this disease was a disease of the past, anxieties were renewed when outbreaks were reported in several areas around the country. Although the etiology still eludes us, insight has been gained. Environmental and genetic factors are believed to play a role in the epidemiology of this disease. Additionally, the implicated organism, the group A streptococcus, has many strains, and differences in its many proteins may determine their potential for rheumatic fever. The mechanisms leading to disease are not clear, but the streptococcus has been implicated as a source of antigens with cross-reactivity with human tissues and has been shown to modify immune mechanisms. Clinical aspects are briefly reviewed and physicians are reminded to consider rheumatic fever as a diagnostic possibility in the appropriate settings.

REFERENCES

1. Markowitz, M and Kaplan, DL: Reappearance of rheumatic fever. Adv Pediatr 36:39, 1989.
2. Stollerman, G: The return of rheumatic fever. Hosp Pract Nov. 15:100, 1988.
3. Stollerman, G: Rheumatogenic group A streptococci and the return of rheumatic fever. Adv Intern Med 35:1, 1990.
4. Bisno, AL: The resurgence of acute rheumatic fever in the United States. Annu Rev Med 41:319, 1990.
5. Dobson, SRM: Group A streptococci revisited. Arch Dis Child 64:977, 1989.
6. Lerner, PI: Turning back group A streptococci. Cleveland Clinics Journal of Medicine 57:316, 1989.
7. Wallace, MR, Garst, PD, Papadimos, TJ, et al: The return of acute rheumatic fever in young adults. JAMA 262:2557, 1989.
8. Quinn, RW: Comprehensive review of morbidity and mortality trends for rheumatic fever, streptococcal disease, and scarlet fever: The decline of rheumatic fever. Rev Infect Dis 11:928, 1989.
9. Zabriskie, JB: Rheumatic fever: The interplay between host, genetics and microbe. Circulation 71:1077, 1985.
10. Mason, TM, Fisher, M, and Kujala, G: Acute rheumatic fever in West Virginia: Not just a disease of children. Arch Intern Med 151:133, 1991.
11. Veasy, LG, Wiedmeier, SE, Orsmond, GS, et al: Resurgence of acute rheumatic fever in the intermountain area of the United States. N Engl J Med 316:421, 1987.
12. Papadimos, T, Escamilla, J, Garst, P, et al: Acute rheumatic fever at the Navy Training Center—San Diego, California. JAMA 259:1782, 1988.
13. Sampson, GL, Williams, RG, Wetzel, NE, et al: Acute rheumatic fever among army trainees—Fort Leonard Wood, Missouri, 1987–1988. JAMA 260:2185, 1988.
14. Hosier, DM, Craenen, J, Teske, DW, et al: Resurgence of rheumatic fever. Am J Dis Child 141:730, 1987.
15. Congeni, B, Rizzo, L, Congeni, J, et al: Outbreaks of rheumatic fever in Northeast Ohio. J Pediatr 111:176, 1987.
16. Wald, ER, Dashefsky, B, Feidt, C, et al: Acute rheumatic fever in Western Pennsylvania and the tri-state area. Pediatrics 80:371, 1987.
17. Agarwal, BL: Rheumatic heart disease unabated in developing countries. Lancet 2:910, 1981.

18. Public Health Board of Denmark: Reported rheumatic fever incidence in Denmark, 1862–1962. In DiSciasco, G and Taranta, A: Rheumatic fever in children. Am Heart J 99:635, 1980.

19. Hoffman, S, Henrichsen, J, and Schmidt, K: Incidence and diagnosis of acute rheumatic fever in Denmark, 1980 and 1983. Acta Med Scand 224:587, 1988.

20. Imamoglu, A and Ozen, S: Epidemiology of rheumatic heart disease. Arch Dis Child 63:1501, 1988.

21. Robinson, SJ: Incidence of rheumatic fever in San Francisco children: A 10-year study. J Pediatr 49:272, 1956.

22. Levinson, SS, Bearfield, JL, Ausbrook, DK, et al: The Chicago Rheumatic Fever Program: A 20-plus year history. J Chronic Dis 35:199, 1982.

23. Gordis, L: Studies in the epidemiology and preventability of rheumatic fever: I. Demographic factors and the incidence of acute attacks. J Chronic Dis 21:645, 1969.

24. Land, MA and Bisno, AI: Acute rheumatic fever: A vanishing disease in suburbia. JAMA 249:895, 1983.

25. Holmberg, SD and Faich, GA: Streptococcal pharyngitis and acute rheumatic fever in Rhode Island. JAMA 250:2307, 1983.

26. Schwartz, RH, Hepner, SI, and Ziai, M: Incidence of acute rheumatic fever: A suburban community hospital experience during the 1970s. Clin Pediatr 22:798, 1983.

27. Gordis, L: The virtual disappearance of rheumatic fever in the United States: Lessons in the rise and fall of disease. Circulation 72:1155, 1985.

28. Lancefield, RC: Differentiation of group A streptococci with a common R antigen into three serologic types, with special reference to the bacteriocidal test. J Exp Med 106:525, 1957.

29. Rammelkamp, CH: The Lewis A. Conner Memorial Lecture. Rheumatic heart disease—A challenge. Circulation 17:842, 1958.

30. Siegel, AC, Johnson, EE, and Stollerman, GH: Controlled studies of streptococcal pharyngitis in a pediatric population. I. Factors related to the attack rate of rheumatic fever. N Engl J Med 265:559, 1961.

31. Kass, EH and Seastone, CV: The role of mucoid polysaccharide (hyaluronic acid) in the virulence of group A hemolytic streptococci. J Exp Med 79:319, 1944.

32. Stollerman, GH: The relative rheumatogenicity of strains of group A streptococci. Mod Concepts Cardiovasc Dis 44:35, 1975.

33. Whitnack, E and Beachey, EH: Inhibition of complement mediated opsonization and phagocytosis of streptococcus pyogenes by D fragments of fibrinogen and fibrin bound to cell surface M proteins. J Exp Med 162:1983, 1985.

34. Dajani, AS, Bisno, AL, Chung, KJ, et al: Prevention of rheumatic fever. Circulation 78:1082, 1988.

35. Kutter, AG and Krumweide, E: Observations on the effect of streptococcal upper respiratory infections on rheumatic children: A 3-year study. J Clin Invest 20:273, 1941.

36. Majeed, HA, Faisal, FA, Yousof, AM, et al: The rheumatogenic and nephritogenic strains of the group A streptococcus: The Kuwait experience. NZ Med J 101:398, 1988.

37. Bessen, D, Jones, KF, and Fischetti, VA: Evidence for two distinct classes of streptococcal M protein and their relationship to rheumatic fever. J Exp Med 169:269, 1989.

38. Kraus, W, Dale, JB, and Beachey, EH: Identification of an epitope of type 1 streptococcal M protein that is shared with a 43-kDa protein of human myocardium and renal glomeruli. J Immunol 145:4089, 1990.

39. Taranta, A, Torosdag, S, Metrakos, JD, et al: Rheumatic fever in monozygotic and dizygotic twins. Circulation 20:778, 1959.

40. Caughey, DE, Douglas, R, Wilson, W, et al: HLA antigens in Europeans and Maoris with rheumatic heart disease. J Rheumatol 2:319, 1975.

41. Patarroyo, ME, Winchester, RJ, Vejerano, A, et al: Association of a B-cell alloantigen with susceptibility to rheumatic fever. Nature 278:173, 1979.

42. Ayoub, EM, Barrett, DJ, Maclaren, NK, et al: Association of class II human histocompatibility leukocyte antigens with rheumatic fever. J Clin Invest 77:2019, 1986.

43. Zabriskie, JB, Lavenchy, D, and Williams, RC: Rheumtic fever-associated B cell alloantigens as identified by monoclonal antibodies. Arthritis Rheum 28:1047, 1985.

44. Khanna, AK, Buskirk, DR, Williams, RC, et al: Presence of a non-HLA B-cell antigen in rheumatic fever patients and their families as defined by a monoclonal antibody. J Clin Invest 83:1710, 1989.

45. Taneja, V, Mehra, NK, and Reddy, KS: HLA-DR/DQ antigens and reactivity to B-cell alloantigen D8/17 in Indian patients with rheumatic heart disease. Circulation 80:335, 1989.

46. Rich, SS, Gray, ED, Talbot, R, et al: Cell surface markers and cellular immune response associated with rheumatic heart disease: Complex segregation analysis. Genet Epidemiol 5:463, 1988.

47. Frank, PF, Stollerman, GH, and Miller, LF: Protection of a military population from rheumatic fever: Routine administration of benzathine penicillin G to healthy individuals. JAMA 193:119, 1965.

48. Massell, BF, Chute, CG, Walker, AM, et al: Penicillin and the marked decrease in morbidity and mortality from rheumatic fever in the United States. N Engl J Med 318:280,1988.

49. Gordis, L: Effectiveness of comprehensive care programs in preventing rheumatic fever. N Engl J Med 289:331, 1973.

50. Budetti, P, Butler, J, McManus, P, et al: Federal health programs reforms: Implications for children's healthcare. Milbank Mem Fund Q 60:155, 1981.

51. Kaplan, EL, Johnson, DR, and Cleary, PP: Group A streptococcal serotypes isolated from patients and sibling contacts during the resurgence of rheumatic fever in the United States in the mid-1980s. J Infect Dis 159:101, 1989.

52. Marcon, MJ, Hribar, MM, Hosier, DM, et al: Occurrence of mucoid M-18 streptococcus pyogenes in a central Ohio pediatric population. J Clin Microbiol 26:1539, 1988.

53. Kaplan, EL and Wannamaker, LW: Streptolysin O: Suppression of its antigenicity by lipids extracted from skin. Proc Soc Exp Biol Med 146:205, 1974.

54. Hafez, M, El-Battoty, MF, Hawas, S, et al: Evidence of inherited susceptibility of increased streptococcal adherence to pharyngeal cells of children with rheumatic fever. Br J Rheumatol 28:304, 1989.

55. Gray, ED, Regelmann, WR, Abdin, Z, et al: Compartmentalization of cells bearing "rheumatic" cell surface antigens in peripheral blood and tonsils in rheumatic heart disease. J Infect Dis 155:2471, 1976.

56. Alarcon-Riquelme, ME, Alarcon-Sequvia, D, Loredo-Abdala, A, et al: T-lymphocyte subsets, suppressor and contrasuppressor cell functions, and production of interleukin-2 in the peripheral blood of rheumatic fever patients and their apparently healthy siblings. Clin Immunol Immunopathol 55:120, 1990.

57. Hafez, M, El-Shannaway, F, El-Salab, SH, et al: Studies of peripheral blood T-lymphocytes in assessment of disease activity in rheumatic fever. Br J Rheumatol 27:181, 1988.

58. Cairns, LM: The immunology of rheumatic fever. NZ Med J 101:388, 1988.

59. Raizada, V, Williams, RC, Chopra, P, et al: Tissue distribution of lymphocytes in rheumatic heart valves as defined by monoclonal anti-T cell antibodies. Am J Med 74:90, 1983.

60. Miller, LC, Gray, ED, Mansour, M, et al: Cytokines and immunoglobulin in rheumatic heart disease: Production by blood and tonsillar mononuclear cells. J Rheumatol 16:1436, 1989.

61. van de Rijn, I, Fillit, H, and Brandeis, WE: Serial studies on circulating immune complexes in poststreptococcal sequelae. Clin Exp Immunol 34:318, 1978.

62. Gupta, RC, Badhwar, AK, Bisno, AL, et al: Detection of C-reactive protein, streptolysin O, and antistreptolysin O antibodies in immune complexes isolated from the sera of patients with acute rheumatic fever. J Immunol 137:2173, 1986.

63. Svartman, M, Potter, EV, Poon-King, T, et al: Immunoglobulins and complement components in synovial fluid of patients with acute rheumatic fever. J Clin Invest 56:111, 1975.

64. Kaplan, MH, Bolande, R, Rakita, L, et al: Presence of bound immunoglobulins and complement in the myocardium in acute rheumatic fever. N Engl J Med 271:637, 1964.

65. Barnert, AL, Terry, EE, and Persellin, RH: Acute rheumatic fever in adults. JAMA 232:925, 1975.

66. Dale, JB and Beachey, EH: Multiple heart cross-reactive epitopes of streptococcal M proteins. J Exp Med 161:113, 1985.

67. Cunningham, MW, Krisher, K, and Graves, DC: Murine monoclonal antibodies reactive with human heart and group A streptococcal membrane antigens. Infect Immun 46:34, 1984.

68. Dorling, J, Kingston, D, and Webb, JA: Antistreptococcal antibodies reacting with brain tissue. Br J Exp Pathol 57:255, 1976.

69. Husby, G, van de Rijn, I, and Zabriskie, JB: Antibodies reacting with cytoplasm of subthalamic and caudate nuclei neurons in chorea and acute rheumatic fever. J Exp Med 144:1094, 1976.

70. Kingston, D and Glynn, LE: Antistreptococcal antibodies reacting with brain tissue. I. Immunofluorescent studies. Br J Exp Pathol 57:114, 1976.

71. Cunningham, MW, McCormack, JM, Talaber, LR, et al: Human monoclonal antibodies reactive with antigens of the group A streptococcus and human heart. J Immunol 141:2760, 1988.

72. Dale, JB and Beachey, EH: Epitopes of streptococcal M proteins shared with cardiac myosin. J Exp Med 162:583, 1985.

73. Cunningham, MW, McCormack, Fenderson, PG, et al: Human and murine antibodies cross-reactive with streptococcal M protein and myosin recognize the sequence GLN-LYS-SER-LYS-GLN in M protein. J Immunol 13:2677, 1989.
74. Kingston, D and Glynn, LE: A cross-reaction between streptococcus pyogenes and human fibroblasts, endothelial cells and astrocytes. Immunology 21:1003, 1971.
75. Lancefield, RC: Current knowledge of the type specific M antigens of group A streptococci. J Immunol 89:307, 1962.
76. Kaplan, MH: Immunologic relation of streptococcal and tissue antigens. J Immunol 90:595, 1963.
77. Froude, J, Gibofsky, A, Buskirk, DR, et al: Cross-reactivity between streptococcus and human tissue: A model of molecular mimicry and autoimmunity. Curr Top Microbiol Immunol 145:5, 1989.
78. van de Rijn, I, Zabriskie, JB, and McCarty, M: Group A streptococcal antigens cross-reactive with myocardium: Purification of heart-reactive antibody and isolation and characterization of the streptococcal antigen. J Exp Med 146:579, 1977.
79. Dale, JB and Beachey, EH: Protective antigenic determinant of streptococcal M protein shared with sarcolemmal membrane protein of human heart. J Exp Med 156:1165, 1982.
80. Sargent, SJ, Beachey, EH, Corbett, CE, et al: Sequence of protective epitopes of streptococcal M proteins shared with cardiac sarcolemmal membranes. J Immunol 139:1285, 1987.
81. Dale, JB and Beachey, EH: Epitopes of streptococcal M proteins shared with cardiac myosin. J Exp Med 162:583, 1985.
82. Dale, JB and Beachey, EH: Localization of protective epitopes of the amino terminal of type 5 streptococcal M protein. J Exp Med 163:1191, 1986.
83. Bronze, MS, Beachey, EH, and Dale, JB: Protective and heart cross-reactive epitopes located within the NH2 terminus of type 19 streptococcal M protein. J Exp Med 167:1849,1988.
84. Bessen, D and Fischetti, VA: Influence of intranasal immunization with synthetic peptides corresponding to conserved epitopes of M protein on mucosal colonization by group A streptococci. Infect Immunol 56:2666, 1988.
85. Goldstein, I, Halpern, B, and Robert, L: Immunologic relationship between streptococcal A polysaccharide and structural glycoproteins of heart valve. Nature 213:44, 1967.
86. Dudding, BA and Ayoub, EM: Persistence of streptococcal group A antibody in patients with rheumatic valvular disease. J Exp Med 128:1081, 1968.
87. Freimer, EH: Studies of L forms and rotoplasts of group A streptococci. J Exp Med 117:377, 1963.
88. Zabriskie, JB and Freimer, EH: An immunologic relationship between the group A streptococcus and mammalian muscle. J Exp Med 124:661, 1966.
89. O'Connor, SP and Cleary, PP: Localization of the streptococcal C5a peptidase to the surface of group A streptococci. Infect Immun 53:432, 1986.
90. Waller, BF: Rheumatic and nonrheumatic conditions producing valvular heart disease. Cardiovasc Clin 16:3, 1986.
91. Taranta, A and Stollerman, GH: The relationship of Sydenham's chorea to infection with group A streptococci. Am J Med 20:170, 1956.
92. Perry, BC: Erythema marginatum (rheumaticum). Arch Dis Child 12:233, 1937.
93. Massell, BF, Fyler, DC, and Rey, SB: The clinical picture of rheumatic fever: Diagnosis, immediate prognosis, course and therapeutic implications. Am J Cardiol 1:436, 1958.
94. Stollerman, GH, Lewis, AJ, Shcultz, I, et al: Relationship of immune response to Group A streptococci to the course of acute, chronic and recurrent rheumatic fever. Am J Med 20:163, 1956.
95. Kaplan, EL: Rapid detection of group A streptococcal antigen for the clinician and the epidemiologist: Accurate? Cost-effective? Useful? NZ Med J 101:401, 1988.
96. Jones, TD: The diagnosis of rheumatic fever. JAMA 126:481, 1944.
97. Denny, FW: T. Duckett Jones and rheumatic fever in 1986. Circulation 76:963, 1987.
98. Massell, BF, Warren, GE, Sturgis, GE, et al: Clinical response of rheumatic fever and acute carditis to ACTH. N Engl J Med 242:641, 1950.
99. Feinstein, AR and Spagnuolo, M: Mimetic features of rheumatic fever recurrences. N Engl J Med 262:533, 1960.
100. Bland, EF and Jones, TD: Rheumatic fever and rheumatic heart disease: A 20-year report on 1000 patients followed since childhood. Circulation 4:836, 1951.
101. Hodes, RM: Recurrence of rheumatic fever after valve replacement. Cardiology 76:465, 1989.
102. Poirier, TP, Kehoe, MA, and Beachey, EH: protective immunity evoked by oral administration of attenuated aroA *Salmonella typhimurium* expressing cloned streptococcal M protein. J Exp Med 168:25, 1988.

CHAPTER 2

Valvular Heart Disease of Congenital Origin

William C. Roberts, M.D.

This chapter focuses on congenital conditions affecting one or more cardiac valves. A congenital condition may or may not cause cardiac dysfunction at birth. When delayed the dysfunction often is the result of an acquired condition affecting the congenitally malformed or improperly formed valve. The order of discussion will be mitral, aortic, pulmonic, and tricuspid valves. One congenital systemic condition that causes abnormality of one or more cardiac valves also will be discussed.

MITRAL VALVE

Congenital conditions that affect the mitral valve include mitral valve prolapse, cleft anterior mitral leaflet associated with atrioventricular canal, the parachute mitral valve syndrome, abnormalities of the left-sided atrioventricular valve associated with corrected transposition of the great arteries, double orifice mitral valve, and anomalous origin of the left main coronary artery from the pulmonary trunk.

MITRAL VALVE PROLAPSE

Although recognized earlier,[1-4] delineation of the click-late systolic murmur syndrome as a consequence of mitral valve prolapse was not appreciated until the 1960s.[5-9] It is now apparent that the click-late systolic murmur is common, probably occurring in 5% or more of persons older than 15 years of age.[10-12] Although generally not considered as such, the click-systolic murmur syndrome, probably in most persons, is a form of congenital heart disease, and, therefore, is the most common congenital heart disease.[13] The auscultatory manifestations, however, are usually not evident until adulthood.

The click-murmur syndrome may be viewed from both auscultatory and morphologic standpoints as manifesting three stages (1) systolic click(s) only, (2) click(s) plus a mid- to late-systolic murmur, and (3) pansystolic murmur only. Although progression from stage 1 to 3 has been documented in relatively few patients, it appears likely that this is the natural sequence of events in some patients. In others, there may be no progression from stage 1; patients in stage 2 may revert to stage 1; patients in stage 1 may lose their click(s) altogether; and patients appearing in stage 3 (pansystolic murmur) may have had no documentation of stages 1 and 2. With rare exception, stages 1 and 2 are unassociated with symptomatic evidence of cardiac dysfunction. The exception includes patients with arrhythmias and/or chest pain. Patients in stage 3 have congestive heart failure because of the associated severe mitral regurgitation. The stage 3 floppy mitral valve is the major cause of *pure* (i.e., no element of stenosis) *severe, isolated* (i.e., aortic valve normal anatomically and functionally) mitral regurgitation requiring valve replacement or repair.[14] As a consequence, considerable anatomic information is available on the floppy mitral valve that produces a pansystolic murmur (stage 3) and causes severe mitral regurgitation.[15] In contrast, less anatomic information is available in patients with only a systolic click(s) (stage 1) or those with both a click(s) and a late-systolic murmur (stage 2).[16]

Several names applied to this syndrome describe to some extent what the valve looks like anatomically, thus the names "prolapsing posterior mitral leaflet," "prolapsing mitral valve," "billowing or ballooning mitral leaflet syndrome," "overshooting or hooded mitral valve," "floppy mitral valve," and "myxomatous or mucinous degeneration of the mitral valve." I prefer the term *mitral valve prolapse.*

Defining mitral valve prolapse morphologically has not been easy. Pomerance[17] defined the entity as a ballooning deformity of the mitral leaflets, the affected portions of which were increased in area and protruded into the left atrium in ventricular systole. Waller and associates[14] also used either a focal or a diffuse increase in mitral area as a criterion but also required an increased length, either focal or diffuse, from basal attachment of the leaflet to its distal margin. Lucas and Edwards[18] listed the following features for diagnosis: (1) interchordal hooding involving both the rough and the clear zones of the involved leaflet or leaflets, (2) height of the interchordal hooding >4 mm, (3) interchordal hooding involving >50% of the anterior leaflet of >67% of the posterior leaflet. Dollar and Roberts[16] used 2 criteria for mitral valve prolapse: (1) elongation of a portion of posterior mitral leaflet such that the distance from distal margin to its attachment at the mitral anulus was >1.5 cm or (2) presence of mitral leaflet protrusion toward the left atrium, usually also associated with missing chordae tendineae, and the prolapsed portion of the leaflet involving >50% of the anterior leaflet and >33% of the posterior leaflet. Others have referred to this leaflet prolapse as "interchordal hooding."

Other useful anatomic findings in identifying mitral valve prolapse include the following:

(1) *An increase in the transverse dimension of the leaflets such that the length of the mitral circumference measured on a line corresponding to the distal margin of the posterior leaflet is much larger than the circumference measured at the level of the mitral anulus.* In the normal valve, the two are the same. The result is analogous to an accordion not fully extended, or better, a skirt gathered at the waist. The leaflets of the opened mitral valve are flat or smooth (like the mucosa of the ileum), whereas those of the opened floppy mitral valve are undulating (like those of the duodenum or jejunum).

(2) *Excessive thinning and lengthening of chordae tendineae.* Chordal elongation, however, is rare without concomitant leaflet elongation. The chordae also occasionally may be shorter than normal.

(3) *Dilation of the mitral anulus.* This does not occur to any significant degree in the absence of the mitral valve prolapse.[19] Anular dilation is the major cause of development of severe mitral regurgitation in the presence of mitral valve prolapse (the other is rupture of chordae tendineae).[15] Normally, the mitral anulus in adults averages approximately 9 cm in circumference. In patients with left ventricular dilation from any cause with or without mitral regurgitation, the circumference of the mitral anulus usually dilates slightly, to approximately 11 cm or <25% above normal. Among patients with mitral valve prolapse associated with severe mitral regurgitation, the circumference of the mitral anulus generally increases >50% above normal or to circumferences of 14 to 18 cm. When the anulus dilates to this extent, the leaflets may "stretch" or flatten transversely, and this stretching diminishes the amount of scalloping. In addition, the left ventricular dilation may cause longitudinal stretching of the leaflets. The amount of scalloping in the stage 3 valves, therefore, appears to be less than that observed in the stage 2 valves. Roberts and coworkers[15] examined operatively excised mitral valves in 83 patients (aged 26–79 years [mean 60]; 26 women [31%] and 57 men [69%]) with mitral valve prolapse and mitral regurgitation severe enough to warrant mitral valve replacement. All 83 operatively excised valves were examined by the same person, and all excised valves had been purely regurgitant (no element of stenosis). No patients had hemodynamic evidence of dysfunction of the aortic valve. In each valve, a portion of the posterior mitral leaflet was elongated such that the distance from the distal margin to basal attachment of this leaflet was similar to the distance from the distal margin of the anterior leaflet to its basal attachment to the left atrial wall. Two major mechanisms for the severe mitral regurgitation were found: (1) dilation of the mitral anulus with or without rupture of chordae tendineae and (2) rupture of chordae tendineae with or without dilation of the mitral anulus. Of the 83 patients, 48 (58%) had both dilated anuli (>11 cm in circumference) and ruptured chordae tendineae; 16 (19%) had dilated anuli without ruptured chordae; and 16 (19%) had ruptured chordae without significant anular dilation. In 3 patients, the anulus was not dilated, nor were chordae ruptured, and, therefore, the mechanism of the mitral regurgitation is uncertain. Mitral chordal rupture was nearly as frequent in the 64 patients with clearly dilated anular circumferences as in the 19 patients with normal or insignificantly dilated anular circumferences (≤11 cm).

(4) *Focal thickening of mural endocardium of the left ventricle behind the posterior mitral leaflet and the mitral chordae tendineae.* Salazar and Edwards[20] called these fibrous thickenings "friction lesions" to indicate that they are believed to result from friction between the overlying leaflets and chordae and the underlying left ventricular wall. Of the 102 necropsy cases with mitral valve prolapse studied by Lucas and Edwards,[18] 77 (75%) had these friction lesions, and in 3 (3%), the mural endocardial friction lesions had entrapped the overlying chordae. Dollar and Roberts[16] observed these friction lesions in 23 (68%) of 34 patients with mitral valve prolapse in whom each heart was examined specifically for these lesions. The friction lesions, therefore, are common in patients with mitral valve prolapse, and their presence strongly suggests mitral valve prolapse.

(5) *Fibrinous deposits on the atrial surface of the prolapsed portion of the mitral leaflet, particularly at the angle formed between the prolapsed leaflet and left atrial*

wall (mitral valve-left atrial angle). These deposits in the angle may be a source of emboli.

Microscopically, the prolapsed mitral leaflet may or may not contain an excessive amount of acid mucopolysaccharide material. Both the normal and the prolapsed mitral leaflets consist of two elements, the fibrosa and the spongiosa. The *fibrosa* consists of fibrous tissue (collagen), and the *spongiosa,* of mucoid or myxomatous material high in acid mucopolysaccharide material. In most valve diseases, the fibrosa element is increased and may entirely replace the spongiosa element. In the prolapsed mitral leaflet, the spongiosa element, the more central portion of the leaflet, may increase to a greater extent than the fibrosa element. The resulting increased myxoid or myxomatous stroma, however, does not appear abnormal, that is, degenerated. Thus, the term *myxoid* or *myxomatous degeneration* for this condition is not appropriate. The amount of fibrous tissue in the mitral leaflets in mitral valve prolapse also is usually increased, but its increase may be a secondary phenomenon. The fibrosa element may be subdivided into two components, the *auricularis,* which normally is a thin layer forming the atrial or contact aspect of the leaflet, and the *ventricularis,* which normally is a relatively thick layer that covers the ventricular aspect of the leaflet. The atrial aspect of the prolapsed mitral leaflet often is focally thickened. This change probably is secondary to abnormal friction from contact between the prolapsed segment of the leaflet and its "opposite number," that is, the other leaflet, or between two prolapsed segments of the same leaflet.[21,22] The changes on the ventricular surface of the leaflet consist of connective tissue "pads" forming primarily in the interchordal segments. This proliferation of fibrous tissue may extend into adjacent chordae tendineae and onto ventricular endocardium behind the posterior mitral leaflet.[20,22] The interchordal collections of fibrous tissue are considered responses to the tension and stretching that occur at the undersurface of a prolapsed leaflet or segment of leaflet.[22] This increase in fibrous tissue, particularly on the ventricular surface of the leaflet, has caused, I suspect, the floppy valve in years past to be considered rheumatic in origin. Fibrin deposits also may occur on the atrial aspects of the prolapsed mitral leaflet, and they may not be found on gross examination.[17]

Ultrastructural studies of floppy mitral valves have disclosed alterations of the collagen fibers in the leaflets and in the chordae tendineae.[23] These changes have included fragmentation, splitting, swelling, and coarse granularity of the individual collagen fibers, and, in addition, spiraling and twisting of the fibers. Also, some elastic fibers are fragmented and contain cystic spaces. These alterations in the structure of the collagen may be more important than the accumulation of the acid mucopolysaccharide material in that they lead to focal weaknesses in the leaflets. The left ventricular systolic pressure exerted against these weakened areas may lead to prolapse or focal interchordal hooding. Although the actual prolapse of the mitral valve may be acquired and a consequence of the left ventricular systolic (closing) pressure, the focally weak areas of the leaflets are probably most often congenital in origin, and the later bulging with or without rupture is acquired as a consequence of the high intra-arterial pressure. The frequency of mitral valve prolapse also may be higher in persons with elevated left ventricular systolic pressures compared with persons in whom this pressure is at normal levels.[24]

Opportunities for structural study of a mitral valve associated with only a click(s) have been rare. I have studied one such valve. (The child had been examined by John Barlow, M.D., of Johannesburg, South Africa.) The child, who had no symptoms of cardiac dysfunction, died of leukemia and at necropsy had a perfectly competent mitral valve but three distinct foci where leaflet overlapped adjacent leaflet. The leaflets otherwise were smooth and, specifically, devoid of so-called scallops. There are no reported anatomic descriptions, to my knowledge, of mitral valves producing one or more systolic clicks without an associated precordial systolic murmur. Examination at necropsy of mitral valves of patients who during life had documentation of systolic click(s) plus a mid-late systolic murmur (Barlow syndrome) also are infrequent. Death in stage 2 as in stage 1 is usually from a noncardiac cause. In this stage, the most characteristic feature is leaflet scalloping, which represents excessive leaflet owing to an increase in the transverse or commissure-to-commissure dimension of the leaflet.[16] This mitral anulus, as in stage 1, is not dilated. The chordae tendineae may or may not be elongated.

Just as the frequency of mitral valve prolapse varies clinically depending on the age and sex group being examined and in the clinical criteria employed for diagnosis (auscultatory, echocardiographic, angiographic), its frequency at necropsy is quite variable and the variation is determined by several factors: (1) the age and sex group of the population being examined; (2) the type of institution where necropsy is performed (general hospital, referral hospital for cardiovascular disease, or medical examiner's [coroner's] office), (3) the expertise in cardiovascular disease of the physician performing the necropsy or reporting the findings, (4) the percent of total deaths having autopsies at the particular hospital, (5) the presence or absence of evidence of cardiac disease before death, (6) whether or not the patient underwent mitral valve replacement or repair, and (7) whether or not the percentage of patients being examined had a high frequency of the Marfan's syndrome, infective endocarditis, atrial septal defect, and so on. No study better shows how bias alters the findings in necropsy studies than the one performed by Lucas and Edwards.[18] These investigators in one portion of their study determined the frequency of the complications of floppy mitral valves observed at necropsy in one community (nonreferral) hospital for adults. Of 1376 autopsies performed, 7.4% or 102 patients at necropsy had morphologically floppy mitral valves. Their mean age at death was 69 $\pm$ 12 years; 62 (61%) were men and 40 (39%) were women. Of the 102 patients, mitral valve prolapse was the cause of death in only 2. Of the 102 patients, one leaflet had prolapsed in 34 patients, and two leaflets in 68. Only 18 patients had anatomic evidence of previous mitral regurgitation: 7 had infective endocarditis; 7, ruptured chordae tendineae (without infection); 1, the Marfan syndrome; 3, secundum atrial septal defect. No patient died suddenly. In contrast, in the other portion of their study, these authors described complications in 69 necropsy patients whose hearts had been sent to Edwards for his opinion and interest. Among these 69 patients, 16 (23%) had died suddenly and unexpectedly; 19 (28%) had ruptured chordae tendineae (without infection); 7 (10%), infective endocarditis; 20 (29%), the Marfan syndrome; and 9 (13%), secundum type atrial septal defect. Thus, in contrast to their infrequency in their community hospital series, most cases submitted to their cardiovascular registry from other institutions had ruptured chordae, infective endocarditis, sudden unexpected and unexplained death, or the Marfan syndrome.

Two other necropsy studies can be compared with the community hospital series collected by Lucas and Edwards. Pomerance[17] collected from one general hospital 35 cases at necropsy of "ballooning deformity" of the mitral valve: 23 (66%) were men and 12 (34%) were women; their ages ranged from 51 to 98 years (mean 74). Death was attributed to mitral valve prolapse in only 4 patients (11%). Only one leaflet had prolapsed in 12 patients and 2 leaflets in 23 (6%). Eight patients had anatomic evidence of mitral regurgitation, only 1 had atrial septal defect, 9 (26%) had anatomic evidence of tricuspid valve prolapse, 9 (26%) had mitral anular calcific deposits, and 13 (37%) had hearts of increased weight. Davies and associates[25] gathered 90 necropsy cases of the floppy mitral valve from four general hospitals. This number represented 4.5% of autopsies at the four hospitals during the time. Of the 90 patients, 44 (49%) were men and 46 (51%) were women; they ranged in age from <40 to 100 years. Death in 15 was attributed to mitral valve prolapse (the number dying suddenly was not mentioned). The prolapse involved one leaflet in 69 patients (77%) and both mitral leaflets in 21 (23%); 63 (70%) also had anatomic evidence of tricuspid valve prolapse. Only 6 (7%) patients had dilated mitral anuli; only 3 (3%) had mitral anular calcium; and 8 had hearts weighing >300 g.

Dollar and Roberts[16] studied at necropsy 56 patients aged 16 to 70 years (mean 48) with mitral valve prolapse. Of these, 15 patients, aged 16 to 69 years (mean 39), died suddenly, and mitral valve prolapse was the only cardiac condition found at necropsy (hereafter called isolated mitral valve prolapse). The remaining 41 patients had other conditions that were capable of being fatal. Of the latter 41 patients, 7, aged 17 to 59 years (mean 45), had associated congenital heart disease, and 34 patients, aged 17 to 70 years (mean 52), had no associated congenital cardiac abnormalities. Compared with the 34 patients without associated congenital heart disease and with nonmitral valve prolapse conditions capable in themselves of being fatal, the 15 patients who died suddenly with isolated mitral valve prolapse were younger (mean age 39 ± 17 vs. 52 ± 15 years; $p = 0.01$), more often women (67% vs. 26%; $p = 0.008$), and had a lower frequency of mitral regurgitation (7% vs. 38%; $p = 0.02$). The 15 patients dying suddenly with isolated mitral valve prolapse also were less likely to have evidence of ruptured chordae tendineae (29% vs. 67%; $p = 0.04$). The frequency of increased heart weight (67% vs. 59%), a dilated mitral valve anulus (80% vs. 81%), a dilated tricuspid valve anulus (17% vs. 17%), an elongated anterior mitral leaflet (86% vs. 54%), an elongated posterior mitral leaflet (79% vs. 77%), and fibrous endocardial plaque under the posterior mitral leaflet (73% vs. 63%) was similar between the two groups. The severity of the prolapse (mild, 20% vs. 11%; moderate, 27% vs. 58%; severe, 53% vs. 32%) also was similar between the two groups. Thus, persons with mitral valve prolapse dying suddenly without another recognized condition tend to be relatively young women without mitral regurgitation.

The frequency of mitral valve prolapse among patients undergoing mitral valve replacement for *isolated* (aortic valve function normal), *pure* (no element of stenosis), and *severe* mitral regurgitation is high. Indeed, prolapse appears to be the most common etiology of isolated, pure, and severe mitral regurgitation. My associates and I[14] reviewed the records and operatively excised mitral valves of 97 patients (57 men), aged 32 to 78 years (mean 54), who underwent mitral valve replacement because of 3+/4+ or 4+/4+ mitral regurgitation as determined by left ventricular angiography. Of the 97 patients, the cause of the mitral regurgitation was leaflet prolapse in 60 (62%), papillary muscle dysfunction from coronary artery disease in 29 (30%), infective endocarditis involving apparently previously normal mitral valves in 5, and rheumatic heart disease in 3 patients. Of the 60 patients with mitral valve prolapse, 13 had ruptured chordae tendineae, including all 4 patients with infective endocarditis superimposed on mitral valve prolapse. The circumference of the mitral anulus in patients with mitral valve prolapse without ruptured chordae was significantly larger than those in the patients in other groups and in 18 control subjects, both of which were normal. Likewise, the areas of the excised leaflets in the prolapsed valves were much larger than in the other groups and in the control subjects, both of which were normal. The product of the circumference (in cm) multiplied by the area (in cm^2) calculated for the normal valves ranged from 45 to 140 cm^3 (average 91). The average product was 150 cm^3 in the prolapsed valves with ruptured chordae and 273 cm^3 in the prolapsed valves with intact chordae. The products were 87, 91, and 106 cm^3, respectively, in the valves regurgitant because of papillary muscle dysfunction, infective endocarditis, or rheumatic disease; these products did not differ from those of the normal valves.

The correct cause of the mitral regurgitation in the 97 patients was usually predictable from the history alone. Of the 29 patients with papillary muscle dysfunction from atherosclerotic coronary artery disease, all had clinical evidence of myocardial ischemia—history of acute myocardial infarction that had healed in 24, left ventricular aneurysm from a silent infarction in 1, and angina pectoris in 4. Of the 5 patients with mitral regurgitation secondary to infective endocarditis, 4 had well-documented episodes of infection that had been cured by antibiotic therapy; none had evidence of valvular dysfunction before the episode of infective endocarditis. Of the 3 patients with mitral regurgitation secondary to a rheumatic origin, 2 had a history of acute rheumatic fever, whereas this item was positive in only 5 of the other 94 patients. Clinical diagnosis of mitral valve prolapse was by a process of exclusion. Only 2 (3%) of the 60 patients had historic evidence of previous acute myocardial infarction; 5 (8%) had a history of acute rheumatic fever; and 4 (7%) had a history of active infective endocarditis. Compared with the 5 patients classified as having ruptured chordae tendineae on previously normal valves (4 of whom had a history of infective endocarditis), the 4 patients with healed infective endocarditis and mitral valve prolapse were older (mean age 61 vs. 42 years), had previous systolic nurmurs of mitral regurgitation before the episode of infective endocarditis (4 of 4 vs. 0 of 5), and had a longer mean duration of congestive heart failure (11 vs. 4 months). Thus, of the 60 patients with mitral valve prolapse, 51 (85%) had no historic evidence of myocardial ischemia, acute rheumatic fever, or infective endocarditis.

The origin of the mitral regurgitation also was suggested preoperatively by more objective means. All 29 patients with mitral regurgitation secondary to coronary artery disease had abnormal Q waves by electrocardiogram, whereas abnormal Q waves were present in only 4 of the 60 patients with mitral valve prolapse and in none of the 8 patients with mitral regurgitation from either infective endocarditis or rheumatic disease. Atrial fibrillation was significantly more common in the patients in whom the mitral regurgitation resulted from coronary artery disease—in 7 (24%) of these 29 patients, in only 4 (7%) of the 60 patients with mitral valve prolapse, and in 2 of the 8 patients with either infective endocarditis or a rheumatic origin. Of the 60 patients with mitral valve prolapse, 43 had M-mode echocardiograms, and in 32 (74%) mitral valve prolapse was demonstrated.[26] Of the 29 patients with symptomatic coronary artery disease, M-mode echocardiograms were done in 22; only 2 (9%) had mitral valve prolapse. Of the 8 patients with mitral regurgitation from infective endocarditis or rheumatic etiology, 7 had echocardiograms; none had mitral valve prolapse. Left ventriculograms, performed in all 97 patients, indicated mitral valve prolapse in only 16 (27%) of the 60 patients with mitral valve prolapse and in none of the other 37 patients with other causes. Selective coronary angiograms were performed in 53 (55%) of the 97 patients. All 29 with mitral regurgitation secondary to coronary artery disease had significant (>50% diameter reduction) coronary narrowing angiographically in at least two of the three major coronary arteries. Of the 60 patients with mitral valve prolapse, coronary angiograms were performed in 23; only 3 (13%) had significant coronary arterial narrowing, limited in each to one coronary artery. Auscultation and hemodynamic data at cardiac catheterization were not helpful in delineating the origin of the mitral regurgitation. None of the 97 patients—including the 60 classified as having mitral valve prolapse—had systolic clicks, and the systolic precordial murmurs in all 97 patients were holosystolic. The average pulmonary arterial, left atrial (or pulmonary arterial wedge), and left ventricular pressures were similar in the 97 patients irrespective of the origin of the mitral regurgitation. The systolic systemic arterial pressures, however, were significantly higher in the patients with mitral valve prolapse and ruptured chordae tendineae than in those with mitral valve prolapse and intact chordae tendineae.

Mitral valve prolapse appears now to be a more common cause of rupture of mitral chordae tendineae than does infective endocarditis. Among 25 patients having mitral valve replacement for pure mitral regurgitation associated with rupture of chordae tendineae, Jeresaty and associates[27] found mitral valve prolapse (based on "redundancy and marked hooding of the mitral leaflets") to be the cause of the chordal rupture in 23 (92%), only 1 of whom had had infective endocarditis. Four of the 25 patients had auscultatory and angiographic or echocardiographic evidence of mitral valve prolapse before the chordal rupture. Among patients with ruptured chordae tendineae associated with mitral valve prolapse, sometimes identifying ruptured chords is actually difficult. The term *rupture,* however, is commonly applied to those leaflets that no longer have chordal insertions present when clearly chordae should be attached.[15]

In addition to mitral regurgitation, rupture of chordae tendineae, and infective endocarditis, other complications of mitral valve prolapse include *mitral anular calcification.* Pomerance[17] observed mitral anular calcium in 9 (26%) of her 35 necropsy patients with mitral valve prolapse. The cause of the *arrhythmias* and *chest pain* is unclear.[28] No evidence exists to suggest a myocardial or coronary arterial factor. Shrivastava and associates[22] have suggested that the friction between mitral chordae tendineae and the underlying left ventricular mural endocardium may be an arrhythmic stimulus. The cause of the *acute strokes* or *transient cerebral ischemic attacks* that occur in an occasional patient with mitral valve prolapse also is unclear. The small fibrin-platelet thrombi occasionally seen at the mitral valve-left atrial angle may be sources of emboli for either cerebral or myocardial ischemia.[18]

The cause of mitral valve prolapse, as alluded to earlier, almost certainly in most patients is congenital in origin, or at least the connective tissue of the mitral leaflets, chordae, and anulus appears to be congenitally defective. The finding of classic mitral valve prolapse at birth is evidence for the congenital thesis. The occurrence of mitral valve prolapse in certain clearly hereditary conditions, for example, the Marfan syndrome, is evidence of congenitally defective mitral tissue. Its association with aneurysm of the fossa ovale membrane or atrial septal defect and Ebstein's anomaly of the tricuspid valve also may support this thesis.[29-31]

CLEFT ANTERIOR MITRAL LEAFLET

Partial atrioventricular "defect" includes a spectrum of five anatomic anomalies.[32,33] Some patients have all five and others have only one or two. The five are the following: (1) defect in the lower portion of the atrial septum, so-called primum atrial septal defect; (2) defect in, or absence of, the posterobasal portion of ventricular septum; (3) cleft, anterior mitral leaflet; (4) anomalous chordae tendineae from the anterior mitral leaflet to the crest of the ventricular septum; and (5) partial or complete absence of the septal tricuspid valve leaflet. At least four potential functional consequences of these five anatomic anomalies exist. They are (1) shunt at the atrial level, (2) shunt at the ventricular level, (3) mitral regurgitation, and (4) obstruction to left ventricular outflow. More than 95% of patients with partial atrioventricular defect have a primum-type atrial septal defect, and most of those without a primum defect have a shunt at the ventricular level. The occurrence of mitral regurgitation from a cleft in the anterior mitral leaflet unassociated with a defect in either atrial or ventricular septa is rare, but such has been the case in several reported patients.[34–36] Indeed, at least 10 patients have been reported at necropsy to have a cleft in the anterior mitral leaflet unassociated with a defect in either the atrial or ventricular septum.[36] Of these, only 5 were older than 10 years of age. Nine of the 10 patients had mitral regurgitation.

LEFT-SIDED ATRIOVENTRICULAR VALVE REGURGITATION ASSOCIATED WITH CORRECTED TRANSPOSITION OF THE GREAT ARTERIES

Corrected transposition is an entity that has produced much confusion.[37] Corrected transposition and complete transposition are quite different; the only thing they have in common is the word "transposition." Complete transposition is essentially one defect: the great arteries are transposed, so that the aorta arises from the right ventricle and the pulmonary trunk from the left ventricle. In corrected transposition, the great arteries also are transposed, but, in addition, the ventricles, atrioventricular valves, coronary arteries, and conduction system are inverted. Patients with complete transposition die because they have inadequate communications between the two circuits. Patients with corrected transposition theoretically should be able to live a full life span, but usually this is not the case because associated defects—namely, ventricular septal defect or regurgitation of the left-sided atrioventricular valve, or both—cause the heart to function abnormally. Abnormalities of the left-sided atrioventricular valve, a systemic valve but anatomically a tricuspid valve, are the most common associated anomalies in corrected transposition.[37,38] Of the anomalies, the most frequent is the Ebstein-type malformation. These valves are intrinsically regurgitant because the chordae are short and the leaflets are closely adherent to the ventricular endocardium.

Most patients with corrected transposition have a defect in the ventricular septum that is associated with a left-to-right shunt.[37] Thus, most patients with corrected transposition present with evidence of excessive pulmonary blood flow. An occasional patient with corrected transposition, however, may have no defects in the cardiac septa and no ductus.[38] These individuals may present with evidence of pure mitral regurgitation and some of these patients during life have been considered to have rheumatic mitral regurgitation.[38]

Mitral Regurgitation Resulting from Papillary Muscle Dysfunction Produced by Origin of the Left Main Coronary Artery from the Pulmonary Trunk

When the left main coronary artery arises from the pulmonary trunk, the anterolateral wall of the left venticle including the anterolateral papillary muscle are usually inadequately perfused with arterial blood. As a consequence, the anterolateral papillary muscle atrophies and it may calcify.[32,33] The consequence is mitral regurgitation, which may be severe. Mitral regurgitation may even be the presenting manifestation of anomalously arising left main coronary artery from the pulmonary trunk.

Double-Orifice Mitral Valve

This valve from the left atrium has the appearance similar to looking down the muzzle of a double-barreled shotgun. Generally, both orifices are totally competent.[39]

AORTIC VALVE

Congenital conditions that affect the aortic valve include unicuspid, bicuspid, and quadricuspid valvular malformations, prolapse of one or more aortic valve cusps (usually associated with ventricular septal defect), atresia of the aortic valve, and congenital conditions that primarily affect the aorta (the Marfan syndrome) and secondarily lead to aortic valve dysfunction.

Aortic Valve Stenosis Involving a Congenitally Malformed Valve

If papillary muscle dysfunction is excluded, valvular aortic stenosis is the most common fatal cardiac valve lesion, comprising 49% of 1010 personally studied necropsy patients older than 15 years of age with valvular heart disease.[33] Of the 495 necropsy patients with aortic stenosis (with or without aortic regurgitation), the lesion was isolated in 59%, and in the other 41%, the mitral valve was stenotic or regurgitant or both. The evidence is substantial that the cause of aortic stenosis, when associated with mitral valve disease, is rheumatic.[40,41] In contrast, the evidence is substantial that isolated (mitral valve anatomically normal) aortic stenosis (with or without associated aortic regurgitation) is nonrheumatic in origin.[42-47] This section focuses on patients with isolated aortic stenosis.

In contrast to what was generally believed 30 or so years ago,[48] at least three factors indicate that anatomically isolated aortic valve disease (actually either stenosis or pure regurgitation) is nonrheumatic in origin:[40] (1) The low frequency (about 10%) of a positive history of acute rheumatic fever; (2) the absence of Aschoff bodies; and, most importantly, (3) the frequency of an underlying congenital malformation of the aortic valve.

The structure of the aortic valve in aortic stenosis can be correlated to some extent with the age of the patient. In patients younger than 15 years old, the aortic valve most commonly (60%) is congenitally unicuspid and unicommissural; in patients 15 to 65 years of age, the valve is most commonly (60%) congenitally bicuspid; and in patients older than age 65 years, the valve is most commonly (90%) tricuspid. The stenosis is either due to, or superimposed on, the congenitally malformed aortic valve in virtually all patients younger than 15 years of age, and in about 70% of patients aged 16 to 65 years. A congenitally malformed, in this case congenitally bicuspid, valve appears to be the underlying condition in about 10% of patients older than 65 years with aortic stenosis.

The unicommissural valve, the only type of unicuspid valve observed in the aortic valve position, was described initially by Edwards[49] in 1958. Although this valve, like all other congenitally malformed aortic valves, tends to get progressively more stenotic with time, the unicuspid aortic valve is almost certainly stenotic from the time of birth, whereas this usually is not the case with the congenitally bicuspid valve. Actually, the fewer the number of aortic valve cusps and commissures, the greater the likelihood that the valve is stenotic from birth.

Next to the floppy mitral valve, the congenitally bicuspid aortic valve is the most frequent major congenital malformation of the heart or great vessels.[13] Although its exact frequency is uncertain, this malformation appears to occur in about 1% of human births. Osler[50] found 10 apparently normally functioning congenitally bicuspid aortic valves in 800 autopsies (750 of which were performed by him), a frequency of 1%. Eight additional patients had infective endocarditis involving congenitally bicuspid aortic valves. Thus, 18 (2%) of 800 had either normally functioning or infected congenitally bicuspid aortic valves. Grant and associates[51] found apparently normally functioning congenitally bicuspid aortic valves in 12 (1%) of 1350 necropsy patients. Osler,[50] Lewis and Grant,[52] and Grant and coworkers[51] do not appear to have appreciated that the bicuspid condition of this valve may underlie severe stenosis at this site. Thus, if congenitally bicuspid aortic valves that develop complications (stenosis or regurgitation with or without infection) are added to those that function normally during the entire lifetime, the frequency of congenitally bicuspid aortic valves may exceed 1% of the population.

Among the complications of the bicuspid condition of the aortic valve, stenosis is by far the most frequent followed by pure regurgitation.[53] The latter lesion is most frequently the result of its being the site of infective endocarditis. Among 200 patients (75% male) with congenitally bicuspid aortic valves studied personally at necropsy, 157 (79%) had aortic stenosis, 22 (11%) had pure aortic regurgitation (in 19 from infective endocarditis), and 21 (10%) had normally functioning bicuspid valves. The latter 21 patients died of noncardiac causes, and the presence of the congenitally bicuspid aortic valve was a surprise finding at necropsy. Of the 157 patients with aortic stenosis, calcific deposits were present on both aortic valve cusps in 155 (99%); the 2 patients without calcific deposits were younger than 30 years of age. Calcific deposits, in contrast, were rare in the patients with pure aortic regurgitation. Infective endocarditis occurred in 14 (9%) of the 157 patients with aortic stenosis and in 19 (86%) of the 22 with pure aortic regurgitation. The infection was the prime cause of the regurgitation in all 19 patients. Infective endocarditis usually affects the normally functioning or only mildly dysfunctioning bicuspid aortic valve.[54] It infrequently affects a significantly stenotic aortic valve. The infection usually causes considerable destruction of one or both aortic valve cusps, leading to severe aortic regurgitation. Rarely, perforation of a cusp may occur without superimposed infective endocarditis.[55] The presence of a bicuspid aortic valve in an intravenous drug user is particularly devastating.[56,57]

Congenitally bicuspid aortic valves also are observed commonly in patients having aortic valve replacement for *isolated* (mitral valve function normal) aortic stenosis with or without associated aortic regurgitation, and preoperative detection of the bicuspid valve is reliable by preoperative cross-sectional echocardiography.[58] Among 393 patients aged 17 to 74 years with aortic stenosis with or without aortic regurgitation having aortic valve replacement at the National Heart, Lung, and Blood Institute from 1962 to 1982, 28 (7%) had unicommissural, unicuspid aortic valves; 203 (52%) had congenitally bicuspid aortic valves; 101 (26%) had three-cuspid aortic valves; and in 61 (15%), the number of cusps could not be determined by examination of the operatively excised valve. Subramanian and associates[59] determined the number of aortic valve cusps present in 338 patients (most aged 50 to 70 years) undergoing aortic valve replacement for isolated (I excluded their 36 patients with associated mitral stenosis or regurgitation) "pure" aortic stenosis during 4 different years (1965, 1970, 1975, and 1980). Of the 338 patients, 21 (6%) had unicommissural, unicuspid valves; 171 (51%) had congenitally bicuspid valves; 94 (28%) had tricuspid aortic valves; and in 14 patients (4%), the number of cusps present was not discernible.

Congenitally bicuspid aortic valves also are found commonly among patients undergoing aortic valve replacement for *isolated* (normal mitral valve function), pure (no element of stenosis) aortic regurgitation; the bicuspid status of the purely regurgitant aortic valve also is reliably detected by preoperative cross-sectional echocardiography.[53,60] Of 190 patients having aortic valve replacement for pure, chronic aortic regurgitation (mitral valve normal) at the National Heart, Lung, and Blood Institute, 21 (11%) had congenitally bicuspid aortic valves.[53] Of the 21 patients, 14 (67%) never had infective endocarditis, and, therefore, the regurgitation was on the basis of the congenital malformation only; the other 7 (33%) had infective endocarditis superimposed on the bicuspid condition. Severe aortic regurgitation in each resulted primarily from the infection, which in each was healed by antibiotics. Olson and associates[61] also determined the frequency of bicuspid aortic valves in 145 patients having isolated aortic valve replacement for pure aortic regurgitation or severe regurgitation associated with only mild aortic stenosis. (The basis of the presence or absence of associated aortic stenosis was by "clinical" means, which apparently did not mean hemodynamic studies.) Of the 145 patients, 49 (34%) had congenitally bicuspid aortic valves. Of these 49 patients, 41 (84%) apparently never had infective endocarditis, and the regurgitation primarily was on the basis of the bicuspid state of the valve; the other 8 (16%) had had infective endocarditis, which was the major cause of the regurgitation. Of the remaining 96 patients (66%), 94 (65% of total) had three-cuspid aortic valves, and 2 (1% of total) had quadricuspid valves. Of the 94 patients with three-cuspid aortic valves, the cause of the aortic regurgitation in 34 (36%) was "postinflammatory" (presumably rheumatic in at least 31—each of the aortic valve cusps in these patients was diffusely fibrotic with or without cuspal retraction and/or commissural fusion); associated with aortic root dilation in 44 (47%) (idiopathic in 43 [98%] and syphilitic in 1 [2%]); associated with infective endocarditis in 12 (13%); and associated with ventricular septal defect 4 (4%).

The reason one congenitally bicuspid aortic valve becomes stenotic, another purely regurgitant, and another the site of infective endocarditis is unknown. It is clear, however, that stenosis, regurgitation, and infection are complications of the bicuspid condition of the aortic valve, and none of them are present at birth. It appears likely that a congenitally bicuspid aortic valve becomes stenotic only as its cusps become fibrotic and calcified; neither cusp of a congenitally bicuspid aortic valve is severely thickened by fibrous tissue or calcific deposits at the time of birth.

The frequency of development of stenosis or pure regurgitation at the site of a congenitally bicuspid aortic valve also is unknown. Lewis and Grant[52] concluded that vegetations develop at these sites in about 23% of adults (16 of 69) with congenitally bicuspid valves. Of 31 patients with "subacute infective endocarditis" studied at necropsy by Lewis and Grant,[52] 8 (26%) had congenitally bicuspid aortic valves. Two (9%) of 22 patients studied at necropsy by Fulton and Levine[62] had congenitally bicuspid aortic valves. None of these investigators apparently was aware that congenitally bicuspid aortic valves also could become stenotic.

The mechanism by which a congenitally bicuspid aortic valve becomes stenotic or purely regurgitant is uncertain. No evidence exists to suggest that the valve is stenotic or regurgitant at birth. Likewise, there is no evidence that superimposed rheumatic fever or rheumatic heart disease is the cause of the stenosis or pure regurgitation. The explanation advanced by Edwards[63] is attractive. He proposed that it is not mechanically possible for a congenitally bicuspid aortic valve to open and close properly. The distances between the lateral attachments of normal aortic valvular cusps along their free margins are curved lines. The extra length allows the cusps to move freely during opening and closing of the orifice. In contrast, the distances between the lateral attachments of congenitally bicuspid aortic valves along their free margins approach straight lines. If these distances were exactly straight lines, the valve could not open during ventricular systole. Consequently, at least one cusp is larger than the other. But the excessive length of one or both cusps of a congenitally bicuspid aortic valve produces abnormal contact between the cusps. This abnormal contact, in turn, causes focal fibrous thickening that with time becomes diffuse, and dystrophic calcification thereafter occurs. Thus, stenosis of a congenitally bicuspid aortic valve may be the result of trauma to these cusps produced by their abnormal contact with each other. Although this explanation is appealing, it does not explain why one congenitally bicuspid aortic valve becomes stenotic, another becomes entirely regurgitant with or without infection, and another remains free of complications.

It is well recognized that patients with aortic isthmic coarctation often have congenitally bicuspid aortic valves. Of 200 patients with aortic isthmic coarctation studied at necropsy by Abbott,[64] 27% had congenitally bicuspid aortic valves. Of 104 patients with aortic isthmic coarctation studied at necropsy by Reifenstein and associates,[65] 62% had congenitally bicuspid aortic valves. These authors also pointed out that ascending aortic tears with or without dissection also were common (about 20%) in patients with aortic isthmic coarctation, but similar aortic lesions have an increased frequency among patients with congenitally bicuspid aortic valves unassociated with aortic isthmic coarctation. Less well appreciated is an occasional patient who may present with clinical features of aortic stenosis but by aortogram be found to have aortic isthmic coarctation. Among 157 personally studied necropsy patients with stenotic congenitally bicuspid aortic valves, 7 (4%) had aortic isthmic coarctation.

Patients with bicuspid aortic valves have an increased frequency of aortic dissection compared with persons with a tricuspid aortic valve. A bicuspid aortic valve was found in 11 (13%) of 85 patients with aortic dissection reported by Gore and Seiwert,[66] in 11 (9%) of 119 cases reported by Edwards and coworkers,[67] and in 14 (7.5%) of 186 necropsy patients with aortic dissection reported by Roberts and

Roberts.[68] Aortic dissection was found in 8 (5%) of 152 necropsy patients aged 20 years and older with a bicuspid aortic valve by Fenoglio and colleagues.[69] Larson and Edwards[70] observed aortic dissection in 18 (6%) of 293 necropsy patients with a bicuspid aortic valve and in 141 (0.67%) of 21,105 persons with a tricuspid aortic valve, a nine-fold difference. Roberts and Roberts[68] found aortic dissection in 14 (4%) of 328 patients studied at necropsy with a congenitally bicuspid aortic valve. Of the 16 patients with congenitally malformed aortic valves (14 bicuspid and 2 unicuspid) studied by Roberts and Roberts,[68] the entrance tear was in the ascending aorta in all 16. The aortic valve was stenotic in 6, and 2 had associated aortic isthmic coarctation. Histologic sections of aorta disclosed severe degeneration of the elastic fibers of aortic media in 90% of the patients studied. Thus, a congenitally malformed aortic valve appears to be present at least five times more frequently in adults with aortic dissection than in those without dissection.

The use of echocardiography and magnetic resonance imaging allows detection of the presence of a bicuspid aortic valve before symptoms or signs of cardiac dysfunction appear. In a person found to have a bicuspid aortic valve, the following advice may be useful in preventing or delaying the development of complications:[71]

(1) *Avoid infection.* Prophylactic antibiotics obviously are required during dental and other operative procedures. Sir William Osler was the one who pointed out in 1885 the extreme propensity of the bicuspid aortic valve to be the site of infective endocarditis.[72] Certainly one with a bicuspid aortic valve should not use illicit drugs intravenously.

(2) *Maintain a normal systemic blood pressure.* Although the bicuspid aortic valve probably is not affected adversely by the left ventricular systolic pressure irrespective of its level, the level of the valve's closing pressure, that is, the aortic diastolic pressure, probably plays a prominent role in determining whether the bicuspid valve becomes stenotic, purely regurgitant (without superimposed infective endocarditis), or functions normally throughout life.

(3) *Keep the heart rate relatively slow.* If the aortic valve closes only 55 times a minute rather than 75 times a minute (a 27% heart rate reduction), then the wear and tear received by the aortic valve from the aorta's closing pressure would be reduced. The best way to produce a relatively slow heart rate is by various aerobic exercises. Although the heart rate increases during exercise, the total 24-hour heart beats probably would be reduced substantially. Beta-blocker therapy could be useful to achieve this objective.

(4) *Keep the serum total cholesterol level relatively low.* The major reason a bicuspid aortic valve becomes stenotic is because large calcific deposits develop on the aortic aspects of the cusps, and these deposits impart an immobility to the cusps that prevents their opening adequately during ventricular systole. Thus, prevention of calcific deposits is essential for prevention of stenosis. Older persons in the Western world commonly develop calcific deposits on the aortic aspects of the aortic valve cusps, on the ventricular aspects of the posterior mitral leaflet (mitral "anular" calcium), and in atherosclerotic plaques in the coronary arteries (as well as in plaques in other arteries). The development of calcific deposits on the aortic valve, mitral anulus, and coronary arteries with age occurs only in those populations with serum total cholesterol levels >150 mg/dl and usually in those persons with levels >200 mg/dl. Thus, maintaining a low serum total cholesterol level prevents calcific deposits on a normally formed aortic valve, and therefore maintaining a low level should have a similar effect on a bicuspid aortic valve. Calcific deposits are never

present on the aortic valve at birth; they are always acquired. Calcific deposits are less common on stenotic mitral valves (rheumatic origin) in persons residing in the undeveloped nations of the world (where the serum total cholesterol levels often are <150 mg/dl) than in persons in the Western world where these levels are usually >150 mg/dl. Thus, maintaining relatively low serum total cholesterol level might deter calcific deposition on a bicuspid aortic valve. If there is no calcium, then there is usually no stenosis. Preventing calcific deposits, however, would not prevent the development of pure aortic regurgitation of infective endocarditis.

(5) *Try to forget that the aortic valve is bicuspid.* As long as the bicuspid valve functions normally, there is nothing to worry about. No one can predict which bicuspid aortic valve will function normally for a full lifetime and which one will become stenotic, purely regurgitant (without superimposed infective endocarditis), or infected. In other words, the natural history of a congenitally bicuspid aortic valve is unknown. About 1% of live births have a congenitally bicuspid valve. This means that about 50 million (of 5 billion) persons on planet earth have a congenitally bicuspid aortic valve, and about 2.5 million persons in the United States have a bicuspid aortic valve. What percentage of them in a lifetime will develop stenosis, pure regurgitation, infection, or no complications is unknown. Thus, clinicians must focus on areas other than the bicuspid aortic valve. Even with the worst scenario, aortic valve replacement is usually highly successful.

In contrast to the congenitally bicuspid aortic valve, the congenitally *unicuspid aortic valve* is far less common (about 15 times less common). At least two varieties of the unicuspid aortic valve exist. In one type, the orifice is located in the center of the cusp and there are no attachments or only rudimentary ones to the wall of the aorta. Edwards[49] referred to this valve as the *simple-dome* type. Another name might be *acommissural* valve. This type of valve is commonly found in patients with congenitally pulmonic stenosis. Indeed, it is the most frequent type of valve seen in that setting but is exceedingly uncommon in the aortic valve position. A second type of unicuspid valve is the *unicommissural* one. This valve, described by Edwards[49] in 1958, is characterized by an eccentrically located orifice and only one lateral attachment to the aortic wall, which is at the level of the orifice. From above, this valve has the appearance of an exclamation mark. In contrast to the bicuspid aortic valve, the unicuspid valve is nearly always stenotic from the time of birth.

The tricuspid aortic valves rarely appear to be stenotic at birth. If stenosis is present at birth and the aortic valve has three cusps, the stenosis is usually the result of a very small aortic "anulus" rather than the result of fusion of the cusps. Acquired stenosis of a three-cusp aortic valve, in contrast, is common. Of the necropsy patients aged 16 to 65 years that I studied with clinically isolated aortic stenosis (with or without regurgitation), 25% had tricuspid valves; among those older than 65 years of age, 90% had tricuspid valves. In the age group 16 to 65 years, about 50% of these patients with clinically isolated aortic stenosis and three-cuspid aortic valves also had diffuse fibrous thickening of the mitral leaflets. The associated diffuse mitral leaflet thickening is strong evidence that the etiology of the aortic stenosis in this group is rheumatic.[33,40] Also, nearly 75% of this group had positive histories[40] of acute rheumatic fever, whereas 10% of the other group, that is, those with anatomically normal mitral valves with aortic stenosis, had positive histories. The etiology of the aortic stenosis in patients 65 years of age and younger with three-cuspid aortic valves and anatomically normal mitral valves is unsolved. Possibly, minor abnormalities in the sizes of the aortic valve cusps from birth set the stage for abnormal contact of the cusps with one another with resultant fibrosis and finally stenosis.[45,73]

The least commonly seen congenitally malformed aortic valve is the *quadricuspid* one.[74,75] It rarely causes valvular dysfunction, and therefore most commonly is observed as an incidental finding at necropsy. Diagnosis of this valve type, however, has been made by echocardiogram. Prophylactic antibiotic therapy is not likely to be necessary for prevention of infective endocarditis in this circumstance.

AORTIC VALVE REGURGITATION ASSOCIATED WITH VENTRICULAR SEPTAL DEFECT

Among patients with isolated ventricular septal defect producing a significant left-to-right shunt and in whom the defect is not operatively closed, about 4% develop aortic regurgitation, which usually appears after the age of 5 years. The regurgitation in this circumstance results from prolapse of one or two aortic valve cusps into the ventricular septal defect.[76,77] As the degree of aortic regurgitation worsens, the degree of left-to-right shunt diminishes (because the prolapsed cusp(s) progressively "close" the defect in the ventricular septum). Strictly speaking, the aortic regurgitation is not congenital, but it occurs in the setting of congenital heart disease, namely the presence of ventricular septal defect. The degree of aortic regurgitation may be severe, and the combination of aortic regurgitation complicating ventricular septal defect may lead to the largest hearts encountered in humans.[78]

THE MARFAN SYNDROME AND FORME FRUSTE VARIETIES

The Marfan syndrome generally involves the bones, joints, eyes, heart, and blood vessels. The extremities are long and thin (dolichostenomelia), the ligaments and joint capsules are redundant, the lenses are dislocated (ectopia lentis), the ascending aorta often is dilated, and one or both left-sided cardiac valves frequently are regurgitant. Cardiovascular disease is by far the most common cause of death in patients with the Marfan syndrome. Of the 18 necropsy patients that I studied who fulfilled McKusick's criteria for this syndrome, all died from cardiovascular disease, and death in each was premature (mean age = 34 years [range 15 to 52]).[79] Of 56 deceased patients with this syndrome studied during life by Murdoch and associates,[80] cardiovascular disease was the cause of death in 52 (93%), and the mean age at death was 32 years. Of the 151 previously reported necropsy patients with the Marfan syndrome, the mean age at death was 23 years and ranged from stillbirth to 65 years. (The 91 articles in which these 151 patients were described are listed in the article by Roberts and Honig.[79])

A variety of cardiovascular lesions has been observed in the great arteries and hearts of patients with the Marfan syndrome. The 18 necropsy patients that I studied who had this syndrome could be readily separated into three groups on the basis of their cardiovascular lesions. Group 1 included 13 patients with *fusiform aneurysms of the ascending aorta*. All 13 patients had aortic regurgitation, and 6 also had associated mitral regurgitation. In each, the aneurysm involved the sinus and the proximal tubular portions of ascending aorta; 2 also had fusiform aneurysms in the descending thoracic aorta. Histologic study of the wall of the ascending aorta disclosed the typical lesion of this syndrome, that is, massive loss of elastic fibers and increased amounts of mucoid material in the media. Group 2 included 3 patients with *dissection* of the entire aorta. Before dissection, the aorta in each was of normal size, and, histologically, the wall of the aorta was normal. None of these 3 patients had either aortic or mitral regurgitation before the aortic dissection. Two, however, had had systemic hypertension. Group 3 included 2 patients with isolated mitral regurgitation with floppy mitral leaflets and markedly dilated mitral anuli. In each, the aortic lumen was of normal size, and its wall was normal histologically.

In contrast to the predominant occurrence of fusiform ascending aortic aneurysm in the patients I studied (13 of 18) and the relatively infrequent occurrence of aortic dissection (3 of 18), aortic dissection was the most frequent gross cardiovascular abnormality observed in the previously reported necropsy patients with the Marfan syndrome (57 [38%] of 151 patients), followed by aortic root aneurysm without dissection (53 [38%] patients), then mitral regurgitation without aortic root aneurysm or dissection (33 [22%] patients). Finally, 8 patients (5%) did not have aortic dissection, root aneurysm, or mitral regurgitation and were placed in a miscellaneous group. Analysis of the previously reported necropsy patients disclosed that those with either fusiform ascending aortic aneurysm or aortic dissection had similar mean ages (28 and 27 years), men were slightly more frequent in both groups (3:2), and only 10% of the 110 patients were aged 15 years or younger (nearly 70%). Sisk and associates[81] observed similar findings in 15 patients with the Marfan syndrome diagnosed at younger than 15 years of age.

As in all my 13 patients with fusiform ascending aortic aneurysms (or "anul-aortic ectasia"), evidence of aortic regurgitation was present in almost all (95%) of the previously reported necropsy patients with fusiform ascending aortic aneurysm. As an indication of the severity of the aortic regurgitation in the reported patients with fusiform ascending aortic aneurysm, the average indirect peak systolic systemic arterial pressure in the 29 (of the 53) patients in whom this information was available was 146 mm Hg (range 100 to 195), and the average end-diastolic systemic arterial pressure was 43 mm Hg (range 0 to 90), yielding an average pulse pressure of a little more than 100 mm Hg (range 40 to 170). Of the 29 patients with fusiform root aneurysm and reported blood pressure measurements, 18 (62%) had systemic arterial systolic pressures <140 mm Hg, 26 (90%) had systemic diastolic pressures <60 mm Hg, and 23 (79%) had pulse pressures >60 mm Hg.

In contrast to their frequent recording in the reported necropsy patients with fusiform ascending aortic aneurysms, blood pressure values *before the dissection occcurred* were virtually unreported in the 57 previously reported necropsy patients with aortic dissection (see Roberts and Honig[79]). Nevertheless, evidence of the presence of aortic regurgitation before the aortic dissection was rare. The reason that aortic regurgitation before dissection is rare in the patients with aortic dissection is because dissection is infrequent in the patients with fusiform ascending aortic aneurysm, and it is the latter that primarily is responsible for the severe aortic regurgitation (in the absence of healed dissection). With few exceptions, aortic dissection in patients with the Marfan syndrome tends to affect the previously normal-sized aorta or the aorta that is only slightly dilated. None of 13 necropsy patients that I studied with fusiform ascending aortic aneurysm had aortic dissection, and none of the 3 patients that I studied with dissection of the entire aorta had evidence of fusiform ascending aortic aneurysm or aortic regurgitation before the dissection. Of the reported patients with aortic dissection, those with dilated ascending aortas over a long period of time usually had healed dissections, and the dilation in them appeared to be the result of aneurysm of the false channel. In at least 14 of the 57 previously reported patients with aortic dissection, the dissection had healed (see Roberts and Honig[79]).

The reason that fusiform ascending aortic aneurysm occurs in some patients with the Marfan syndrome and aortic dissection in others appears to lie in the status of the aortic media. In each of the 13 necropsy patients that I studied with fusiform aneurysm of the ascending aorta, histologic study of the wall of the aorta disclosed severe degrees of "cystic medial necrosis." In contrast, none of 3 patients with dissection involving the entire aorta had cystic medial necrosis by histologic examination. Furthermore, in 44 of the 53 previously reported necropsy patients with fusiform ascending aortic aneurysm, cystic medial necrosis was described, and in the other 9 patients, its presence or absence was simply not mentioned. It was not mentioned as being absent in any patient, and in those in whom photomicrographs were illustrated, the degree of cystic medial necrosis was nearly always severe. Among the 57 previously reported necropsy patients with aortic dissection, cystic medial necrosis was described as being present in 35 and as being absent in 7. In the patients, however, in whom photomicrographs of aorta were illustrated, the degree of cystic medial necrosis was usually minimal or mild, and rarely was the degree of cystic medial necrosis as severe as that observed routinely in the patients with fusiform ascending aortic aneurysm.

Thus, the aortic media appears to be quite different in the patient with fusiform ascending aortic aneurysm and in those with aortic dissection, particularly when the latter involves the entire aorta. In the patients with fusiform ascending aortic aneurysm, "massive" degeneration or loss of the elastic fibers of the media and increased quantities of collagen and mucoid material usually occur. The increased quantities of collagen would appear to prevent longitudinal aortic dissection. The aortic media in the patients with aortic dissection, in contrast, tends to be normal or to have only a mild degree of cystic medial necrosis, just as in patients with aortic dissection and systemic hypertension who do not have the Marfan syndrome.[82-85] Of the 3 patients I studied with aortic dissection, 2 had evidence of diastolic systemic hypertension, whereas none of the other 16 patients had diastolic hypertension.

In none of the previous reports describing necropsy patients with the Marfan syndrome was the degree of cystic medial necrosis graded. In 1970, however, Carlson and associates[82] graded the severity of cystic medial necrosis from 1 to 4 among patients with systemic hypertension and among others with normotension. They found that the frequency of cystic medial necrosis increased progressively from 10% in the first 2 decades of life to 60% and 64% in the seventh and eighth decades, respectively. The frequency and extent of cystic medial necrosis were higher in the hypertensive than in the normotensive patients of similar age. Schlatmann and Becker[83] confirmed the observation that certain degrees of cystic medial necrosis are observed in the normal aorta and that the degrees of cystic medial necrosis increase with age. Schlatmann and Becker[83] also compared the ascending aortic media in patients with dilated aortas with those in patients with complete or incomplete dissection and found only quantitative differences between the normal aging aorta and the overtly abnormal aorta. Thus, these newer observations regarding the frequency, extent, and significance of cystic medial necrosis must be taken into account when evaluating its presence in patients with the Marfan syndrome. Probably many of the patients with Marfan syndrome with aortic dissection have no more cystic medial necrosis than might be expected for the patient's age or level of systemic arterial pressure.

The term *cystic medial necrosis,* incidentally, has certain defects because "cysts" are relatively infrequent and "necrosis" is difficult to identify. Furthermore, the striking histologic aortic lesion, when full blown, is massive degeneration of elastic fibers, and this feature is ignored by the term *cystic medial necrosis.* When Gsell[86] in 1928 first used the term *medionecrosis* and a year later Erdheim,[87,88] the term *cystic medial necrosis,* stains for elastic fibers were apparently infrequently employed, and loss or degeneration of elastic fibers may be difficult to appreciate on hematoxylin-eosin–stained sections.

When elastic fibers disappear from the aortic wall in this condition, the space previously occupied by them appears to be replaced by collagen fibrils and mucoid material. Although the increased acid mucopolysaccharide material has been considered an inherent defect in this condition, this material may serve simply as "a filler" for the lost elastic fibers. Normally, the media of aorta in the ascending portion contains approximately 58 elastic lamellae.[89] Whether or not the numbers of the elastic lamellae are normal or decreased at the time of birth in the patients with the Marfan syndrome is not clear. Whether normal or decreased, however, fusiform ascending aortic aneurysm, with or without tears, has not been described in newborns with this syndrome. Thus, it appears that although the composition of the aortic media may be defective at birth, the aneurysms form later, presumably the consequence of the intra-aortic pressure's effect on an inherently weak wall.

Although most fusiform aneurysms in the Marfan syndrome involve the ascending aorta (both sinus and tubular portions), aneurysm also may involve the descending thoracic aorta (as it did in two patients I studied) and, as reported by others, the abdominal aorta. Because the numbers of elastic fibers in the abdominal aorta are only about ½ of those present in the ascending aorta with intermediate numbers in between,[89] and because the major histologic finding in the medial portion of the aneurysmal wall is massive loss of elastic fibers, it follows that the ascending aorta is the most common location of fusiform aneurysm in the Marfan syndrome. The ascending portion also moves ("stretches") the most with each heartbeat ("hypermobile aorta"), and this factor also may play a role in this preferential location of aneurysms in this syndrome.[90]

Although the major consequence of fusiform ascending aortic aneurysm in Marfan syndrome is aortic regurgitation (100% of 13 patients I studied and 95% of 42 previously reported patients in whom this information was recorded), rupture of the aneurysm, of course, is also a danger. This event occurred in 2 of 13 patients I studied and in at least 14 (25%) of the 57 previously reported necropsy patients with aortic dissection. Thus, treatment of patients with Marfan syndrome with fusiform ascending aortic aneurysms must be directed at elimination or prevention of aortic regurgitation and at prevention of aneurysmal rupture, not at prevention of dissection, because the latter is an infrequent complication in such patients.

Mitral regurgitation also is frequent in patients with the Marfan syndrome. At least six factors may be important in causing mitral regurgitation: (1) dilation of mitral anuli, (2) floppiness or prolapse of mitral leaflets and/or elongation of chordae tendineae, (3) calcification of mitral anuli, (4) rupture of mitral chordae tendineae, (5) infective endocarditis; and (6) papillary muscle dysfunction. Of these six factors, numbers 1, 2, 3, and 5 appear most important in causing severe degrees of mitral regurgitation. Of the 18 necropsy patients I studied, 9 had mitral regurgitation, isolated in 2 and combined with aortic regurgitation in 7. Of these nine patients, four had floppy mitral valves, whereas none of the nine patients without mitral regurgitation had floppy valves. The "floppiness" involved the posterior mitral leaflet in all four patients. Of the nine patients with mitral regurgitation, the circumference of the mitral anulus ranged from 10 to 17 cm (mean = 15; normal = 9), and of the nine patients without mitral regurgitation, the circumference ranged from 9 to 13 cm (mean = 11). Thus, the mean circumference of the mitral anulus in the nine patients with mitral regurgitation was dilated 67% above normal (15 compared with 9), and that in the nine patients without mitral regurgitation, only 22% above normal (12 compared with 9). Thus, both mitral leaflet prolapse and anular dilation play significant roles in causing mitral regurgitation in these patients.

Calcification of the mitral anulus is known to cause or at least to be associated with mitral regurgitation. The degree of regurgitation produced by this mechanism alone, however, is nearly always mild or minimal, and, in addition, the mitral anuli in patients without Marfan syndrome with mitral anular calcification are nearly always of normal or near-normal circumference. Of the 18 necropsy patients I studied, 5 had mitral anular calcific deposits; all 5 had associated mitral regurgitation, but, in addition, 4 had prolapsing mitral leaflets and in 4 the circumference of the mitral anulus was quite dilated (range 13 to 17 cm [mean = 15]). Evidence for rupture of mitral chordae tendineae was found in five of nine patients I studied with, and in none of the nine patients without, mitral regurgitation. Two of these five patients had histories of infective endocarditis that had healed. All five patients with evidence of mitral chordal rupture had prolapsing mitral leaflets, and four had dilated mitral anuli (range 15 to 17 cm [mean = 16]).

The role played by papillary muscle dysfunction in causing mitral regurgitation in these patients is less clear. Among the 18 patients I studied, the left ventricle was dilated in each and the left ventricular mass was increased in each. The hearts of the 18 patients ranged in weight from 375 to 850 g (mean = 654). In 13 of the 18 patients, the mitral leaflets were increased in length from their basal attachments to their distal margins. This "stretching" probably in part was the result of the elongation (apex to base) of the left ventricular cavities, resulting primarily from the associated aortic regurgitation. The resulting left ventricular dilation may have altered the normal angulation between the papillary muscles and mitral leaflets. Whether or not mitral regurgitation was increased in any patient by this mechanism, however, is uncertain.

In contrast to fusiform ascending aortic aneurysm and dissection, which generally become manifest after childhood, mitral valve abnormalities in the Marfan syndrome may be present at birth. I have studied at necropsy the heart of a 2-day-old child who at birth was found to have a loud murmur typical of mitral regurgitation and, at necropsy, floppy mitral and tricuspid valve leaflets. Although this child had the typical musculoskeletal features of the Marfan syndrome, the eyes were not examined, and there was no family history of the Marfan syndrome in other family members; therefore, this child was not included among the 18 necropsy patients I studied because the definition of the syndrome was not fulfilled. Nevertheless, it is likely that the child did have the Marfan syndrome. Others also have described abnormalities of the mitral or tricuspid valves in patients younger than 1 year of age with the Marfan syndrome.

Although most reports describing necropsy observations in patients with the Marfan syndrome have not mentioned the status of the mitral or tricuspid valves, one must recall that the floppy or prolapsing mitral valve was not recognized clinically until 1963[5] and at necropsy not until a year or so later. Thus, morphologic descriptions of floppy or prolapsing mitral or tricuspid valves would not be expected in the patients with Marfan syndrome until about 1965, and most of the detailed reported necropsy descriptions were before that date. Nevertheless, it is now clear that prolapse of one or both mitral leaflets is common at necropsy in the Marfan syndrome and that clicks, late systolic murmurs, and echocardiographic evidence of prolapse are common in these patients. Spangler and associates[91] found mitral valvular abnormalities by echocardiogram in 16 (62%) of 26 patients with the Marfan syndrome, and late or pansystolic apical murmurs and/or clicks or both in 16 (62%). Of 50 consecutive patients with the Marfan syndrome examined and reported by Pyeritz and McKusick,[92] 24 (48%) had midsystolic clicks with or without late systolic murmurs, and 29 (58%) had echocardiographic evidence of mitral valve prolapse. Although necropsy studies demonstrate abnormalities of the aorta with or without aortic regurgitation to be the most frequent cardiovascular abnormality in the Marfan syndrome, recent clinical and echocardiographic studies show that mitral valve dysfunction is even more common. Even among the previously reported necropsy patients aged 15 years or younger, however, mitral regurgitation was the most frequent type of cardiovascular dysfunction.

Relatively little information on the circumference of the mitral and tricuspid valve anuli has been provided in the previously reported necropsy patients with the Marfan syndrome with or without mitral regurgitation. Of the reported patients with mitral regurgitation, the mitral or tricuspid anular circumference was described as "increased" in several patients. In the 21-year-old man with severe mitral regurgitation reported by Van Buchem,[93] the mitral anulus was reported to be 18 cm and the tricuspid anulus, 23 cm in circumference. These are the largest anular circumferences encountered.

Patients with Marfan syndrome with fusiform ascending aortic aneurysms also may have mitral valvular abnormalities with or without mitral regurgitation. Seven of 13 patients I studied with fusiform ascending aortic aneurysms had mitral regurgitation. Of the 53 previously reported necropsy patients with fusiform ascending aortic root aneurysms, at least 9 (17%) had anatomic mitral valve abnormalities, but only 1 definitely had evidence of mitral regurgitation and that patient was only 7 months old, by far the youngest of any of the reported patients with aortic root aneurysm and the Marfan syndrome. (see 79). Of the 57 reported necropsy patients with aortic dissection, 9 (16%) had anatomic abnormalities of the mitral valve with mitral regurgitation in at least 3.

The Marfan syndrome may be associated with mitral anular calcium at a young age. Mitral anular calcific deposits were described in 5 of the 151 previously reported necropsy patients with the Marfan syndrome, and their ages ranged from 15 to 35 years (mean = 27)[102]; 3 were female and 2 were male; only 2 definitely had evidence of mitral regurgitation (see 79).

Infective endocarditis involving the mitral valve was described in 6 and possibly 7 of the 151 previously reported necropsy patients with the Marfan syndrome (see 79). Five of the 6 definite cases were among the 33 patients in the mitral regurgitation group. In all 7 patients, the infection involved the mitral valve, and in 1, also the aortic valve. Thus, the mitral valve is the usual site of vegetations when infective endocarditis occurs in patients with the Marfan syndrome. The floppy or prolapsing valve is the one most likely to be the site of infection. Because rupture of chordae tendineae is a frequent complication of infection involving the mitral valve, the degree of mitral regurgitation resulting from the infection can be severe.[94,95]

Although the heretofore discussion concerned only patients with typical features of the Marfan syndrome, the cardiovascular features described in them also occur in patients without skeletal or ocular features of this syndrome or histories of this syndrome in other family members.[96] In addition, the characteristic histologic features in the wall of ascending aorta also have been observed in the aorta of patients with congenitally malformed aortic valves, particularly the bicuspid condition, and in patients with aortic stenosis superimposed on a congenitally malformed valve.[67,68,97]

AORTIC VALVE ATRESIA

Aortic valve atresia, the worst of all types of heart diseases, that is, the one with the shortest survival, is the most common cause of death from heart disease in the first week of life.[98,99] It also is the most common cause of congestive heart failure and cardiomegaly in the first week of life. The hearts of patients with aortic valve atresia, with few exceptions, are uniform in appearance. No remnant of the aortic valve exists so that the ascending aorta, which is always hypoplastic, acts simply as a common coronary artery. Likewise, the left ventricle is markedly hypoplastic, and the ventricular septum is intact. The mitral valve is either hypoplastic or atretic. The left atrium is small. Some type of defect is nearly always present in the atrial septum, most commonly a valve-incompetent patent foramen ovale. Because both systemic and pulmonary venous blood empty into the right side of the heart, the right atrium, right ventricle, and the major pulmonary arteries are quite dilated. The systemic arteries are supplied entirely through a patent ductus arteriosus, which is usually large.

Roberts and associates[98] described 73 necropsy patients with aortic valve atresia. The mean age at death was 5 days; 80% died during the first week of life, and 70% were boys. Of the 73 patients, 69 (95%) had a hypoplastic left ventricle with intact ventricular septum and either an atretic (25 patients) or hypoplastic (44 patients) mitral valve. The other 4 patients had a well-developed left ventricle with one or more defects in the ventricular septum and either an atretic (1 patient) or well-developed (3 patients) mitral valve. (A well-developed left ventricle or ventricular septal defect in association with absence of the aortic valve is rare.[100])

TRICUSPID VALVE

The major congenital condition of the tricuspid valve unassociated with defects in the cardiac septa other than valvular competent or incompetent patent foramen ovale is Ebstein's anomaly.

EBSTEIN'S ANOMALY

This condition is characterized by caudal displacement of both septal and posterior tricuspid valve leaflets—or at least portions of them—such that the basal attachment of these leaflets is directly to the right ventricular myocardial wall rather than to the tricuspid valve anulus.[76,101,102] In addition, the anterior tricuspid valve leaflet is elongated, its area is increased, and the circumference of the junction of right atrial and right ventricular walls—the site of the true tricuspid valve anulus—is increased. The extent of the caudal displacement of the septal and posterior tricuspid valve leaflets is variable but may be so extreme that one or both of these leaflets attach to the ventricular septum rather than to the right ventricular wall. The tricuspid valve orifice as a consequence is usually incompetent. Cardiac dysfunction in these patients (in the absence of associated pulmonic valve stenosis) appears to result primarily from inadequate pumping of the right ventricle because the atrialized portion of the right ventricle has a thin wall which contracts poorly. The functioning mass of right ventricular muscle may be reduced to outflow portion. As a result, pulmonary blood flow may decrease, and the right atrial and systemic venous pressures may rise. Prognosis in patients with Ebstein's anomaly depends, in general, on the degree of caudal displacement of the tricuspid leaflets and the magnitude of associated valvular incompetency. The average life expectancy is 37 years. In its most severe form, Ebstein's anomaly has been the presumed cause of intrauterine and perinatal death, but survival into the seventh and eighth decades may occur.[101] Death most frequently (about 40%) results from congestive cardiac failure, another 20% from supraventricular arrhythmias, and the remainder from miscellaneous causes. About 75% of these patients have an atrial septal defect with some right-to-left shunting. Most defects are valvular-incompetent patent foramen ovale.

The clinical features of Ebstein's anomaly were first well described in 1950 by Engle and colleagues.[103] The typical patient is fatigued, dyspneic, often cyanotic, and has a large, "quiet" globular heart, gallop rhythm, systolic and scratchy diastolic murmurs, right bundle-branch block, and occasionally atrioventricular conduction delay (Wolff-Parkinson-White [type B] in 10%). Diagnosis of this anomaly may be difficult. Some patients may be acyanotic, asymptomatic, and devoid of diagnostically useful physical findings. In this situation, the electrocardiogram may be helpful. Diagnosis in patients surviving past the fourth decade may be confused with more common forms of acquired heart disease. The echocardiogram is very helpful in diagnosis. Diagnosis, if unsuspected, may be missed at catheterization.

PULMONIC VALVE

Congenital conditions affecting the pulmonic valve include pulmonic valve stenosis (with or without associated regurgitation) and pure pulmonic regurgitation.

PULMONIC STENOSIS

Congenital valvular pulmonic stenosis with intact ventricular septum is the most common form of isolated right ventricular outflow obstruction and comprises about 10% of all major congenital cardiovascular anomalies in patients surviving beyond infancy. The stenotic valve usually has a domed shape or funnel shape with a small (<5 mm) opening at the apex.[76] Three raphes extend from the valve to the pulmonary trunk, and these probably represent vestigial commissures. Rarely, three separate cusps are identifiable, but when this occurs, additional developmental defects usually are present. The mean age of death in unoperated patients with isolated pulmonic stenosis is 25 years.[104] Older patients with this malformation may develop calcific deposits in the valve.[105,106] About 25% of patients with pulmonic stenosis and intact ventricular septum have a shunt at the atrial level—right-to-left in two thirds and entirely left-to-right in the other third.[107,108]

Congenitally bicuspid pulmonic valves are rare in comparison with the frequency of congenitally bicuspid aortic valves. Although they are commonly associated with other congenital cardiovascular malformations, particularly Fallot's tetralogy, congenitally bicuspid pulmonic valves are rare in patients with isolated pulmonic stenosis. No reports, to my knowledge, have described isolated pulmonic stenosis complicating the congenitally bicuspid valve. Pulmonic valve stenosis with a dome-shaped pulmonic valve, however, has been observed in association with aortic valve stenosis complicating a bicuspid aortic valve.[109]

PURE PULMONIC REGURGITATION

Isolated pure congenital pulmonary regurgitation is rare. It may complicate idiopathic dilation of the pulmonary trunk, hypoplasia or aplasia of the pulmonic cusps, congenitally bicuspid or quadricuspid valves, or malformed tricuspid valves. Of 158 patients reported with congenitally quadricuspid pulmonic valves, only 4 appeared incompetent.[76]

The natural history of congenital pulmonic regurgitation is unclear. When secondary to an aplastic valve, congestive heart failure and death have occurred in infancy. Evidence of right ventricular dysfunction without symptoms of congestive cardiac failure may occur in adults. Most reported patients are young and asymptomatic. Although they may have abnormal right ventricular and pulmonary arterial pulsations and enlarged pulmonary trunks, the right ventricular and pulmonary arterial pressures are usually normal.

REFERENCES

1. Griffith, JP: Midsystolic and late-systolic mitral murmurs. Am J Med Sci 104:285, 1892.
2. Levine, SA and Thompson, WP: Systolic gallop rhythm. A clinical study. N Engl J Med 213:1021, 1935.
3. Brigden, W and Leatham, A: Mitral incompetence. Br Heart J 15:55, 1953.
4. Reid, JVO: Midsystolic clicks. S Afr Med J 35:353, 1961.
5. Barlow, JB, Pocock, WA, Marchand P, et al: The significance of late-systolic murmurs. Am Heart J 66:443, 1963.
6. Segal, BL and Likoff, W: Late-systolic murmur of mitral regurgitation. Am Heart J 67:757, 1964.
7. Barlow, JB and Bosman, CK: Aneurysmal protrusion of the posterior leaflet of the mitral valve. An auscultatory-electrocardiograph syndrome. Am Heart J 71:166, 1965.
8. Criley, JM, Lewis, KB, Humphries, JO, et al: Prolapse of the mitral valve: Clinical and cine-angiocardiographic findings. Br Heart J 28:488, 1966.
9. Barlow, JB, Bosman, CK, Pocock, WA, et al: Late-systolic murmurs and nonejection ("midlate") systolic clicks. An analysis of 90 patients. Br Heart J 30:203, 1968.
10. Markiewicz, W, Stoner, J, London, E, et al: Mitral valve prolapse in 100 presumably healthy young females. Circulation 53:464, 1976.
11. Procacci, PM, Savran SV, Schreiter, SL, et al: Prevalence of clinical mitral-valve prolapse in 1169 young women. N Engl J Med 294:1086, 1976.
12. Savage, DD, Garrison, RJ, Devereux, RB, et al: Mitral valve prolapse in the general population. I. Epidemiologic features. The Framingham study. Am Heart J 106:571, 1983.
13. Roberts, WC: The two most common congenital heart diseases. Am J Cardiol 53:1198, 1984.
14. Waller, BF, Morrow, AG, Maron, BJ, et al: Etiology of clinically isolated severe, chronic, pure mitral regurgitation: Analysis of 97 patients over 30 years of age having mitral valve replacement. Am Heart J 104:276, 1982.
15. Roberts, WC, McIntosh, CL and Wallace, RB: Mechanisms of severe mitral regurgitation in mitral valve prolapse determined from analysis of operatively excised valves. Am Heart J 113:1316, 1987.
16. Dollar, AL and Roberts, WC: Morphologic comparison of patients with mitral valve prolapse who died suddenly with patients who died from severe valvular dysfunction or other conditions. J Am Coll Cardiol 17:921, 1991.

17. Pomerance, A: Ballooning deformity (mucoid degeneration) of atrioventricular valves. Br Heart J 31:343, 1969.
18. Lucas, RV, Jr and Edwards, JE: The floppy mitral valve. Curr Prob Cardiol 7:1, 1982.
19. Bulkley, BH and Roberts, WC: Dilatation of the mitral anulus. A rare cause of mitral regurgitation. Am J Med 59:457, 1975.
20. Salazar, AE and Edwards, JE: Friction lesions of ventricular endocardium. Relation to chordae tendineae of mitral valve. Arch Pathol 90:364, 1970.
21. Guthrie, RB and Edwards, JE: Pathology of the myxomatous mitral valve: Nature, secondary changes and complications. Minn Med 59:637, 1976.
22. Shrivastava, S, Guthrie, RB, and Edwards, JE: Prolapse of the mitral valve. Mod Concepts Cardiovasc Dis 46:57, 1977.
23. Renteria, VG, Ferrans, VJ, Jones, M, et al: Intracellular collagen fibrils in prolapsed ("floppy") human atrioventricular valves. Lab Invest 35:439, 1976.
24. Roberts, WC: Mitral valve prolapse and systemic hypertension. Am J Cardiol 56:703, 1985.
25. Davies, MJ, Moore, BP, and Baimbridge, MV: The floppy mitral valve. Study of incidence, pathology, and complications in surgical, necropsy, and forensic material. Br Heart J 40:468, 1978.
26. Waller, BF, Maron, BJ, Del Negro, AA, et al: Frequency and significance of M-mode echocardiographic evidence of mitral valve prolapse in clinically isolated pure mitral regurgitation. Analysis of 60 patients having mitral valve replacement. Am J Cardiol 53:139, 1984.
27. Jeresaty, RM, Edwards, JE, and Chawla, SK: Mitral valve prolapse and ruptured chordae tendineae. Am J Cardiol 55:138, 1985.
28. Savage, DD, Levy, D, Garrison, RJ, et al: Mitral valve prolapse in the general population. 3. Dysrhythmias: The Framingham study. Am Heart J 106:582, 1983.
29. Roberts, WC, Glancy, DL, Seningen, RP, et al: Prolapse of the mitral valve (floppy valve) associated with Ebstein's anomaly of the tricuspid valve. Am J Cardiol 38:377, 1976.
30. Cabin, HS and Roberts, WC: Ebstein's anomaly of the tricuspid valve and prolapse of the mitral valve. Am Heart J 101:177, 1981.
31. Roberts, WC: Aneurysm (redundancy) of the atrial septum (fossa ovale membrane) and prolapse (redundancy) of the mitral valve. Am J Cardiol 54:1153, 1984.
32. Roberts, WC and Perloff, JK: Mitral valvular disease. A clinicopathologic survey of the conditions causing the mitral valve to function abnormally. Ann Intern Med 77:939, 1972.
33. Roberts, WC: Morphologic features of the normal and abnormal mitral valve. Am J Cardiol 51:1005, 1983.
34. Braunwald, E, Ross, RS, Morrow, AG, et al: Differential diagnosis of mitral regurgitation in childhood. Ann Intern Med 54:1223, 1961.
35. Brockenbrough, EC, Braunwald, E, Roberts, WC, et al: Partial persistent atrioventricular canal simulating pure mitral regurgitation. Am Heart J 63:9, 1962.
36. Barth, CW, III, Dibdin, JD, and Roberts, WC: Mitral valve cleft without cardiac septal defect causing severe mitral regurgitation but allowing long survival. Am J Cardiol 55:1229, 1985.
37. Berry, WB, Roberts, WC, Morrow, AG, et al: Corrected transposition of the aorta and pulmonary trunk. Clinical, hemodynamic and pathologic findings. Am J Med 36:35, 1964.
38. Roberts, WC, Ross, RS, and Davis, FW, Jr: Congenital corrected transposition of the great vessels in adulthood simulating rheumatic valvular disease. Bull Johns Hopkins Hosp 114:157, 1964.
39. Rosenberg, J and Roberts, WC: Double orifice mitral valve. Study of the anomaly in two calves and a summary of the literature in humans. Arch Pathol 86:77, 1968.
40. Roberts, WC: Anatomically isolated aortic valvular disease. The case against its being of rheumatic etiology. Am J Med 49:151, 1970.
41. Roberts, WC and Virmani, R: Aschoff bodies at necropsy in valvular heart disease. Evidence from an analysis of 543 patients over 14 years of age that rheumatic heart disease, at least anatomically, is a disease of the mitral valve. Circulation 57:803, 1978.
42. Roberts, WC and Morrow, AG: Congenital aortic stenosis produced by a unicommissural valve. Br Heart J 27:505, 1965.
43. Roberts, WC and Elliott, LP: Lesions complicating the congenitally bicuspid aortic valve. Anatomic and radiographic features. Radiol Clin North Am 6:409, 1968.
44. Roberts, WC: The congenitally bicuspid aortic valve. A study of 85 autopsy cases. Am J Cardiol 26:72, 1970.
45. Roberts, WC: The structure of the aortic valve in clincially isolated aortic stenosis. An autopsy study of 162 patients over 15 years of age. Circulation 42:91, 1970.
46. Roberts, WC, Perloff, JK, and Constantino, T: Severe valvular aortic stenosis in patients over 65 years of age. A clinicopathologic study. Am J Cardiol 27:497, 1971.

47. Falcone, WM, Roberts, WC, Morrow, AG, et al: Congenital aortic stenosis resulting from unicom-
    missural valve. Clinical and anatomic features in 21 adult patients. Circulation 44:272, 1971.
48. Karsner, HT and Koletsky, S: Calcific Disease of the Aortic Valve. JB Lippincott, Philadelphia, p
    111, 1947.
49. Edwards, JE: Pathologic aspects of cardiac valvular insufficiencies. Arch Surg 77:634, 1958.
50. Osler, W: The bicuspid condition of the aortic valves. Trans Assoc Am Physicians 2:185, 1886.
51. Grant, RT, Wood, JE, and Jones, TD: Heart valve irregularities in relation to subacute bacterial
    endocarditis. Heart 14:247, 1928.
52. Lewis, T and Grant, RT: Observations relating to subacute infective endocarditis. Part 1. Notes on
    the normal structure of aortic valve. Part 2. Bicuspid aortic valves of congenital origin. Part
    3. Bicuspic aortic valves in subacute infective endocarditis. Heart 10:21, 1923.
53. Roberts, WC, Morrow, AG, McIntosh, CL, et al: Congenitally bicuspid aortic valve causing severe,
    pure aortic regurgitation without superimposed infective endocarditis. Analysis of 13 patients
    requiring aortic valve replacement. Am J Cardiol 47:206, 1981.
54. Arnett, EN and Roberts WC: Active infective endocarditis: A clinicopathologic analysis of 137
    necropsy patients. Curr Probl Cardiol 1:1, 1976.
55. Roberts, WC, McIntosh, CL, and Wallace, RB: Aortic valve perforation with calcific aortic stenosis
    and without infective endocarditis or significant aortic regurgitation. Am J Cardiol 59:476,
    1987.
56. Dressler, FA and Roberts, WC: Infective endocarditis in opiate addicts: Analysis of 80 cases studied
    at necropsy. Am J Cardiol 63:1240, 1989.
57. Dressler, FA and Roberts, WC: Modes of death and types of cardiac diseases in opiate addicts:
    Analysis of 168 necropsy cases. Am J Cardiol 64:909, 1989.
58. Brandenburg, RO, Jr, Tajik, AJ, Edwards, WD, et al: Accuracy of two-dimensional echocardio-
    graphic diagnosis of congenitally bicuspid aortic valve. Echocardiographic-anatomic correla-
    tion in 115 patients. Am J Cardiol 51:1469, 1983.
59. Subramanian, R, Olson, LJ, and Edwards, WD: Surgical pathology of pure aortic stenosis: A study
    of 374 cases. Mayo Clin Proc 59:683, 1984.
60. Stewart, WJ, King, ME, Gillam, LD, et al: Prevalence of aortic valve prolapse with bicuspid aortic
    valve and its relation to aortic regurgitation: A cross-sectional echocardiographic study. Am J
    Cardiol 54:1277, 1984.
61. Olson, LJ, Subramanian, R, and Edwards, WD: Surgical pathology of pure aortic insufficiency: A
    study of 225 cases. Mayo Clin Proc 59:835, 1984.
62. Fulton, MN and Levine, SA: Subacute bacterial endocarditis, with special reference to the valvular
    lesions and previous history. Am J Med Sci 183:60, 1932.
63. Edwards, JE: The congenital bicuspid aortic valve. Circulation 34:485, 1961.
64. Abbott, ME: Coarctation of the aorta of the adult type. II. A statistical study and historical retro-
    spect of 200 recorded cases, with autopsy, of stenosis or obliteration of the descending arch in
    subjects above the age of 2 years. Am Heart J 3:392, 1928.
65. Reifenstein, GH, Levine, SA, and Gross, RE: Coarctation of the aorta. A review of 104 autopsied
    cases of "adult type," 2 years of age or older. Am Heart J 33:146, 1947.
66. Gore, I and Seiwert, VJ: Dissecting aneurysm of the aorta: Pathologic aspects. An analysis of 85
    fatal cases. Arch Pathol 53:121, 1952.
67. Edwards, WD, Leaf, DS, and Edwards, JE: Dissecting aortic aneurysm associated with congenital
    bicuspid aortic valve. Circulation 57:1022, 1978.
68. Roberts, CS and Roberts, WC: Dissection of the aorta associated with congenital malformation of
    the aortic valve. J Am Coll Cardiol 17:712, 1991.
69. Fenoglio, JJ, Jr, McAllister, HA, Jr, DeCastro, CM, et al: Congenital bicuspid aortic valve after
    age 20. Am J Cardiol 39:164, 1977.
70. Larson, EW and Edwards WD: Risk factors for aortic dissection: A necropsy study of 161 cases.
    Am J Cardiol 53:849, 1984.
71. Roberts, WC: Living with a congenitally bicuspid aortic valve. Am J Cardiol 64:1408, 1989.
72. Osler, W: Malignant endocarditis. Lancet 1:415, 1885.
73. Silver, MA and Roberts, WC: Detailed anatomy of the normally functioning aortic valve in hearts
    of normal and increased weight. Am J Cardiol 55:454, 1985.
74. Hurwitz, LE and Roberts, WC: Quadricuspid semilunar valve. Am J Cardiol 31:623, 1973.
75. Fernicola, DJ, Mann, JM, and Roberts, WC: Congenitally quadricuspid aortic valve: Analysis of
    six necropsy patients. Am J Cardiol 63:136, 1989.
76. Roberts, WC, Dangel, JC, and Bulkley, BH: Nonrheumatic valvular cardiac disease. A clinico-

pathologic survey of 27 different conditions causing valvular dysfunction. Cardiovasc Clin 5:333, 1973.

77. Roberts, WC: Left ventricular outflow tract obstruction and aortic regurgitation. In Edwards, JE, Lev, M, and Abell, MR (eds): The Heart. Williams & Wilkins, Baltimore, 1974, p 110.

78. Roberts, WC and Podolak, MJ: The king of hearts: Analysis of 23 patients with hearts weighing 1,000 grams or more. Am J Cardiol 55:485, 1985.

79. Roberts, SC and Honig, MS: The spectrum of cardiovascular disease in the Marfan syndrome: A clinico-morphologic study of 18 necropsy patients and comparison to 151 previously reported necropsy patients. Am Heart J 104:115, 1982.

80. Murdoch, JL, Walker, BA, Halpern, BL, et al: Life expectancy and causes of death in the Marfan syndrome. N Engl J Med 286:804, 1972.

81. Sisk, HE, Zahka, KG, Pyeritz, RE, et al: The Marfan syndrome in early childhood: Analysis of 15 patients diagnosed at less than 4 years of age. Am J Cardiol 52:353, 1983.

82. Carlson, RG, Lillehei, CW, and Edwards, JE: Cystic medial necrosis of the ascending aorta in relation to age and hypertension. Am J Cardiol 25:411, 1970.

83. Schlatmann, TJM and Becker, AE: Histologic changes in the normal aging aorta: Implications for dissecting aortic aneurysm. Am J Cardiol 39:13, 1977.

84. Schlatmann, TJM and Becker, AE: Pathogenesis of dissecting aneurysm of aorta. Comparative histopathologic study of significance of medial changes. Am J Cardiol 39:21, 1977.

85. Roberts, WC: Aortic dissection: Anatomy, consequences, and causes. Am Heart J 101:195, 1981.

86. Gsell, O: Wandnekrosen der aorta als selbständige Erkrankung und ihre Beziehung zur spontan-ruptur. Virchows Arch Pathol Anat Physiol 270:1, 1928.

87. Erdheim, J: Medionecrosis aortae idiopathica. Virchows Arch Pathol Anat Physiol 273:454, 1929.

88. Erdheim, J: Medionecrosis aortae idiopathica cystica. Virchows Arch Pathol Anat Physiol 276:187, 1930.

89. Wolinsky, H and Glagov, S: A lamellar unit of aortic medial structure and function in mammals. Circ Res 20:99, 1967.

90. Benchimol, A, Dresser, KB, and Neese, TC: Hypermobility of the aorta in Marfan's syndrome. Angiology 23:103, 1972.

91. Spangler, RD, Nora, JJ, Lortscher, RH, et al: Echocardiography in Marfan's syndrome. Chest 69:72, 1976.

92. Pyeritz, RE and McKusick, VA: The Marfan syndrome: Diagnosis and management. N Engl J Med 300:772, 1979.

93. Van Buchem, FSP: Cardiovascular disease in arachnodactyly. Acta Med Scand 161:197, 1958.

94. Roberts, WC, Braunwald, E, and Morrow, AG: Acute severe mitral regurgitation secondary to ruptured chordae tendineae. Clinical, hemodynamic, and pathologic considerations. Circulation 33:58, 1966.

95. Roberts, WC: Characteristics and consequences of infective endocarditis (active or healed or both) learned from morphologic studies. In Rahimtoola, SH (ed): Infective Endocarditis. Grune & Stratton, New York, 1978, p 55.

96. Waller, BF, Reis, RL, McIntosh, CL, et al: Marfan cardiovascular disease without the Marfan syndrome. Fusiform ascending aortic aneurysm with aortic and mitral valve regurgitation. Chest 77:533, 1980.

97. Fukuda, T, Tadavarthy, SM, and Edwards, JE: Dissecting aneurysm of aorta complicating aortic valvular stenosis. Circulation 53:169, 1976.

98. Roberts, WC, Perry, LW, Chandra, RS, et al: Aortic valve atresia: A new classification based on necropsy study of 73 cases. Am J Cardiol 37:753, 1976.

99. Roberts, WC: The worst heart disease. Am J Cardiol 54:1169, 1984.

100. Perry, LW, Scott, LP, III, Shapiro, SR, et al: Atresia of the aortic valve with ventricular septal defect. A clinicopathologic study of four newborns. Chest 72:757, 1977.

101. Cabin, HS, Wood, TP, Smith, JO, et al: Ebstein's anomaly in the elderly. Chest 80:218, 1981.

102. Silver, MA, Cohen, SR, McIntosh, CL, et al: Late (5 to 132 months) clinical and hemodynamic results after either tricuspid valve replacement or anuloplasty for Ebstein's anomaly of the tricuspid valve. Am J Cardiol 54:627, 1984.

103. Engle, MA, Payne, TPB, Bruins, C, et al: Ebstein's anomaly of the tricuspid valve. Report of three cases and analysis of the clinical syndrome. Circulation 1:1246, 1950.

104. Fontana, RS and Edwards, JE: Congenital Cardiac Disease: A Review of 357 Cases Studied Pathologically. WB Saunders, Philadelphia, 1962.

105. Roberts, WC, Mason, DT, Morrow, AG, et al: Calcific pulmonic stenosis. Circulation 37:973, 1968.
106. Covarrubias, EA, Sheikh, MU, Isner, JM, et al: Calcific pulmonic stenosis in adulthood. Treatment by valve replacement (porcine xenograft) with postoperative hemodynamic evaluation. Chest 75:399, 1979.
107. Roberts, WC, Shemin, RJ, and Kent, KM: Frequency and direction of interatrial shunting in valvular pulmonic stenosis with intact ventricular septum and without left ventricular inflow or outflow obstruction. An analysis of 127 patients treated by valvulotomy. Am Heart J 99:142, 1980.
108. Arnett, FN, Aisner, SC, Lewis, KB, et al: Pulmonic valve stenosis, atrial septal defect and left-to-right interatrial shunting with intact ventricular septum. A distinct hemodynamic-morphologic syndrome. Chest 78:759, 1980.
109. Shemin, RJ, Kent, KM, and Roberts, WC: Syndrome of valvular pulmonary stenosis and valvular aortic stenosis with atrial septal defect. Br Heart J 42:442, 1979.

PART 2

Electrocardiography

CHAPTER 3

The Electrocardiogram in Valvular Heart Disease

Mark A. Goldstein, M.D.
Eric L. Michelson, M.D.
Leonard S. Dreifus, M.D.

Valvular heart disease, whether acquired or congenital, can have a variety of clinical presentations. The electrocardiogram (ECG) may reflect some of the multifaceted aspects of valvular heart disease, although not always quantitatively and occasionally not even qualitatively. Valvular heart disease is a dynamic process, reflecting both the nature and extent of anatomic and hemodynamic alterations. Important factors include the etiology, severity, and chronicity of pathophysiologic and structural derangements, as well as the presence of superimposed acute decompensation, concomitant cardiac disease, or comorbid conditions.

The ECG can be affected by valvular heart disease through several general mechanisms, including chamber dilation and hypertrophy, scarring (e.g. rheumatic heart disease), ischemia, and pressure phenomena. The ECG is the sum of its parts. Therefore, these mechanisms can affect the heart rate and rhythm; the amplitude, duration, axis, and morphology of the P wave, QRS complex, and T and U waves; intervals (PR, QT); and the ST and TP segments. However, the ECG and its various components are at best indirect indicators of the complexities of the underlying pathophysiology of valvular heart disease or its clinical manifestations.

In the past, limited diagnostic modalities were available to follow the patient with valvular heart disease. The ECG aided in following the natural history of these patients, but it was never very predictive and never replaced the clinical evaluation. Nowadays, although the history and physical examination are still very important, newer noninvasive tests, most notably echocardiography (particularly 2-D and color-flow Doppler techniques), have supplanted the ECG in the quantitative and qualitative assessment of valvular heart disease, as well as in directing invasive and therapeutic interventions.

The ECG has therefore become of secondary importance in following the patient with valvular heart disease, with the notable exception of identifying and managing patients with rhythm and conduction disorders. Yet, the ECG is a universally available tool, and invariably these patients will have serial ECGs done during the course of their disease. Accordingly, the clinician should recognize the usual ECG manifestations of valvular heart disease and integrate these findings into the overall diagnostic and therapeutic plan.

As patients with valvular heart disease survive into more advanced years, the likelihood of concomitant hypertensive cardiovascular disease, coronary artery disease, and other cardiac disorders increases. The ECG may be valuable in the diagnosis of such common concomitant or incidental events as acute myocardial infarction. Conversely, the ECG diagnosis or other cardiac conditions may be confounded by the presence of advanced valvular heart disease.

This chapter will highlight some of the common ECG manifestations of several of the major valvular lesions in the adult. The ECG in its broader sense can include the resting ECG, ambulatory ECG monitoring, and the signal-averaged ECG, and in its broadest sense intracardiac recordings such as those obtained with electrode catheters.

MITRAL STENOSIS

Isolated mitral stenosis in the adult is most commonly caused by rheumatic heart disease. The functional consequences of the obstruction of mitral flow are initially an increase in left atrial and pulmonary venous pressures. As the disease progresses, pulmonary arterial hypertension and, ultimately, elevated right ventricular pressure ensue. The structural consequences of progressive mitral stenosis are left atrial enlargement, and, if pulmonary hypertension develops, right ventricular hypertrophy (RVH).

The ECG in mitral stenosis commonly demonstrates left atrial enlargement as

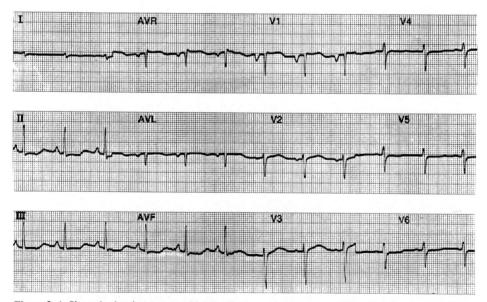

Figure 3–1. Sinus rhythm is present at 75 bpm. P waves are tall and peaked in leads 2, 3, and AVF and deeply inverted in V1. Mild right axis deviation is present with an S wave greater than R wave in leads 1, V5, and V6. Minimal evidence of right ventricular hypertrophy is present, as well as marked left atrial enlargement. This patient had combined mitral stenosis and tricuspid regurgitation.

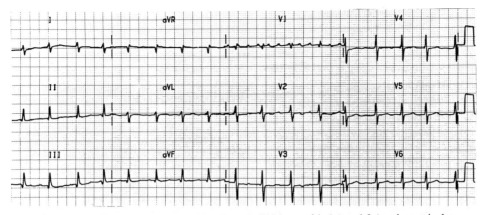

Figure 3–2. Atrial flutter is present at approximately 280 bpm with 4:1 and 3:1 atrioventricular conduction ratios. Right axis deviation is present. S waves are greater than R waves in leads I and AVL, with terminal S waves in leads V4–V6. A QR pattern is seen in lead V1 with a prominent R′ wave and incomplete RBBB. Right ventricular hypertrophy is evident in this patient with pure mitral stenosis.

a wide notched P wave ("P-mitrale," best seen in lead II) and a biphasic P wave in V_1 with a prominent terminal trough. With disease progression and the development of pulmonary hypertension, evidence of RVH may be seen on the ECG; RVH can manifest as right axis deviation of the frontal QRS axis, a tall R wave in V_1 (R/S ratio > 1), and secondary ST-T changes, or the findings may be more subtle (Fig. 3–1). Incomplete or complete right bundle branch block can also develop (Fig. 3–2). Rarely, left atrial membranes and other congenital or acquired

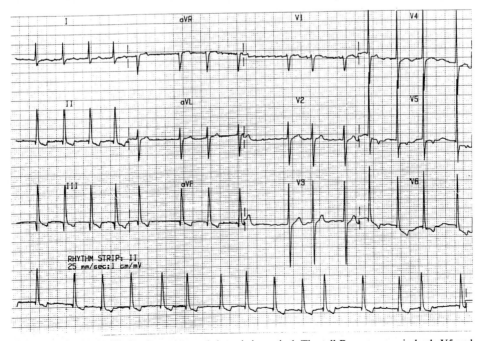

Figure 3–3. Atrial fibrillation is present and the axis is vertical. The tall R waves seen in leads V5 and V6 are discordant with the small S waves in lead V1. Combined ventricular hypertrophy is present in this patient with combined mitral stenosis and aortic stenosis.

anomalies (e.g., myxoma) may mimic mitral stenosis, with or without associated ECG findings.

Investigators have demonstrated that the ECG is not a sensitive indicator of RVH or the degree of pulmonary hypertension. In fact, some patients with severe mitral stenosis at cardiac catheterization may have a "borderline" or normal ECG.[1]

Atrial flutter or fibrillation may develop in individuals with mitral stenosis, associated with increasing left atrial pressure and left atrial enlargement, and may lead to marked hemodynamic decompensation as well as thromboembolic complications (see Fig. 3–2).

Frequently, multivalvular disease may be present due to rheumatic valvulitis. Consequently, combined ventricular hypertrophy can be identified on the ECG, as seen in Figure 3–3, in a patient with both mitral and aortic stenosis. Conversely, marked right atrial or right ventricular dilation and RVH may mask concomitant left ventricular hypertrophy (LVH) in patients with multivalvular disease.

MITRAL REGURGITATION

The ECG manifestations of mitral regurgitation, as with other lesions, are dependent upon the etiology, severity, and duration of the insufficiency. Etiologies of chronic mitral regurgitation include rheumatic heart disease and infective endocarditis, but the most common causes of mitral regurgitation in adults currently are mitral valve prolapse[2,3] and coronary artery disease.

In chronic mitral regurgitation, volume overload of the left heart leads to left atrial and left ventricular dilation, and ultimately LVH. The ECG may demonstrate these progressive changes.[4-6] The various criteria of LVH have in common high QRS voltage, but all have their limitations when attempts are made to correlate ECG findings with necropsy data. Echocardiography is a more sensitive and specific technique than the ECG for diagnosing LVH.[7]

Acute mitral regurgitation is not accompanied by immediate dilation of the left atrium and left ventricle. The ECG may therefore be normal or only show nonspecific findings including sinus tachycardia and ST-T wave alterations. ECG changes of a myocardial infarction may be noted when acute mitral regurgitation is related to coronary artery disease. Such changes are more commonly noted in the inferior leads.[8] In acute mitral regurgitation associated with myocardial infarction, the other most common ECG finding is first-degree atrioventricular (AV) block.[9]

Complex ventricular arrhythmias including runs of nonsustained ventricular tachycardia may be noted on the 12-lead ECG and on ambulatory ECG recordings in patients with chronic mitral regurgitation, especially those with left ventricular dysfunction. Such a finding may identify a particularly high-risk group with a poorer prognosis and increased risk of sudden death.[10]

MITRAL VALVE PROLAPSE

Mitral valve prolapse is best recognized noninvasively by physical examination and echocardiography.[11,12] Echocardiography when combined with Doppler technology is particularly valuable in determining the presence of concomitant mitral regurgitation and its severity.

In the majority of individuals with mitral valve prolapse, especially those who are asymptomatic, the resting ECG is normal. Classic mitral valve prolapse (Barlow's syndrome) may include palpitations, chest discomfort, fatigue, and anxiety. The ECG in these symptomatic individuals may demonstrate a variety of ST-T wave changes particularly in the inferolateral leads. These changes may include T-wave inversion and sometimes ST-segment depression.[12] QT prolongation may also be seen. Arrhythmias may occasionally be observed on ambulatory ECG recordings, including premature atrial contractions, premature ventricular contractions, supraventricular tachycardia, AV block, and bradyarrhythmias. Rarely, ventricular tachyarrhythmias may be potentially life-threatening, and in such cases, aggressive management is warranted.

Atypical chest pain may prompt evaluation by exercise testing in patients with mitral valve prolapse. Patients with mitral valve prolapse may have an abnormal response to exercise testing (false–positive test) with ST-segment depression observed with exercise in the absence of coronary artery disease. Chest pain in young adults with mitral valve prolapse fails to correlate with ischemic changes on stress testing. However, exercise testing can be used to determine whether or not their pain is associated with exercise and to establish the presence or absence of exercise-induced arrhythmias.[13,14]

AORTIC STENOSIS

Aortic stenosis in younger adults is often related to a congenitally stenotic aortic valve,[15] and in middle-aged adults, particularly men, to a bicuspid aortic valve. In some middle-aged individuals, rheumatic heart disease can be identified as the causative factor; rheumatic aortic stenosis is almost always associated with rheumatic involvement of the mitral valve. In elderly individuals, degenerative calcification of a tricuspid aortic valve is the most common etiology of aortic stenosis.[16,17]

The ECG in aortic stenosis does not readily distinguish between valvular aortic stenosis or the supravalvular or discrete subvalvular form. The ECG in patients with mild-to-moderate aortic stenosis is often normal. Aortic stenosis leads to pressure overload of the left ventricle and progressively to LVH, and ultimately to left ventricular dysfunction. In moderate and severe aortic stenosis, the ECG usually demonstrates changes of LVH (Fig. 3–4), but in some cases, such as young adults with congenital aortic stenosis, the ECG may remain remarkably normal despite marked ventricular hypertrophy. Even in cases of acquired aortic stenosis, the ECG may not reliably reflect the severity of aortic stenosis or progression of disease.

The ECG in advanced aortic valve disease may reveal associated conduction system disease or arrhythmias. The degenerative calcific process involved in many cases of aortic valvular disease can extend to involve the conduction system. This can lead to various degrees of AV heart block, left anterior fascicular block, left bundle branch block, and less commonly right bundle branch block. The onset of atrial fibrillation is typically associated with marked decompensation and may be encountered very late in the course of aortic stenosis. The combination of the loss of atrial kick and rapid irregular rates with inadequate ventricular filling can be devastating. Atrial fibrillation is more common in older individuals and in the presence of combined mitral and aortic disease. Combined ventricular hypertrophy is characteristic of such multivalvular lesions.

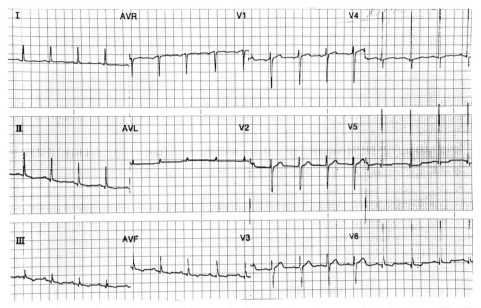

Figure 3–4. Sinus rhythm is present with normal axis. Tall R waves are seen in leads V5 and V6. ST segments are depressed with inverted T waves in the lateral precordial leads. These findings are consistent with "systolic overload" of the left ventricle as seen in aortic stenosis.

AORTIC REGURGITATION

Aortic regurgitation has a variety of causes including association with a bicuspid aortic valve, calcific degeneration of the aortic valve in the elderly, rheumatic heart disease, infective endocarditis, Marfan's syndrome, syphilis, collagen vascular disease (e.g., ankylosing spondylitis), and hypertensive aortic disease. Aortic regurgitation may occur in isolation, combined with aortic stenosis, or in association with involvement of other valves. The ECG only rarely gives a clue to the etiology.

The ECG in acute aortic regurgitation (e.g., endocarditis or aortic root dissection) may be normal or may show ST-T wave changes related to ischemia. Chronic aortic regurgitation is often a longstanding condition that leads progressively to left ventricular volume overload and to LVH. The T waves in the left precordial leads are frequently upright ("diastolic overload") (Fig. 3–5) as opposed to inverted, which is observed in aortic stenosis ("pressure overload") (see Fig. 3–4). The ECG may demonstrate more advanced LVH over time. Evidence of conduction system abnormalities, including left axis deviation, usually occur later in the course of aortic regurgitation.

PULMONIC STENOSIS

Pulmonic stenosis is a relatively common form of congenital heart disease. The natural history of pulmonic stenosis is related to the severity of the obstruction. Severe stenosis may lead to heart failure in childhood whereas individuals with mild stenosis may have a normal life expectancy.

The ECG may be normal in the presence of mild pulmonic stenosis. Severe stenosis may lead to ECG evidence of RVH, right axis deviation, and right atrial

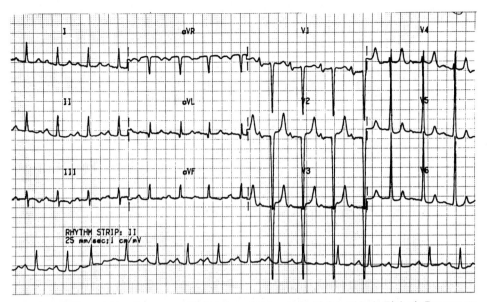

Figure 3–5. Sinus rhythm is present with first degree atrioventricular heart block. Biphasic P waves are seen in lead V1 suggesting combined atrial hypertrophy. Tall R waves are seen in leads V5 and V6 and deep S waves in V1. Importantly, T waves are upright in V4–V6, suggesting "diastolic overload" of the left ventricle as seen in aortic regurgitation.

enlargement. If the pulmonary hypertension is secondary to mitral stenosis, left atrial enlargement may be observed on the ECG.

TRICUSPID STENOSIS

The most common cause of tricuspid stenosis is rheumatic fever. Rheumatic involvement of the tricuspid valve is usually associated with concomitant involvement of the mitral valve. The rheumatic tricuspid valve is usually both stenotic and regurgitant. Isolated tricuspid stenosis can be encountered: for example, in the carcinoid syndrome. Mechanical obstruction of the tricuspid valve can occur due to right atrial myxoma, tumor, or right atrial thrombi.

Tricuspid stenosis leads to elevated right atrial pressure and, ultimately, may cause a reduction in cardiac output. The hemodynamic abnormalities of tricuspid stenosis also may be worsened by the frequent presence of mitral stenosis. The ECG in tricuspid stenosis may show right atrial enlargement in the absence of RVH. Atrial fibrillation is common. The ECG also may reflect the presence of concomitant mitral stenosis.

TRICUSPID REGURGITATION

Tricuspid regurgitation is often due to right ventricular dilation and failure.[18] The most common etiology of isolated tricuspid regurgitation is infective endocarditis in the intravenous drug abuser. Tricuspid regurgitation also can be produced by trauma, myocardial infarction, carcinoid syndrome, and congenital abnormal-

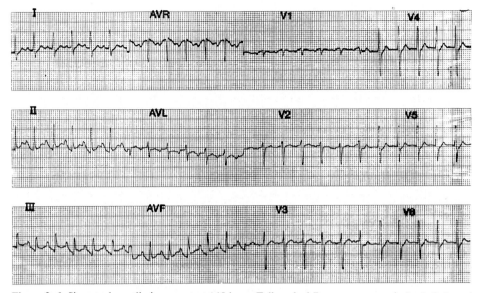

Figure 3–6. Sinus tachycardia is present at 145 bpm. Tall peaked P waves are seen in leads 2, 3, and AVF. S waves are present in 1, AVL, V5, V6, and V1. Right atrial enlargement is suggested in this patient with tricuspid regurgitation.

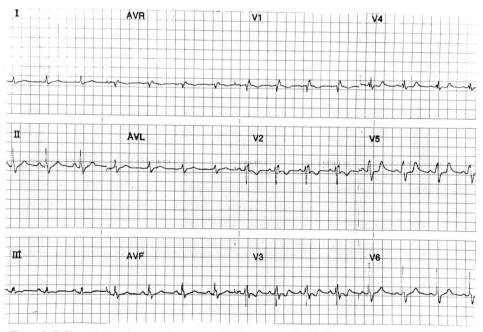

Figure 3–7. Sinus rhythm is present at a rate of 78 bpm. A small wide S wave is seen in leads AVL and V6 with small QR wave in V1, a manifestation of incomplete RBBB. Right atrial enlargement is present with subtle evidence of right ventricular hypertrophy. Low amplitude fractionated QRS complexes with an incomplete RBBB pattern are characteristic of Ebstein's anomaly. Evidence of ventricular preexcitation via a right-sided bypass tract may also be present in some cases.

ities such as Ebstein's anomaly and atrial septal defect.[19] Rheumatic fever is a rare cause of tricuspid regurgitation.

Tricuspid regurgitation leads to volume overload of the right atrium and right ventricle and, ultimately, produces right atrial and right ventricular enlargement. Figure 3–6 shows an example with right atrial enlargement associated with a right terminal conduction delay. The ECG may show RVH, and right bundle branch block may be present. Atrial fibrillation is common when hemodynamically advanced disease is present.

EBSTEIN'S ANOMALY

In Ebstein's anomaly, portions of the posterior and septal leaflets of the tricuspid valve are displaced downward into the right ventricular cavity and attach to the ventricular wall below the annulus. A patent foramen ovale is most often present.

Ebstein's anomaly results in obstruction to right ventricular filling due to a small right ventricle. The tricuspid valve is frequently insufficient. There is usually an initially large right-to-left shunt through the patent foramen ovale.

The ECG commonly shows right atrial enlargement. The PR interval is often prolonged with first-degree AV block. An incomplete or complete right bundle branch block may be present (Fig. 3–7). Ten percent of patients with Ebstein's anomaly may have evidence of AV preexcitation and a right-sided bypass tract.[19] Paroxysms of atrial fibrillation with rapid anomalous AV conduction in such cases can be catastrophic and mandate definitive ablative therapy.

ACKNOWLEDGMENT

We gratefully acknowledge the assistance of Marchia T. Stukes with manuscript preparation.

REFERENCES

1. Cosby, RS, Levinson, DC, Dimitroff, SP, et al: The electrocardiogram in congenital heart disease and mitral stenosis. A correlation of electrocardiographic patterns with right ventricular pressure, flow, and work. Am Heart J 46:670, 1953.
2. Silverman, ME and Hurst, JW: The mitral complex. Interaction of the anatomy, physiology, and pathology of the mitral anulus, mitral valve leaflets, chordae tendineae, and papillary muscles. Am Heart J 76:399, 1968.
3. Barlow, JB and Pocock, WA: The problem of nonejection systolic clicks and associated mitral systolic murmurs: Emphasis on the billowing mitral leaflet syndrome. Am Heart J 90:637, 1975.
4. Surawicz, B: Electrocardiographic diagnosis of chamber enlargement. J Am Coll Cardiol 8:711, 1986.
5. Romhilt, DW, Bove, KE, Norris, RJ, et al: A critical appraisal of the electrocardiographic criteria for the diagnosis of left ventricular hypertrophy. Circulation 40:185, 1969.
6. Murphy, ML, Thenabadu, PN, De Soyza, N, et al: Reevaluation of electrocardiographic criteria for left, right, and combined cardiac ventricular hypertrophy. Am J Cardiol 53:1140, 1984.
7. Levy, D, Garrison, RJ, Savage, DD, et al: Prognostic implications of echocardiographically determined left ventricular mass in the Framingham Heart Study. N Engl J Med 322:1561, 1990.
8. Heikkila, J: Mitral incompetence complicating acute myocardial infarction. Br Heart J 29:162, 1967.
9. Gahl, K, Sutton, R, Pearson, M, et al: Mitral regurgitation in coronary heart disease. Br Heart J 39:13, 1977.

10. Hochreiter, C, Niles, N, Devereux, RB, et al: Mitral regurgitation: Relationship of noninvasive descriptors of right and left ventricular performance to clinical and hemodynamic findings and to prognosis in medically and surgically treated patients. Circulation 73:900, 1986.

11. Crawley, IS, Morris, DC, and Silverman, BD: Valvular heart disease. In Hurst, JW, Logue, RB, Schlant, RC, et al (eds): The Heart, ed 4. McGraw-Hill, New York, 1978, p 992.

12. Devereux, RB, Kramer-Fox, R, and Kligfield, P: Mitral valve prolapse: Causes, clinical manifestations, and management. Ann Intern Med 111:305, 1989.

13. Winkle, RA, Lopes, MG, Fitzgerald, JW, et al: Arrhythmias in patients with mitral valve prolapse. Circulation 52:73, 1975.

14. DeMaria, AN, Amsterdam, EA, Vismara, LA, et al: Arrhythmias in the mitral valve prolapse syndrome. Prevalence, nature, and frequency. Ann Intern Med 84:656, 1976.

15. Glancy, DL and Epstein, SE: Differential diagnosis of type and severity of obstruction of left ventricular outflow. Prog Cardiovasc Dis 14:153, 1971.

16. Roberts, WC: The structure of the aortic valve in clinically isolated aortic stenosis. An autopsy study of 162 patients over 15 years of age. Circulation 42:91, 1970.

17. Roberts, WC, Perloff, JK, and Constantino, T: Severe valvular aortic stenosis in patients over 65 years of age. A clinicopathologic study. Am J Cardiol 27:497, 1971.

18. McMichael, J and Shillingford, JP: The role of valvular incompetence in heart failure. Br Med J 1:537, 1957.

19. Watson, H: Natural history of Ebstein's anomaly of tricuspic valve in childhood and adolescence. An international cooperative study of 505 cases. Br Heart J 36:417, 1974.

CHAPTER 4

Arrhythmias in Valvular Heart Disease

Leonard S. Dreifus, M.D.

The association of cardiac dysrhythmias and valvular heart disease is clearly linked to the resultant pathophysiology of the myocardium. The incidence, severity, and significance of the cardiac arrhythmias will depend on the degree of myocardial and hemodynamic abnormalities and other contributing factors such as the association of coronary artery disease, hypertension, drugs, and electrolyte imbalance.[1] Furthermore, valvular heart disease can be associated with important abnormalities of the specialized tissues of the heart.[2-5] The sinoatrial and atrioventricular nodes as well as the Purkinje system may become involved by the primary disease such as rheumatic fever or become secondarily involved by subsequent calcification of the valves and contiguous structures.

Almost any cardiac dysrhythmia can be associated with valvular heart disease although congenital or degenerative diseases can affect the valvular structures and produce specific cardiac arrhythmias. This discussion will focus on the cardiac arrhythmias most frequently encountered in the presence of specific valvular pathology. Unfortunately, correction of the valvular dysfunction may not prevent further cardiac arrhythmias in the postoperative period.[6]

MITRAL VALVE PROLAPSE

Arrhythmias associated with mitral valve prolapse have been studied since the early 1970s.[7-15] However, the criteria for diagnosis of the mitral valve prolapse syndrome have changed considerably during the ensuing years. More precise echocardiographic technology and the addition of color-flow Doppler has clarified many important diagnostic criteria. Hence, the earlier studies relating ventricular arrhythmias to the mitral valve prolapse syndrome can account for the variations in the incidence and severity of these arrhythmias. Several authors related the frequency of both supraventricular and ventricular arrhythmias with mitral valve prolapse.[7-10] Whereas some authors simply state the diagnosis of mitral valve prolapse can be made with superior systolic displacement of the mitral valve leaflets on the echocardiogram, other investigators have attempted to correlate the presence of leaflet thickening and displacement in multiple imaging planes or specifically report the quantitative degree of displacement with the presence or absence of serious cardiac arrhythmias.[16,17] Sanfilippo and associates[16] studied 49 patients with mitral valve prolapse. Both ventricular arrhythmias and mitral regurgitation were found to occur with significantly greater frequency in patients with leaflet displacement than the normal matched population. These authors also found that the best echocardiographic predictor of either ventricular arrhythmias or mitral regurgitation was the quantitative degree of leaflet displacement. However, they concluded that most patients with echocardiographic evidence of leaflet displacement actually had a very low incidence of ventricular arrhythmias as well as associated mitral regurgitation.

Hawakawa and Inoh[17] classified mitral valve prolapse as mild, moderate, or severe. They found that ventricular couplets or triplets (Lown grade IV) were found in <10% of patients in the group aged 15 to 17 years. In patients aged 18 to 20 years, a 33% incidence of these ventricular arrhythmias were found, but they did not further increase with age.

Inoh and coworkers[18] reported 84 cases with idiopathic mitral valve prolapse and followed these individuals for a mean of 3.1 years (1–6 years). The incidence of ventricular arrhythmias in this group was 70%, which included about 10% each of Lown grades III, IVA, and IVB. There was one sudden death reported in this group. Mason and colleagues[19] studied 31 patients with mitral valve prolapse in normal subjects. These authors found that supraventricular tachyarrhythmias occurred almost as frequently as those of ventricular origin in the presence of mitral valve prolapse. Supraventricular arrhythmias were encountered in 35% of patients with mitral valve prolapse while observed in only 10% of normal subjects. On the other hand, ventricular arrhythmias were found in 58% of mitral valve prolapse patients compared with only 25% of normal subjects. They concluded that ventricular and supraventricular arrhythmias as well as bradyarrhythmias occurred significantly more frequently in patients with mitral valve prolapse syndrome as compared with normal persons.

Kramer and coworkers[20] compared ambulatory arrhythmias in 63 patients with mitral valve prolapse as well as 28 symptom-matched controlled subjects. They concluded that populations of highly symptomatic individuals regardless of the presence or absence of mitral valve prolapse have a high prevalence of cardiac arrhythmias.

Kligfield and colleagues[21] demonstrated that complex arrhythmias were more common in patients with nonischemic mitral regurgitation irrespective of etiology. Furthermore, these arrhythmias were more strongly associated with hemodynamically important mitral regurgitation than simply with mitral valvular prolapse alone. Similarly, subgroups of their patients suggested that atrial and ventricular complexity and Lown grade IVA or IVB occurred in 65% of patients with mitral valve prolapse who had mitral regurgitation but in only 8% of patients with mitral valve prolapse alone.

Dollar and Roberts[22] compared 15 patients who died suddenly without associated congenital heart disease and with nonmitral prolapse conditions capable in themselves of being fatal with 34 other patients with mitral valve prolapse and comorbidities. The patients with isolated mitral valve prolapse were younger (mean age 39 ± 17 vs. 52 ± 15 years; $p = 0.01$), more often women (67% vs. 26%; $p = 0.008$), and had a lower frequency of mitral regurgitation (7% vs. 38%; $p = 0.02$). The 15 patients dying suddenly with isolated mitral valve prolapse also were less likely to have evidence of ruptured chordae tendineae (29% vs. 67%; $p = 0.04$).

An increased incidence of prolonged QT intervals as well as electrocardiographic evidence of Wolff-Parkinson-White ECG abnormalities is seen in patients with mitral valve prolapse.[23]

Although ventricular arrhythmias appear to increase with age in the general population, no such correlation was found in any of the series associated with mitral valve prolapse. There appears to be an increased incidence of supraventricular mechanisms in the older age group, but this could possibly be attributed to comorbidities, coronary artery disease, and further development of mitral valvular regurgitation, which is associated with the aging process.

MANAGEMENT

Treatment of premature ventricular arrhythmias as well as nonsustained ventricular tachycardia in the absence of symptoms or significant hemodynamic effects is not indicated in these patients. However, symptomatic patients should receive beta-blocking agents as the initial approach to management. Type I antiarrhythmics should be administered only when beta-blocking agents prove ineffective to control symptoms. Although there is a reported increased incidence of sudden death with mitral valve prolapse,[13,22] documented ventricular tachycardias as the sole etiology is still unfounded. Patients with nonsustained ventricular tachycardia should be subjected to an electrophysiologic study and a treatment program initiated in those individuals in whom sustained monomorphic ventricular tachycardia can be induced by this method. The significance of late potentials in the signal-averaged ECG in these patients is still unknown.

Appropriate antiarrhythmic drug therapy in those individuals at risk for sustained monomorphic ventricular tachycardia or sudden death should be offered using electrophysiologic-directed therapy, and in extreme cases implantation of an implantable cardoverter defibrillator (ICD). Patients with an associated Wolff-Parkinson-White syndrome and a short refractory period (<250 ms) of the anomalous pathway should either undergo catheter or surgical ablation of the accessory pathway or appropriate antiarrhythmic drug therapy. Those individuals with the long QT syndrome should be given long-term beta-blocking drug therapy.

RHEUMATIC MITRAL VALVULAR DISEASE

Whereas the predominant cause of mitral stenosis is rheumatic fever, the cardiac arrhythmias associated with acute rheumatic fever are unusual. However, any variety of the atrial arrhythmias, including atrial premature complexes, atrial tachycardia, atrial flutter/fibrillation, or nonparoxysmal junctional tachycardia, can be observed. Notably, arrhythmias originating on the atrial side of the mitral valvular apparatus have been identified using ultramicroelectrode techniques.[24] The etiology for an arrhythmia substrate in the mitral valve apparatus is unknown, but delayed after-potentials and triggered activity have been observed.[24] The rheumatic process results in scarring and calcification of the mitral valve apparatus leading to stenosis. Thickened leaflets also may become adherent or rigid and lead to combined valvular disease of mitral stenosis and regurgitation. The rheumatic process also results in scarring and fibrosis of the atria, which also produce a substrate for the development of atrial arrhythmias. Enlargement of the left atrium due to the mitral stenotic process and regurgitant jet further compromises the structure of the left atria, leading to the development of atrial arrhythmias. The increased pressure within the left atrium and the increased volume of this chamber due to stenosis and/or regurgitant jet also further destroys the atrial tissue.

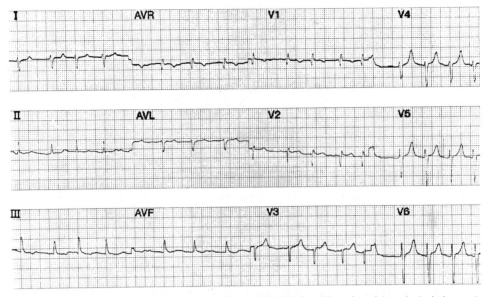

Figure 4–1. A 12-lead electrocardiogram showing atrial fibrillation. There is a right axis deviation and incomplete right bundle branch system block with a QR pattern in lead V1 and S waves in 1, AVL and V5, and V6. Right ventricular hypertrophy is present in the presence of severe mitral stenosis.

Both with mitral stenosis and mitral regurgitation, frequent premature atrial contractions are commonly observed for several years prior to the development of more serious atrial arrhythmias. Finally, atrial fibrillation and/or flutter ensue (Figs. 4–1 and 4–2).

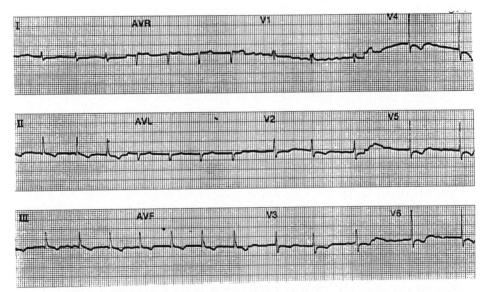

Figure 4–2. Atrial fibrillation is present. There is a right axis deviation present, as well as an rSr prime in V1. An inappropriately small S wave is present in V1 compared with the tall R wave in V5 and V6. Combined ventricular hypertrophy is present, which is produced by mitral stenosis and mitral insufficiency.

MANAGEMENT

Management of these arrhythmias should be directed to maintaining a sinus rhythm. Atrial fibrillation or flutter leads to the development of systemic embolization in at least 2% of these individuals. Consequently, long-term anticoagulation should be instituted once atrial fibrillation is present permanently or even in the presence of oscillations between sinus rhythm and atrial fibrillation. The most effective agents in maintaining sinus rhythm are quinidine and more recently the type 1C agents including propafenone and flecainide. Amiodarone has been successful in converting atrial fibrillation to sinus rhythm and maintaining sinus rhythm for long periods, although this agent has significant toxic side effects. Electric cardioversion may be used to maintain sinus rhythm but should not be employed once atrial fibrillation becomes recurrent and antiarrhythmic drugs fail to maintain the sinus mechanism.

Following a successful commissurotomy or repair of the mitral valve by either a valvuloplasty or the replacement of the mitral valve with a prosthesis, atrial fibrillation may become permanent. It is generally difficult to reestablish a sinus rhythm following these surgical procedures inasmuch as surgery is usually reserved for the advanced manifestations of the mitral valve process, and the mitral valve architecture has been severely compromised. Maintenance of sinus rhythm under these circumstances is extremely difficult.

Frequently, pulmonary edema ensues following the onset of atrial flutter with a rapid ventricular rate. Tachycardia will augment the transmitral valvular pressure gradient, and it further elevates left atrial pressures.[26] By slowing the ventricular rate using cardiac glycosides, beta-adrenergic receptor blocking agents, or verapamil, the hemodynamics and symptoms of pulmonary congestion will markedly improve. Rapid and dramatic slowing of the ventricular rate can frequently be achieved by the administration of an intravenous bolus injection of 6 to 12 mg of adenosine.

Specific patterns of atrial fibrillation can be observed in the presence of mitral valvular disease. Second- or third-degree AV block may ensue in advanced cases of

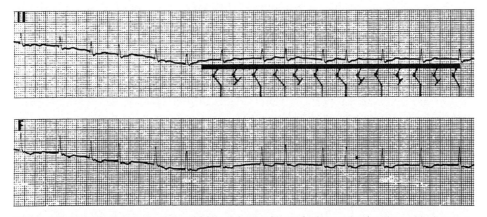

Figure 4–3. Atrial fibrillation is present with impaired atrioventricular conduction due to block. A nonparoxysmal junctional tachycardia is present (cycle length = 400 msec) with varying nodal-ventricular conduction ratios. The pseudobigeminy can be seen due to second-degree block below the accelerated AV junctional pacemaker.

mitral valvulitis and require cardiac pacing. On the other hand, regularization of the ventricular rate in the presence of atrial fibrillation should suggest AV dissociation and acceleration of an AV nonparoxysmal junctional pacemaker, which is invariably due to hypokalemia or digitalis excess (Fig. 4–3). Furthermore, the presence of mitral valve disease and the combination of an atrial arrhythmia and digitalis excess can result in significant, life-threatening ventricular arrhythmias.[27]

Electrophysiologic studies offer a useful approach to risk stratification in patients with sustained and nonsustained ventricular tachycardia. Notably, electrophysiologic-directed antiarrhythmic therapy or the supplemental use of an ICD may be indicated in some circumstances.

AORTIC STENOSIS

The natural history of adults with aortic stenosis embraces a long latency period during which the obstruction and pressure load on the left ventricular myocardium gradually increases. Consequently, the onset of cardiac arrhythmias can be sporadic and occur rather late in the history of the disease process. The symptoms which often commence in the sixth decade of life are angina pectoris, syncope, and finally heart failure.[28] Dilation of the left ventricle and increased fibrosis and scarring with or without the association of coronary artery disease result in serious ventricular arrhythmias. Obviously, in those patients in whom the obstruction remains unrelieved once symptoms become manifest, the prognosis is poor. Survival from the onset of the symptoms to the time of death is approximately 2 years in those individuals who develop congestive heart failure. Furthermore, aortic stenosis is frequently associated with significant coronary artery disease.[29] Therefore, cardiac arrhythmias related to the coronary artery pathology impart an additive risk to the aortic stenotic process. Clearly, the combination of increased oxygen needs by the hypertrophied myocardium and reduction in oxygen delivery also lead to excessive compression of the coronary vessels and ischemic syndromes, which are associated with serious ventricular arrhythmias. However, it is the low ejection fractions, particularly those <40%, that are associated with the most severe ventricular arrhythmias in these patients.

Whereas atrial fibrillation is often present with concomitant rheumatic mitral valvular or coronary artery disease, this arrhythmia is not commonly observed in isolated aortic stenosis. In fact, the presence of atrial fibrillation should alert the clinician to other causes or comorbidities associated with the aortic stenosis (Fig. 4–4).

Syncope is frequently associated with aortic stenosis and is commonly attributed to reduced cerebral perfusion that occurs during exertion when arterial pressure declines subsequent to systemic vasodilation in the presence of a fixed cardiac output.[28] Syncope may be engendered by prolonged supraventricular or ventricular arrhythmias. Syncope also has been identified with transient ventricular fibrillation from which the patient can recover spontaneously. Transient atrial fibrillation with loss of the atrial kick and a marked sudden decline in cardiac output also may produce syncope.

MANAGEMENT

Because aortic valvular stenosis commonly is associated with severe calcification of the aortic valve ring and the summit of the septum, left anterior fascicular

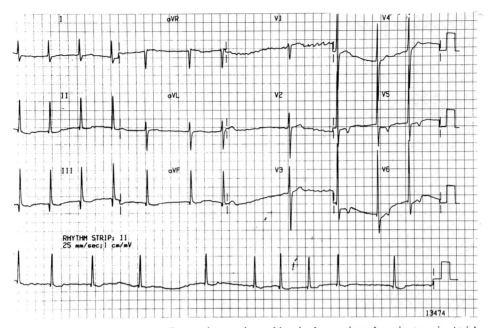

Figure 4–4. A 12-lead electrocardiogram in a patient with mitral stenosis and aortic stenosis. Atrial fibrillation is unusual in patients with aortic stenosis alone. The vertical position of the heart is seen as well as tall R waves in V5 and V6 with inappropriate small S waves in V1 suggesting combined ventricular hypertrophy.

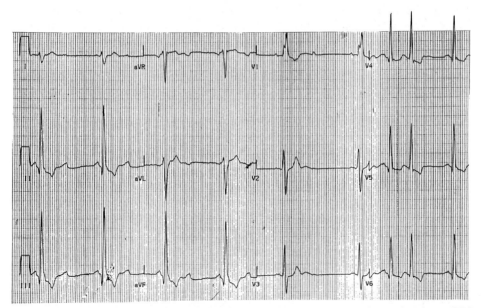

Figure 4–5. A 12-lead electrocardiogram. A sinus rhythm is present at a rate of 73 beats/minute. QRS complexes are widened to 130 msec. A marked right axis deviation is present with right bundle branch block. Significant Q waves are present in leads II, III, and in AVF. Second-degree Mobitz type II block is present. A bifascicular block alternating with trifascicular block (right bundle branch block plus left posterior hemiblock) can be seen. Occasional atrial premature beats are present, with conduction occurring in the supernormal period (V_4–V_6). This patient had severe aortic stenosis with calcification of the summit of the septum.

block or right bundle branch block may be encountered. Consequently, bifascicular block is not uncommon in aortic stenosis, and this may lead finally to complete AV block (Fig. 4–5). In fact, emergence of high-grade subjunctional AV block (Mobitz type II) progressing to complete AV block is frequently found in postoperative aortic stenosis patients. The AV conduction pathology may be due in part to the underlying calcification of the summit of the septum and the calcific process encroaching on the cardiac conduction skeleton. Furthermore, the surgical trauma in and around the AV transmission system also contributes to the development of high-grade AV subjunctional block. Permanent left bundle branch block is not uncommon following replacement of the aortic valve. Consequently, it may be necessary to implant a permanent cardiac pacemaker if AV conduction block persists more than 10 to 12 days after valve replacement.

AORTIC REGURGITATION

Aortic regurgitation, as opposed to isolated aortic stenosis, is commonly caused by rheumatic fever. The aortic cusps become infiltrated with fibrous tissue and retract, a process preventing cusp opposition and closure. Frequently, both aortic stenosis and aortic insufficiency coexist due to associated fusion of the commissures, which restricts the opening of the valve. Trauma, prolapse of the aortic valve, or a congenital unicuspid or a bicuspid valve are not uncommon in the younger child. Congenital aortic bicuspid valves are occasionally associated with the Marfan syndrome.

Although chronic aortic regurgitation may be associated with a generally favorable prognosis for many years, the left ventricle progressively dilates and ejection fraction decreases. Serious ventricular arrhythmias are frequently associated with these nonischemic dilated cardiomyopathies. When rheumatic valvulitis involves both the aortic and mitral valves, combined ventricular hypertrophy and atrial fibrillation are often present (see Fig. 4–4).

MANAGEMENT

Ventricular arrhythmias can be classified as benign, potentially lethal, and lethal. In the presence of valvular heart disease, all ventricular arrhythmias can be potentially lethal. Clearly, the prognosis is linked to the degree of myocardial damage and, more specifically, to the left ventricular ejection fraction. The highest incidence of malignant ventricular arrhythmias is associated with ejection fractions <40%. Consequently, recommendations for valvular repair or replacement should be made when the left ventricular ejection fraction is <50% even in the absence of significant symptoms.

The detection of sustained monomorphic ventricular tachycardia requires prompt therapy. Electrophysiologically directed antiarrhythmic drug therapy or the implantation of an antitachycardia/antifibrillatory device may be required in those individuals in whom the ventricular tachycardia is inducible by programmed stimulation.

Nonsustained ventricular tachycardia is a confounding problem when associated with valvular heart disease. The arrhythmia is potentially lethal, and the clinician is frequently insecure as to whether or not the dysrhythmia will become sustained or evolve into ventricular fibrillation and death. Thus, patients with ejection fraction <40% require electrophysiologic studies and electrophysiologically directed therapy.

TRICUSPID STENOSIS AND REGURGITATION

Invariably, the cause of tricuspid stenosis is related to rheumatic fever. It rarely occurs as an isolated lesion but generally accompanies mitral valve disease. Traditionally, the P waves are in keeping with right atrial enlargement and appear narrow and tall in lead V_1 with widening and increased amplitude in leads II, III, and AVF. P-wave amplitude in leads II and V_1 usually exceeds 0.2 mV. The resulting enlargement of the right atrium is frequently associated with supraventricular tachycardias, some of which are incessant and intractable to management. Eventually atrial fibrillation ensues.

Tricuspid regurgitation usually results secondarily from mitral and aortic valvular disease. An increase in pulmonary artery pressure invariably leads to tricuspid insufficiency, and left ventricular and pulmonary artery pressures between 60 and 80 mm Hg are not unusual. Although other specific arrhythmias are not encountered with marked tricuspid regurgitation, atrial fibrillation is usually present due to other associated valvular pathology. Frequently, correction of the aortic and mitral valvular pathology will reduce pulmonary artery pressure with a consequent reduction in tricuspid regurgitation. However, atrial fibrillation seems to persist in the postoperative period despite correction of the valvular pathology.

MANAGEMENT

Surprisingly, sinus rhythm is present for many years in the presence of right atrial enlargement either due to tricuspid stenosis or insufficiency. However, once atrial fibrillation ensues, the usual management strategies as outlined under mitral valve disease should be prudently exercised. Characteristically, these patients show evidence of digitalis-excess arrhythmias, such as atrial tachycardia with block and accelerated AV junctional tachycardia with or without block, with very small or modest doses of digoxin and even in the presence of serum digoxin levels <1.5 μg/ml. Sinus rhythm can be maintained using the newer type 1C drugs such as propafenone or flecainide. Amiodarone also has been efficient in the maintenance of sinus rhythm in these individuals. Slowing of the ventricular rate in the presence of atrial fibrillation may require the use of verapamil or large doses of diltiazem. Excessively rapid ventricular rates in the presence of these supraventricular arrhythmias may necessitate the use of ablative procedures, such as modifying the AV node to slow the ventricular rate in response to the supraventricular tachycardias or actual complete ablation of the AV nodal transmission system and the insertion of a cardiac pacemaker.

REFERENCES

1. Olshausen, KV, Schwartz, F, Appelbach, J, et al: Determinants of the incidence and severity of ventricular arrhythmias in aortic valve disease. Am J Cardiol 51:1103, 1983.
2. Thompson, R, Mitchell, A, Ahmed, M, et al: Conduction defects in aortic valve disease. Am Heart J 98:3, 1979.

 3. Dhingra, RC, Amat-y-Leon, F, and Wyndham, C: Sites of conduction disease in aortic stenosis. Significance of valve gradient and calcification. Ann Intern Med 87:275–280, 1977.
 4. Bharati, S, Granston, AS, Liebson, PR, et al: The conduction system in mitral valve prolapse syndrome with sudden death. Am Heart J 101:667, 1981.
 5. Thompson, R, Mitchell, A, Ahmed, M, et al: Conduction defects in aortic valve disease. Am Heart J 98:3, 1979.
 6. Hoffman, M, Amann, FW, Roth, J, et al: Sudden cardiac death after aortic valve surgery: Incidence and concomitant factors. Clin Cardiol 12:202, 1989.
 7. DeMaria, AN, Amsterdam, EA, et al: Arrhythmias in the mitral valve syndrome. Ann Intern Med 84:656, 1976.
 8. Procacci, PM, Sarvan, MSV, et al: Prevalence of clinical mitral valve prolapse in 1169 young women. N Engl J Med 294:1086, 1976.
 9. Winkle, RA, Lopes, MG, et al: Life-threatening arrhythmias in the mitral valve prolapse syndrome. Am J Cardiol 60:961, 1976.
10. Campbell, RWF, Goodman, MG, et al: Ventricular arrhythmias in syndrome of balloon deformity of mitral valve. Br Heart J 38:1053, 1976.
11. Winkle, RA, Lopes, MG, Fitzgerald, JW, et al: Arrhythmias in patients with mitral valve prolapse. Circulation 52:73, 1975.
12. Schaal, SF, Fontana, ME, and Wooley, CF: Mitral valve prolapse syndrome spectrum of conduction defects and arrhythmias. Circulation 49:III-97, 1974.
13. Jeresaty, RM: Sudden death in the mitral valve prolapse click syndrome. Am J Cardiol 37:317, 1976.
14. Wei, JY, Bulkley, BH, Schaeffer, AH, et al: Mitral valve prolapse syndrome and recurrent ventricular tachycardia. Ann Intern Med 89:6, 1978.
15. Rakowski, H, Waxman, MB, Wald, RW, et al: Mitral valve prolapse and ventricular fibrillation. Circulation 11:93, 1975.
16. Sanfilippo, AJ, Abdollah, H, and Burggraf, GW: Quantitation and significance of systolic mitral leaflet displacement in mitral valve prolapse. Am J Cardiol 64:1349, 1989.
17. Hayakawa, M and Inon, T: Natural history of mitral valve prolapse with respect to the heart size and ventricular arrhythmias. J Cardiol 14 (suppl):81, 1987.
18. Inoh, T, Kumaki, T, and Kurozumi, Y: Prognosis of mitral valve prolapse related to the changes in the grade and ventricular arrhythmias. J Cardiogr 11:105, 1986.
19. Mason, DT, Lee, G, Chan, MC, et al: Arrhythmias in patients with mitral valve prolapse: Types, evaluation, and therapy. Med Clin North Am 68:1039, 1984.
20. Kramer, HM, Kligfield, P, Richard, B, et al: Arrhythmias in mitral valve prolapse. Arch Intern Med 144:2360, 1984.
21. Kligfield, P, Hochreiter, C, Kramer, H, et al: Complex arrhythmias in mitral regurgitation with and without mitral valve prolapse: Contrast to arrhythmias in mitral valve prolapse without mitral regurgitation. Am J Cardiol 55:1545, 1985.
22. Dollar, AL and Roberts, WC: Morphologic comparison of patients with mitral valve prolapse who died suddenly with patients who died from severe valvular dysfunction or other conditions. J Am Coll Cardiol 17:921, 1991.
23. Mirvis, DM and Erwin, SW: Ventricular pre-excitation and prolonged QT interval syndrome in a patient with mitral valve prolapse. Am Heart J 96:529, 1978.
24. Wit, AL, Fenoglio, JJ, Hordof, AJ, et al: Ultrastructure and transmembrane potentials of cardiac muscle in the human anterior mitral valve leaflet. Circulation 59:1284, 1979.
25. Probst, P, Goldschlager, A, and Selzer, A: Left atrial size and atrial fibrillation in mitral stenosis: Factors influencing their relationship. Circulation 48:1281, 1973.
26. Arandi, DT and Carleton, RA: The deleterious role of tachycardia in mitral stenosis. Circulation 36:511, 1967.
27. Driefus, LS, Katz, M, Watanabe, Y, et al: Clinical significance of disorders of impulse formation and conduction in the atrioventricular junction. Am J Cardiol 11:384, 1963.
28. Schwartz, LS, Goldfischer, J, Srague, GJ, et al: Syncope and sudden death in aortic stenosis. Am J Cardiol 23:647, 1969.
29. Hakki, AH, Kimbiris, D, Iskandrian, AS, et al: Angina pectoris and coronary artery diseases in patients with severe aortic valvular disease. Am Heart J 100:441, 1980.

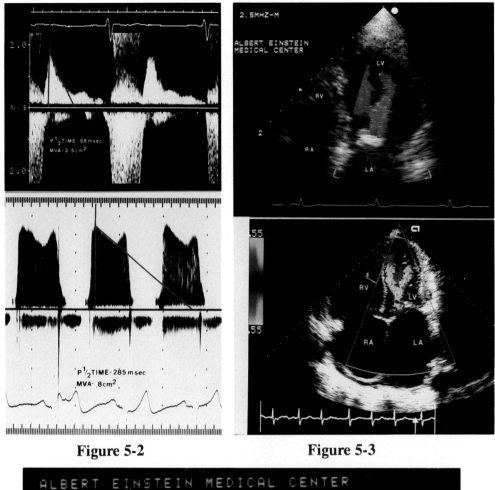

Figure 5-2

Figure 5-3

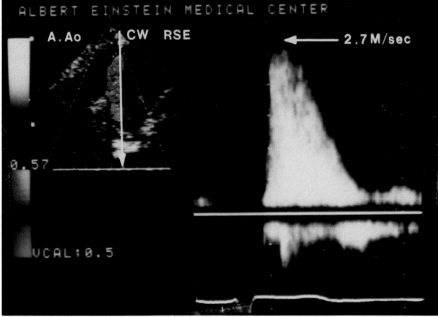

Figure 5-5

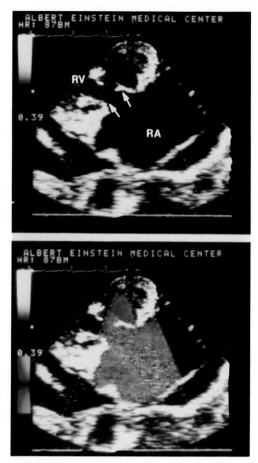

Figure 5-7

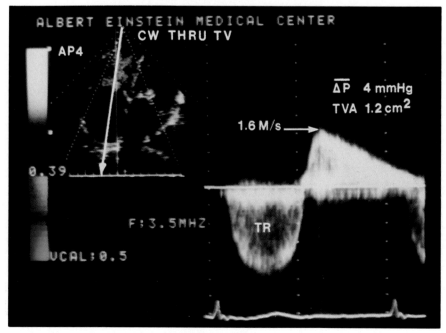

Figure 5-8

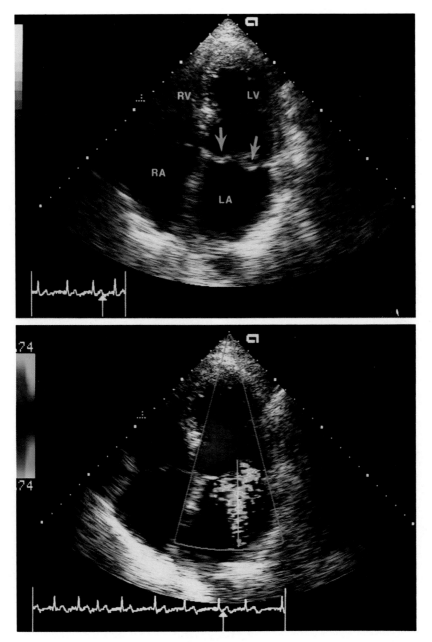

Figure 5-11

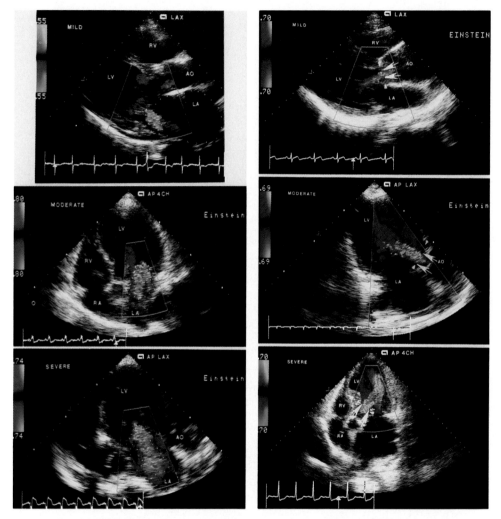

Figure 5-14   **Figure 5-18**

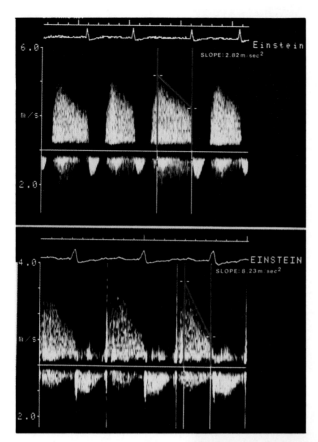

Figure 5-19

Figure 5-21

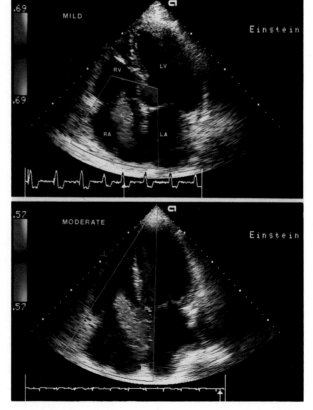

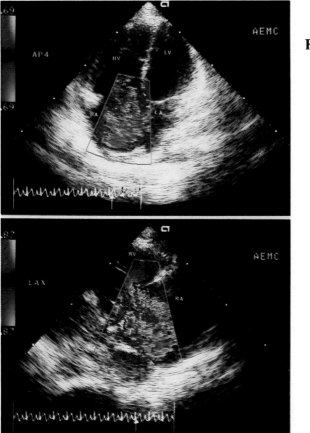

Figure 5-22

Figure 5-23

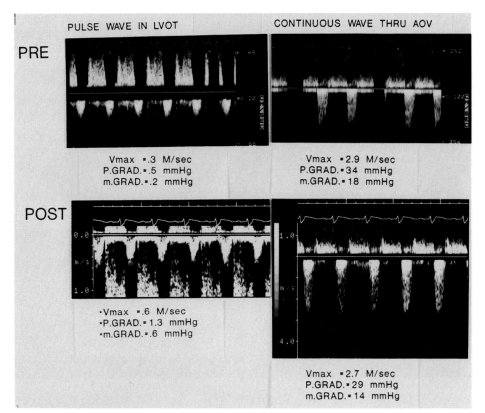

Figure 5-24

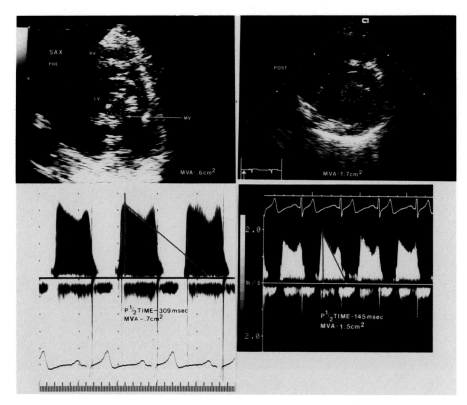

Figure 5-25

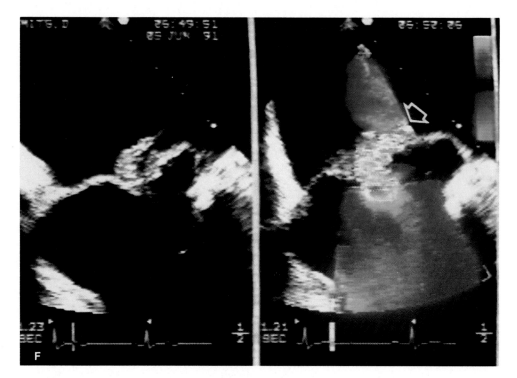

Figure 6-7(f)

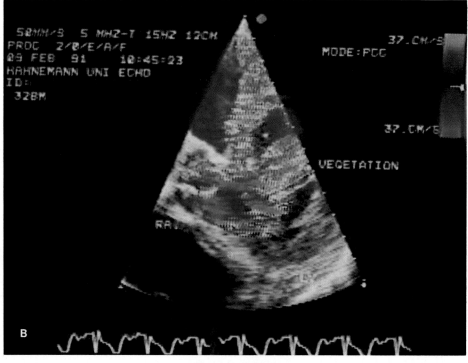

Figure 6-8(b)

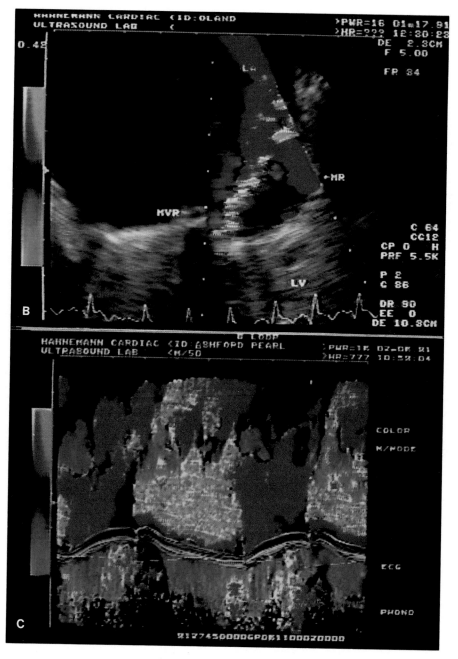

Figure 6-9 (b and c)

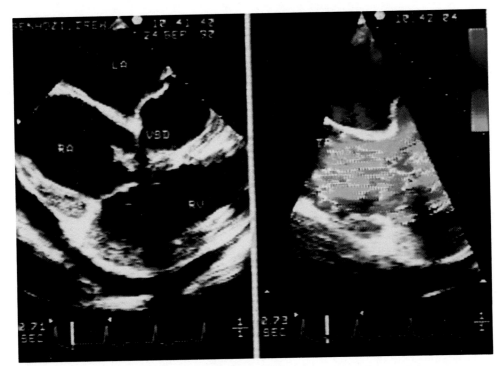

Figure 6-12

Figure 5-2. (*Top*), Pulsed-wave Doppler in a patient with rheumatic heart disease and predominant mitral regurgitation. Increased initial velocity and rapid decay slope (*red lines*) are noted. Mitral valve area (MVA) by pressure half-time (P ½ time) measures 2.5 cm². The MR systolic jet is shown above and below the baseline. (*Bottom*), CW Doppler obtained in a patient with rheumatic mitral stenosis. Initial velocity is increased but decay slope is markedly reduced (*red line*). MVA measures 0.8 cm² by the pressure half-time method (P ½ time).

Figure 5-3. (*Top*), Color flow Doppler echocardiogram obtained in the apical 4-chamber view in a patient with mitral stenosis. The jet is transmitted towards the apex and demonstrates the typical candle flame appearance *(blue within red color)* which occurs due to flow aliasing and velocities exceeding the Nyquist limit. (*Bottom*), Color flow echocardiogram obtained in the apical 4-chamber view in a patient with mitral stenosis. The color jet bifurcates into a medially and laterally directed jet. High velocity of flow is displayed as a mosaic pattern. LA = left atrium; LV = left ventricle; RV = right ventricle; and RA = right atrium.

Figure 5-5. (*Left*), Abnormally directed color flow jet obtained in a 90-year-old patient with senile calcific aortic stenosis obtained from right sternal edge (RSE). By aligning the continuous wave Doppler (CW) signal (*arrow*) through the eccentrically directed jet, the maximal velocity jet can be obtained (*right*). Ao = anterior aortic wall.

Figure 5-7. (*Top*), Two-dimensional echocardiogram obtained in the right ventricular inflow plane in a patient with carcinoid heart disease. During diastole the tricuspid valve leaflets are domed, shortened, and restricted in motion (*arrows*). (*Bottom*), Color flow Doppler study in same patient showing tricuspid regurgitation. RV = right ventricle; RA = right atrium.

Figure 5-8. (*Left*), Color flow Doppler obtained in the apical 4-chamber view in a patient with combined mitral and tricuspid stenosis. Increased turbulence of jet is noted and continuous wave Doppler is aligned through the jet. (*Right*), CW Doppler records a systolic tricuspid regurgitant jet (TR) and a diastolic jet demonstrating an increase in initial diastolic velocity and a reduced diastolic decay slope. Mean pressure gradient (P) measures 4 mmHG and tricuspid valve area (TVA) by the pressure half-time method measures 1.2 cm².

Figure 5-11. (*Top*), Four-chamber view showing prolapse of both anterior and posterior mitral leaflets (*arrows*). RA = right atrium; RV = right ventricle; LV = left ventricle; LA = left atrium. (*Bottom*), Color flow Doppler image of same patient in 4-chamber view. Both leaflets of mitral valve are prolapsing, resulting in a central jet of mitral regurgitation (*arrow*).

Figure 5-14. (*Top*), Parasternal long axis view showing jet of mild mitral regurgitation (MR). MR jet and LA are outlined by white dots. Ratio of MR jet area to LA area is 5%. (*Middle*), Apical 4-chamber view showing moderate MR. MR jet and LA area are outlined by white dots. Ratio of MR jet area to LA area is 35%. (*Bottom*), Apical 4-chamber view showing severe MR. MR jet area and LA area are outlined by white dots. Ratio of MR jet area to LA area is 46%.

Figure 5-18. AR jet width is shown (*arrows*). Left ventricular outflow trace (LVOT) width is shown (*arrow heads*). (*Top*), Mild AR on parasternal long axis view. Ratio of jet width to LVOT width is 30%. (*Middle*), Moderate AR in apical long axis view. Ratio of jet width to LVOT width is 54%. (*Bottom*), Severe AR in apical 5-chamber view. Ratio of jet width to LVOT width is 82%.

Figure 5–19. (*Top*), Continuous wave (CW) spectra of moderate AR with the transducer at the apex of the left ventricle. The slope of the signal is less than $3M/sec^2$ ($2.82 M/sec^2$) and is suggestive of mild to moderate aortic regurgitation. (*Bottom*), Continuous wave spectra of severe AR showing slope greater than $3M/sec^2$ ($8.23M/sec^2$) consistent with severe aortic regurgitation.

Figure 5–21. (*Top*), Mild TR obtained from apical 4-chamber view. (*Bottom*), Moderate TR in same plane. RV = right ventricle; LV = left ventricle; RA = right atrium; LA = left atrium.

Figure 5–22. Severe TR obtained in the apical 4-chamber view (*Top*) and right ventricular (RV) inflow view (*Bottom*). Note the mosaic jet fills most of the right atrium (RA). RV = right ventricle; LV = left ventricle; LA = left atrium.

Figure 5–23. Reversal of flow in hepatic vein. (*Top*), Reversed flow in systole within the hepatic vein consistent with severe tricuspid regurgitation (TR). (*Bottom*), Color M-mode cursor of hepatic vein. During systole there is reversal of flow towards transducer (red) and flow away in diastole (blue).

Figure 5–24. (*Top*), Prevalvuloplasty. Pulse wave (*left*) and continuous wave (*right*) Doppler measurements in a patient with aortic stenosis. The maximal and mean gradients across the aortic valve (AOV) and in the left ventricular outflow tract are listed. Aortic valve area derived by the continuity equation is $0.3cm^2$ and EF measures 10%. Aortic regurgitation is present. (*Bottom*), Postvalvuloplasty. The maximal and mean gradients across the aortic valve (*right*) and in the left ventricular outflow tract (*left*) are listed. Aortic valve area derived by the continuity equation is $0.7cm^2$ and EF measured 20%. Note that there is a very little change in the gradient across the aortic valve. However, with improvement in cardiac output, the flow in the left ventricular outflow tract is considerably increased and aortic valve area has more than doubled.

Figure 5–25. (*Top left*), Prevalvuloplasty. Mitral valve (MV) area (MVA) measures $0.6m^2$ visualized in the parasternal short axis view (SAX). (*Top right*), Postvalvuloplasty. Mitral valve area measures $1.7cm^2$. (*Bottom left*), Prevalvuloplasty. Doppler measured mitral valve area by the pressure half-time (P ½ time) is $0.7cm^2$. (*Bottom right*), Postvalvuloplasty, Doppler measured mitral valve area by the pressure half-time measures $1.5cm^2$.

Figure 5–26. Relationship of echo score to outcome of mitral valvuloplasty. (Adapted from Lefevre et al. [89]).

Figure 6–7. F is the corresponding color flow image demonstrating the eccentric mitral regurgitant jet (*arrow*). LA = left atrium; LV = left ventricle.

Figure 6–8. (*B*) Corresponding color flow image demonstrating severe mitral regurgitation through the perforation. AOV = aortic valve; LA = left atrium; LV = left ventricle; RA = right atrium; RV = right ventricle.

Figure 6–9. (*B*) Perivalvular mitral regurgitation within the left atrium is seen. (*C*) Color flow M-mode demonstrating mosaic pattern of perivalvular mitral regurgitation. LA = left atrium; LV = left ventricle; MR = mitral regurgitation; MV = mitral valve; MVR = mitral valve replacement; RA = right atrium.

Figure 6–12. Transesophageal oblique 4-chamber view of a patient with a ventricular septal defect (VSD). Corresponding color flow image demonstrates severe tricuspid regurgitation. LA = left atrium; RA = right atrium; RV = right ventricle.

PART 3

Newer Diagnostic Methods

CHAPTER 5

Echo-Doppler in Valvular Heart Disease*

Morris N. Kotler, M.D.
Larry E. Jacobs, M.D.
Leo A. Podolsky, M.D.
Colin B. Meyerowitz, M.D.
With Technical Assistance of Alfred Ioli

For many years, cardiac catheterization has been the gold standard for estimating the severity of valvular heart disease. Two-dimensional (2-D) echocardiography provides an accurate noninvasive assessment by delineating valvular anatomic changes; determining left and right ventricular function, chamber enlargement, and wall hypertrophy; and detecting associating pericardial effusion. Doppler echocardiography provides hemodynamic assessment of valvular obstruction, and when combined with color flow, semiquantitation of regurgitation is possible. Because of its versatility, Echo-Doppler techniques have become an indispensable tool in evaluating patients with suspected valve lesions.

MITRAL STENOSIS

The most common cause of mitral stenosis is rheumatic heart disease. Although it is declining in Western nations, it is still prevalent in underdeveloped countries and in migrants from those areas. Congenital mitral stenosis and the parachute mitral valve are rare causes of valvular obstruction. In young patients, commissural fusion occurs, and frequently the leaflets are thin and mobile. In the elderly, calcification and thickening of the leaflets and commissures occur producing a significantly narrowed orifice and a "fish-mouth" appearance.

The echocardiographic features of rheumatic mitral stenosis are best appreciated in the parasternal long axis view and include reduced excursion of the anterior

---

*This study was supported in part by The Women's League for Medical Research, Albert Einstein Medical Center, Philadelphia, PA 19141.

mitral leaflet at the tip with doming of a portion of the leaflet.[1] Frequently, the posterior leaflet is restricted in its motion. In addition, thickening or calcification of the valvular and subvalvular apparatus occurs (Fig. 5–1).[2] The left atrium is generally enlarged as is the right ventricle and right atrium. On rare occasions, a left atrial thrombus can be detected in the posterior portion of the left atrium by transthoracic echocardiography.[3] However, transesophageal echocardiography is frequently required to demonstrate thrombus in the left atrial appendage inasmuch as this portion of the left atrium is not accessible to visualization by the transthoracic route.[4] Assessment of the severity of mitral stenosis by 2-D echocardiography can be performed by measuring the mitral valve orifice area obtained in the parasternal short axis view (see Fig. 5–1). The tip of the mitral valve orifice, which is generally the smallest area, can be obtained by careful scanning in the superior and inferior plane. Imaging of the smallest orifice area by 2-D echocardiography has been shown to correlate with the mitral valve area determined by cardiac catheterization[5–7] as well as with measurements of the mitral valve area obtained during surgery.[5,8] In a small percentage of patients (approximately 10% to 15%), the mitral valve area may not be able to be measured by planimetry as a result of suboptimal image quality, extensive and dense calcification of the leaflets, or predominant subvalvular obstruction.[9] Rheumatic mitral stenosis differs from congenital mitral stenosis in that calcification of the mitral valve apparatus is not encountered in the congenital form. In congenital mitral stenosis, the mitral valve leaflets are fused, the chordae are shortened and fibrotic, and the papillary muscles are occasionally involved as well.[10] The parachute mitral valve is characterized by a single large papillary muscle with normal chordae and valve leaflets. Generally, the obstruction occurs at the subvalvular area as a result of the convergence of the chordae inserting on the single papillary muscle.[11,12] Doppler echocardiography provides hemodynamic assessment of the severity of obstruction to the mitral inflow. By using continuous-wave Doppler, an increased diastolic flow velocity with a reduced diastolic velocity decay slope has been reported (Fig. 5–2).[13,14] Color Doppler allows correct alignment of the jet so that the continuous-wave cursor can be directed parallel to the jet thereby obtaining the maximal velocity of the jet.[15] This technique is especially helpful in patients with abnormally directed jets (Fig. 5–3). Both maximal and mean transvalvular mitral pressure gradients as determined by Doppler echocardiography have been shown to correlate with pressure gradients obtained by cardiac catheterization.[13,16] To obtain the mitral valve area, the pressure half-time method has been employed.[17] The pressure half-time, the time required for the initial diastolic gradient to decline by 50%, is obtained from the Doppler velocity profile by dividing peak velocity by $\sqrt{2}/2$ (0.72) and then measuring the time from the peak velocity to the time velocity has decreased by 72% of peak. The more prolonged the half-time, the more severe the reduction in orifice area[17] (see Fig. 5–2). Thus, using the pressure half-time determination, mitral valve area (MVA) is equal to 220 divided by pressure half-time:

$$MVA = \frac{220}{\text{pressure half-time}}$$

The determination of MVA by the pressure-half time correlates well with MVA obtained by the Gorlin formula at cardiac catheterization.[17,18] The pressure half-time is independent of heart rate and the presence of mitral regurgitation. In

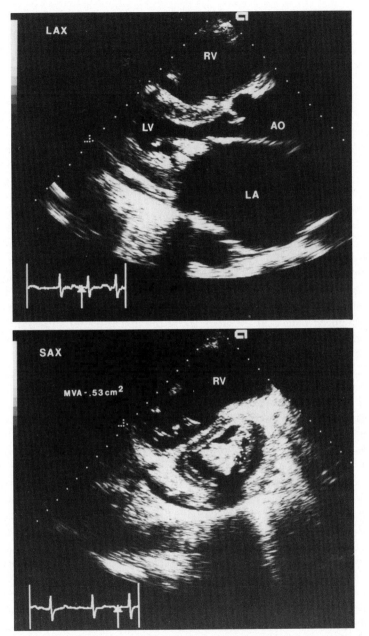

Figure 5–1. *(Top)* Parasternal long axis (LAX) obtained in diastole view in a patient with mitral stenosis. The anterior and posterior mitral leaflets are thickened and heavily calcified with restriction of motion of the tips. The left atrium (LA) and right ventricle (RV) are enlarged. LV = left ventricle; AO = aorta. *(Bottom)* Parasternal short axis view (SAX) obtained in diastole in the same patient. The mitral valve orifice is traced *(dotted lined)* and by planimetry measures 0.53 cm^2 which is significantly reduced. The flattened septum bulges into the left ventricle as a result of an enlarged right ventricle which is caused by pressure and volume overload of the right ventricle.

patients with aortic regurgitation, however, the regurgitant jet may interfere with the calculation of the valve area by the pressure gradient half-time method. Therefore it may be unreliable in patients with combined aortic regurgitation and mitral stenosis.[19]

AORTIC STENOSIS

Two-dimensional echocardiography is helpful in assessing the degree of aortic valve thickness, the presence or absence of calcification, and the degree and extent of restriction of leaflet motion.[9] Additionally, left ventricular function, the extent of left ventricular hypertrophy, and degree of poststenotic dilation of the aorta can be reliably assessed. It is not possible to determine whether the valve is congenitally bicuspid or tricuspid in the presence of extensive and dense calcification. In the absence of severe calcification, the congenitally bicuspid aortic valve is characterized by two leaflets of unequal size with the larger often containing a fibrous ridge (raphe) at the site of congenital fusion. Abnormal commissures are often best seen in the parasternal short axis in diastole, and in systole an oval or circular orifice is observed in the aortic root (circle within a circle).[20] In aortic stenosis, the transvalvular gradient and aortic valvular orifice area can be determined. By aligning the continuous-wave Doppler, the ultrasound can be directed parallel to the flow jet so that the velocity of blood flow distal to the stenotic jet is obtained (Fig. 5–4).[21] The transducer can be placed at the apex using the apical five-chambered view, right parasternal or suprasternal position to obtain the maximum velocity of flow. In older patients with eccentrically directed flow jets, color-flow Doppler is useful in allowing continuous-wave Doppler to be accurately aligned to the abnormally directed flow jet (Fig. 5–5).[22] In a recently reported study, color-flow-guided continuous-wave Doppler allowed more accurate determination of transvalvular gradients.[22] Using the modified Bernoulli equation, the maximal instantaneous and mean transvalvular pressure gradients can be obtained by the formula, $P = 4V^2$, where P is the pressure gradient and V is velocity of transvalvular blood flow as measured by continuous-wave Doppler.[23,24] The Doppler-determined maximal instantaneous gradient generally exceeds the peak-to-peak gradient as obtained by cardiac catheterization.[21] A very elegant study using combined simultaneous continuous-wave Doppler and cardiac catheterization has shown excellent correlation between Doppler-derived gradient measurements and that obtained by cardiac catheterization.[21] The mean gradient is a more reliable estimate of the severity of aortic stenosis as determined by Doppler echocardiography.[21] Determination of gradient alone may be unreliable inasmuch as the gradient is often dependent on the flow and the status of the left ventricle.[23,24] Thus, in severe left ventricular dysfunction, a relatively insignificant gradient can be recorded despite the patient having significant aortic stenosis (Fig. 5–6). The continuity equation is a useful noninvasive test for assessing the severity of aortic stenosis.[25] The continuity equation is represented as follows:

$$A1 \times V1 = A2 \times V2, \text{ where}$$

A1 = cross-sectional area of the left ventricular outflow tract
A2 = cross-sectional area of the stenotic valve
V2 = mean velocity of blood flow at the level of the aortic valve
V1 = mean velocity of blood flow within the ventricular outflow tract

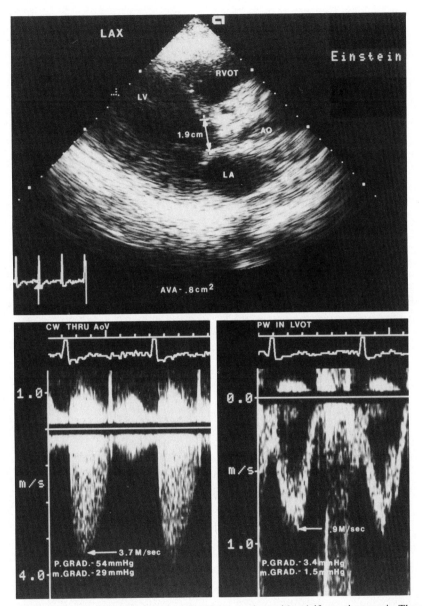

Figure 5–4. *(Top)* Parasternal long axis view (LAX) in a patient with calcific aortic stenosis. The aortic valve leaflets are heavily calcified and are markedly restricted in motion. Left ventricular function was normal in this patient. The left ventricular outflow tract measures 1.9 cm *(arrow). (Bottom Left)* Continuous wave (CW) Doppler obtained in the same patient from the apical 5-chamber view. The maximal gradient measures 54 mmHg and the mean gradient measures 29 mmHg. *(Right)* Pulse wave (PW) Doppler obtained in the left ventricular outflow tract (LVOT). The maximal gradient in two LVOT measures 3.4 mmHg and the mean gradient measures 1.5 mmHg. Aortic valve area (AVA) obtained by the continuity equation measures 0.8 cm^2. See text for description. RVOT = right ventricular outflow tract; AO = aorta; LV = left ventricle; LA = left atrium.

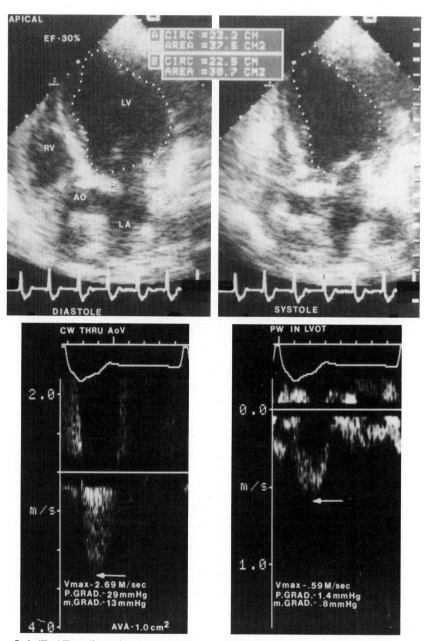

Figure 5–6. *(Top)* Two-dimensional echocardiogram obtained in the apical 5-chamber view during diastole *(left)* and systole *(right)*. The ventricle is markedly dilated and shows significant hypokinesis especially of the postero-lateral wall. The ejection fraction is calculated to be 30%. *(Bottom left)* Continuous Wave (C) Doppler obtained in the apical 5-chamber view with the maximal gradient of 29 mmHg and a mean gradient of 13 mmHg. *(Right)* Pulsed wave (PW) Doppler obtained in the apical 5-chamber view at the level of the left ventricular outflow tract (LVOT). Maximal gradient measures 1.4 mmHg and the mean gradient measures 0.8 mmHg. In this patient with significant left ventricular dysfunction the maximal gradient is only 29 mmHg but the aortic valve area (AVA) measures 1.0 cm^2 by the continuity equation.

With rearrangement of the continuity equation, the true aortic valve area can be determined: A2 = A1 × V1/V2. Continuous-wave Doppler measures the aortic valve velocity, and pulse-wave Doppler measures the mean velocity within the left ventricular outflow tract. A1 is derived from the midsystolic diameter of the left ventricular outflow tract distal to the aortic valve leaflets in the parasternal view. Thus, the continuity equation becomes $A2 = 0.875\ D^2 \times \dfrac{V1}{V2}$. Investigators have used the ratio V1:V2 as a simplified index for predicting the severity of aortic stenosis.[25] If the ratio of V1:V2 is >0.25, then significant aortic stenosis can be reliably excluded. The ratio is thus independent of cardiac output.

A simplified method of determining aortic valve area in patients with clinically significant aortic stenosis has been recently devised. This includes obtaining the fractional shortening velocity ratio.[26] The maximal flow is determined by the continuous-wave Doppler spectral tracing using the modified Bernoulli equation, $P = 4V^2$. Percent fractional shortening (%FS) is calculated as $EDD - \dfrac{ESD}{EDD} \times 100$, where EDD is the end-diastolic and ESD is the end-systolic diameter measurement as obtained by M-mode echocardiography at the midpapillary muscle level. Thus, the fractional shortening velocity equation is represented as follows:

$$\text{aortic area} = \frac{\%FS}{4V^2}$$

Generally, the formula will slightly overestimate the severity of aortic stenosis. However, with appropriate regression formula the fractional shortening velocity ratio has an excellent correlation with that obtained by the Gorlin formula at cardiac catheterization.[26]

TRICUSPID STENOSIS

Generally, rheumatic heart disease is the most common cause of tricuspid stenosis and is characterized by 2-D echocardiography as demonstrating thickening and deformed leaflets, abnormal leaflet motion, and reduced orifice dimension. These echocardiographic manifestations are best appreciated in the right ventricular inflow plane in the long and short axis positions.[9] Generally, tricuspid stenosis is uncommonly accompanied by calcification in contrast to rheumatic mitral stenosis. In addition, abnormal leaflet motion and doming during maximal excursion are evident.[27] In addition to rheumatic causes of tricuspid stenosis, carcinoid disease, methysergide endomyocardial fibrosis, and endomyocardial fibroelastomas can affect the tricuspid valve.[28,29] In severe cases of carcinoid disease, the tricuspid valve may be immobile and fixed in a semiopened position (Fig. 5–7).[30] Carcinoid generally affects right-sided valves and infrequently left-sided valves whereas in rheumatic heart disease, tricuspid stenosis usually occurs in the presence of rheumatic mitral stenosis. To obtain tricuspid inflow signals, the apical four-chamber view or right ventricular inflow is used. Doppler echocardiography, especially continuous-wave, will show increased velocity and decreased decay of the inflow signals not dissimilar from mitral stenosis. However, the velocities are generally not as high as that observed in mitral stenosis (Fig. 5–8). Using the pressure half-time, noninvasive severity of tricuspid stenosis has correlated well with findings obtained by cardiac catheterization.[31]

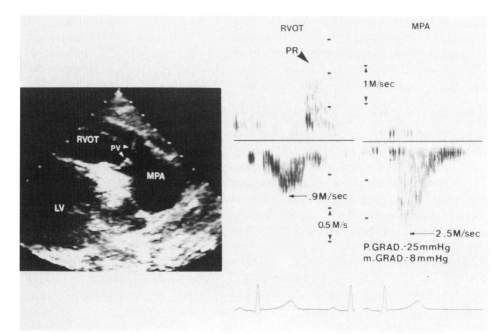

Figure 5–9. *(Left)* Modified parasternal short axis view in a patient with congenital pulmonic stenosis demonstrating domed and restricted leaflet motion during systole. There is poststenotic dilatation of the main pulmonary artery (MPA). PV = pulmonic valve. *(Right)* Continuous wave Doppler showing right pulmonic regurgitation (PR) in the ventricular outflow tract (RVOT) and a maximal (P) gradient of 25 mmHg and mean (M) gradient of 8 mmHg across the stenotic pulmonic valve.

PULMONIC STENOSIS

Pulmonic stenosis generally occurs as a result of congenital heart disease. It is often recognized in childhood but may be missed until adolescence. Rarely, rheumatic heart disease or carcinoid may be associated with combined pulmonic stenosis and regurgitation.[9] Generally, the best view for assessing the pulmonic valve is from the parasternal short axis and subcostal views. Pulmonary valve stenosis should be suspected by 2-D in the presence of systolic doming of the valve (Fig. 5–9).[32,33] When continuous-wave Doppler is appropriately aligned, the pressure gradient obtained in pulmonic valvular stenosis (see Fig. 5–9) can provide accurate hemodynamic assessment and correlates with pressure gradients obtained at cardiac catheterization.[34] Color flow may be used in directing the alignment of the continuous-wave jet to parallel the maximal jet angulation and thus determine the maximal gradient across the pulmonic valve.

MITRAL REGURGITATION

The components of the mitral apparatus necessary for functional competence include the proper interaction of the mitral leaflets, chordae tendineae, papillary muscles, mitral anulus, left atrium, and left ventricle.[35,36] Transthoracic echocardiography yields useful but often incomplete data concerning the interaction of these components. Gross abnormalities of leaflet function often visualized by 2-D echocardiography consist of (1) restricted leaflets secondary to rheumatic involvement (see mitral stenosis); (2) retracted leaflets as a result of localized left ventricular dilation usually in association with inferior myocardial infarction (Fig. 5–10); (3) leaflet destruction by an inflammatory process, such as endocarditis; and (4) myxomatous degeneration with or without leaflet prolapse (Fig. 5–11). Rupture of chordae tendineae results in flail leaflet with characteristic M-mode findings of high-frequency systolic oscillations of the affected leaflet in systole (Fig. 5–12A) and 2-D echocardiographic appearance of a total lack of chordal restraint and motion of the leaflet tip beyond the normal coaptation point deep into the left atrium during systole (Fig. 5–12B). Papillary muscle rupture following myocardial infarction results in severe acute mitral regurgitation (MR). This entity can be recognized by 2-D echocardiography, which visualizes the body of the papillary muscle moving freely within the left ventricle. Dilation of the mitral anulus may be associated with significant MR in patients without leaflet abnormalities.[37,38] The normal mitral anular end-diastolic diameter measures approximately 2.6 cm ($\pm$0.5 cm). An anular diameter of 3.6 cm to 3.8 cm is associated with MR.[38,39] Moderate and severe mitral anular calcification (MAC) but not mild MAC is also associated with significant MR[40] and can be readily diagnosed by transthoracic echocardiography (Fig. 5–13). Both left atrial and left ventricular enlargement are found in association with MR,[37,38] and frequently, the ventricular contraction pattern is associated with a volume overload pattern. It is unclear whether or not left atrium and left ventricular dilation are markers of significant MR or increase the severity of MR by dilating the mitral anulus and distorting leaflet coaptation. Progression of left atrial and left

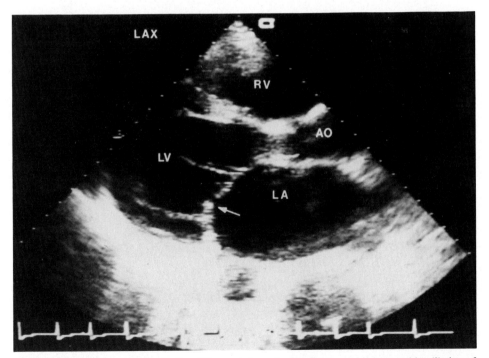

Figure 5–10. Parasternal long axis view. The posterior mitral leaflet *(arrow)* is retracted by dilation of inferior-posterior wall of the left ventricle (LV). This results in an eccentric jet of mitral regurgitation. LA = left atrium; AO = aortic root; RV = right ventricle.

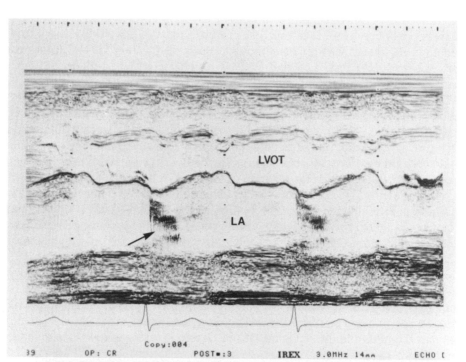

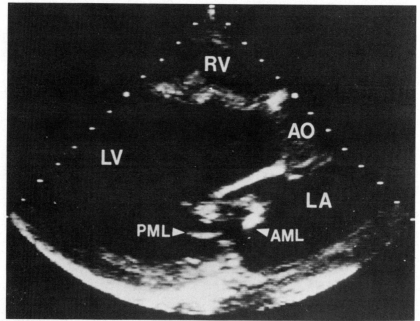

Figure 5–12. *(Top)* M-mode echocardiogram of flail mitrail valve. Note, typical high-frequency oscillation of anterior mitral leaflet *(arrow within left atrium (LA) during systole)*. Abbreviations: LVOT = left ventricular outflow tract. *(Bottom)* Two-dimensional echocardiogram of flail anterior mitral leaflet (AML) protruding deeply into left atrium with loss of normal coaptation point *(arrow)*. Abbreviations: PML = posterior mitral leaflet.

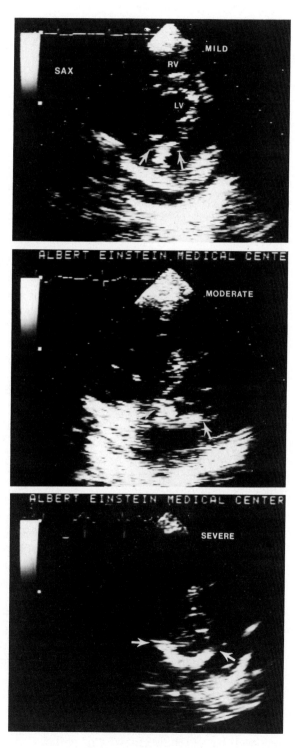

Figure 5–13. Short axis para-sternal views showing differing severity of mitral annulus calcification (MAC). *(Top)* Mild MAC *(arrows)* calcification involves less than one-third of mitral annulus. *(Middle)* Moderate MAC *(arrows)* involves between one-third and two-thirds of annulus. *(Bottom)* Severe MAC *(arrows)* involves greater than two-thirds of annulus.

Table 5–1. Assessment of Mitral Regurgitation by
Color-Flow Doppler

			Sensitivity	Specificity
MJA/LAA	0%–20%	Predicts mild MR	94	100
MJA/LAA	20%–40%	Predicts moderate MR	94	95
MJA/LAA	>40%	Predicts severe MR	93	96
MJA	>8 cm^2	Predicts severe MR	82	94
MJA	<4 cm^2	Predicts mild MR	85	74
AJA	<8 cm^2	Predicts severe MR	82	100
AJA	<4 cm^2	Predicts mild MR	100	63
MJA/LAA	>40%	Predicts severe MR	73	92
MJA/LAA	<20%	Predicts mild MR	65	93

Source: Adapted from Helmcke et al[44] and Spain et al.[45]
MJA = maximal jet area; AJA = average jet area; MJA/LAA = maximal jet area to left atrial
area ratio; MR = mitral regurgitation.

ventricular dilation and decrease in left ventricular function can be accurately followed by M-mode and 2-D echocardiography.

Color-flow Doppler echocardiography is extremely useful for detecting the presence of mitral regurgitation. In those laboratories without color-flow instrumentation, the time-consuming and laborious technique of pulsed-wave Doppler mapping of the regurgitant signal into the left atrial area may be useful.[41–43] Color-flow Doppler integrates velocity at multiple sites within the left atrial area and displays velocity via a color map. Mitral regurgitant velocities are usually well above the Nyquist limit of most color systems and are displayed as a mosaic appearance. Controversy exists as to what constitutes the most clinically useful method of determining MR severity by color flow.

Helmcke and coworkers[44] studied 147 patients with color Doppler using multiple orthogonal planes and compared the color-flow studies to contrast ventriculography. All patients had complete Doppler examinations with careful attention to parasternal short and long axis and apical four-chamber views. The best correlation with angiography was obtained when the regurgitant jet area (maximum obtained from the three planes visualized) was expressed as a percentage of the left atrial area (Fig. 5–14). The left atrial area was obtained in the same plane as the maximal MR jet. Results are tabulated in Table 5–1. Using this method, the ratio of maximal jet area to left atrial area of 0 to 0.2 corresponded to angiographic grade I (mild MR) with a predictive value of 100%, sensitivity of 94%, and specificity of 100%. A ratio of 0.2 to 0.4 corresponded to angiographic grade II (moderate MR) with a predictive value of 85%, sensitivity of 94%, and specificity of 95%. A ratio of >0.4 corresponded to angiographic grade III (severe MR) with a predictive value of 93%, sensitivity of 93%, and specificity of 96%. When maximum MR to left atrial area ratio was compared with the regurgitant fraction, the correlation coefficient was 0.78.

Spain and associates[45] studied 45 patients with color-flow imaging using standard parasternal and apical views and compared the color-flow studies with contrast ventriculography. In contrast to Helmcke's study,[44] Spain and coworkers reported that absolute MR jet area without correction for left atrial size was the best predictor of angiographic MR severity.[45] Results are summarized in Table 5–

1. There was a limited correlation of maximum MR jet area to angiographic regurgitant fraction with the correlation coefficient of only 0.62.

Jet area as displayed by color Doppler is affected by a variety of variables, including hemodynamic factors, such as left ventricular afterload, left atrial contractility and left atrial compliance, and technical factors such as gain setting, variance setting, transducer position, transducer angulation, and jet eccentricity.[46] In addition, the region of the flow disturbance correlates as well with driving pressure as it does to regurgitant volume *in vitro*.

In addition to color-flow mapping, some investigators have determined mitral regurgitant fraction by other Doppler techniques.[47,48] The forward flow across the mitral valve can be calculated by multiplying the mitral anular size by the time velocity integral and comparing that with either flow across the left ventricular outflow tract[47,48] (in the absence of aortic regurgitation) or stroke volume assessed by 2-D echocardiography.[49] Pearson and colleagues[48] found regurgitant fraction to be a useful addition to the assessment of flail postmitral leaflet because of the significant underestimation of MR severity by transthoracic color Doppler in this condition.

AORTIC REGURGITATION

Significant aortic regurgitation (AR) may result from a valvular etiology, such as myxomatous degeneration, rheumatic heart disease, and endocarditis, and is commonly associated with senile calcific aortic stenosis or less commonly with congenitally abnormal aortic valves. In addition, aortic root dilation from any cause may result in abnormal coaptation and significant AR[50] (Fig. 5–15). Significant AR

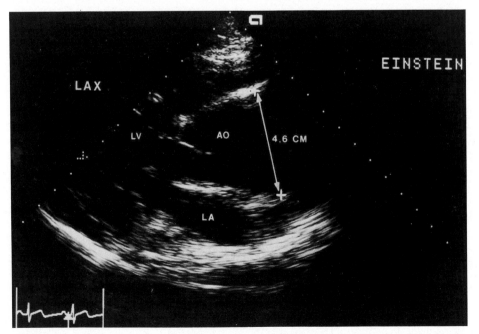

Figure 5–15. Two-dimensional echocardiogram obtained in the parasternal long axis demonstrating moderate dilatation of aortic root measuring 4.6 cm in diameter *(arrow)*. Normal is less than 3.7 cm. Dilated aortic root is commonly associated with aortic regurgitation.

is commonly associated with diastolic flutter of the anterior leaflet of the mitral valve owing to the AR jet impinging on the anterior mitral leaflet (Fig. 5–16). Although fairly specific for AR, it is not useful in grading the severity.[51] Acute severe AR often results in premature closure of the mitral value (Fig. 5–17). This indicates that end-diastolic left ventricular pressure exceeds left atrial pressure, resulting in hemodynamic instability. In acute severe AR, left ventricular cavity size is often normal but systolic function is hyperdynamic.

Doppler echocardiography is extremely useful for assessing AR. Three complementary methods exist for assessing AR severity including: (1) determination of the region of diastolic flow disturbance within the left ventricular outflow tract with pulsed Doppler or, more recently, color Doppler, (2) slope or half-time determination of AR signal by continuous-wave Doppler, (3) assessment of diastolic reversal of flow in the descending or abdominal aorta. Use of all three methods improves the diagnostic yield relative to any single method.

The region of diastolic flow disturbance can be qualitatively assessed using pulsed-wave Doppler techniques by mapping the extent of the regurgitant signal within the left ventricular outflow tract.[52] More recently, color Doppler assessment of AR has emerged as the most useful and practical method for assessing AR jet size because it allows simultaneous assessment of velocity profiles with a single plane. In a study of 29 patients with transthoracic echocardiography and aortog-

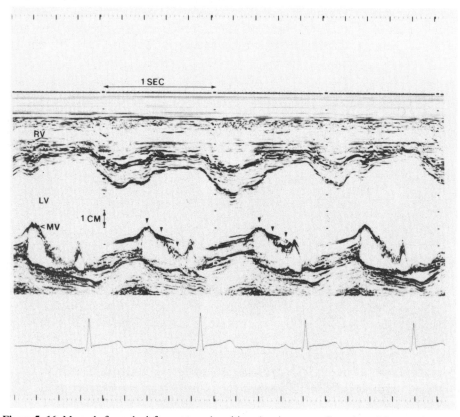

Figure 5–16. M-mode from the left parasternal position showing severe fluttering of the anterior mitral leaflet *(arrowheads)* in association with severe aortic regurgitation.

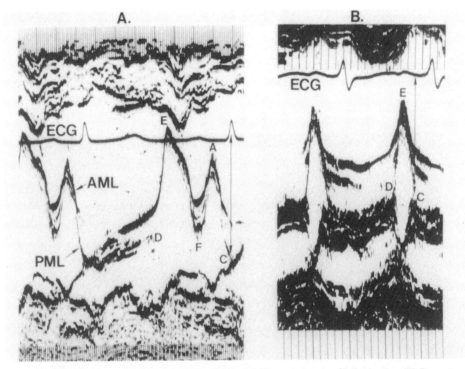

Figure 5–17. M-mode from left parasternal position. (*A*) Normal closure of Mitral valve. (*B*) Premature closure of mitral valve in a patient with acute aortic regurgitation. The valve closes (C-point) before the QRS complex. AML = anterior mitral leaflet. PML = posterior mitral leaflet.

raphy,[53] the width of the AR jet divided by left ventricular outflow tract in the view that demonstrates the maximal jet (usually parasternal or apical views) derived a Spearman correlation coefficient of 0.91 and correctly predicted angiographic severity in 79% of patients. In no case did the method misclassify a patient by more than one grade. Specifically, a ratio of <0.25 is grade I (minimal), 25% to 46% is grade II (mild), 47% to 64% is grade III (moderate), and >65% is grade IV (severe) (Fig. 5–18).

Severe AR causes an elevation in end-diastolic left ventricular pressure and a drop in central aortic pressure resulting in a drop in the central aortic to left ventricular gradient by the end of diastole. Continuous-wave Doppler allows measurements of regurgitant velocity profile, which is directly related by the Bernoulli equation to diastolic aortic left ventricular gradient. Thus, a steep decline in AR velocity spectra in end-diastole correlates with relative equalization of central aortic and the left ventricular pressure. This finding correlates with hemodynamically severe AR.[54]

Generally, a diastolic velocity decay slope of greater than 3 m/sec^2 predicted severe AR with a specificity of 100% but only a sensitivity of 53%[20] (Fig. 5–19). Investigators[55-58] using pressure half-time measurement of regurgitant velocity disagree as to the length of the half-time that predicts severe AR. The maximal half-time predictive of severe AR ranges from 350 to 600 msec.[55] There is significant overlap in deceleration slope and pressure half-times for lesser degrees of AR.

Significant AR causes diastolic reversal of flow within the aorta as well as systolic augmentation of flow within the central aorta. One investigator showed that pandiastolic reversal of flow in the descending aorta (as imaged from the suprasternal notch by pulsed Doppler) (Fig. 5–20) is fairly predictive of significant AR (in absence of patent ductus arteriosus or aortic-pulmonary window). In addition, elevated systolic aortic flow pattern, defined as both peak velocity >0.8 M/sec and

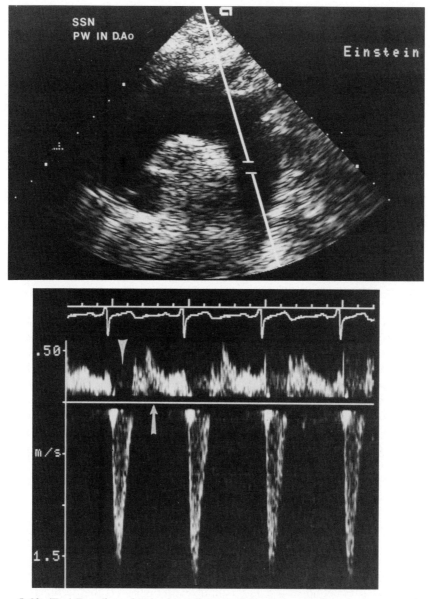

Figure 5–20. *(Top)* Two-dimensional echocardiogram of the aortic arch from the suprasternal notch transducer position. The position of the pulsed-wave sample is demonstrated within the aortic arch. *(Bottom)* Pulsed-wave spectra showing pandiastolic reversal of flow *(arrow)* within aortic arch in a patient with severe AR. Systolic velocity *(arrowhead)* greater than 0.8 M/sec (in this case 1.5 M/sec) is consistent with severe AR.

duration of systolic flow >0.24 seconds was predictive of significant AR.[59] Another investigator[60] has found pandiastolic reversal of flow in the superior abdominal aorta using pulsed Doppler from a subcostal approach as highly specific and sensitive in predicting 3 to $4+$ AR (in the absence of left-to-right shunt).

TRICUSPID REGURGITATION

Tricuspid regurgitation (TR) may result from a leaflet or chordal abnormality in association with tricuspid prolapse, papillary muscle dysfunction, rheumatic disease, Ebstein's anomaly, infective endocarditis, or carcinoid tumor. Anatomically, normal valves are found in up to 47% of patients with pulmonary hypertension, cor-pulmonale, or mitral stenosis.[61] Leaflet abnormalities can be readily appreciated by 2-D echocardiography by viewing the tricuspid valve from multiple planes (i.e., parasternal right ventricular inflow, apical four-chamber view, and subcostal views). Tricuspid regurgitation is commonly associated with tricuspid anular dilation. Specifically, indexed diastolic anular dilation for body surface area >21 mm/m^2 or unindexed anular diameter of >34 mm are highly predictive of severe TR.[62,63]

Pulsed and color Doppler have been used to map the extent of the TR jet in much the same manner as MR is assessed.[62,64,65,66] Unfortunately, because right ventricular contrast ventriculography may induce TR by placement of the catheter across the tricuspid valve, no gold standard for comparison is available. In a study comparing color Doppler with contrast right ventriculography,[65] mild TR was defined as regurgitant flow width of less than half the width of the right atrium, moderate TR as regurgitant flow filling about half the width of the right atrium, and severe TR as regurgitant flow visualized across the entire right atrial cavity (Figs. 5–21 and 5–22). In patients undergoing mitral or aortic repairs, maximal TR flow area to right atrial area ratio of $>34\%$ predicted clinically assessed need for tricuspid anuloplasty during surgery.[62] In addition, reversal of blood flow into hepatic veins during systole as imaged by pulsed Doppler is consistent with significant TR (Fig. 5–23).

Pulmonary artery systolic pressure can be estimated by assessing the peak velocity of the TR signal. Inasmuch as the TR velocity reflects the gradient between the right ventricle and right atrium, the pulmonary artery pressure is equal to this gradient plus right atrial pressure (in the absence of pulmonic stenosis). The right ventricle to right atrium gradient can be calculated by the Bernoulli equation, $P = 4V^2$ (P = pressure gradient, V = velocity of TR). Thus pulmonary artery pressure is estimated by $4V^2$ plus the clinically estimated jugular pressure or an arbitrary right atrial pressure of 14 mm Hg.[67,68]

PULMONIC REGURGITATION

Significant pulmonic regurgitation (PR) is relatively uncommon. However, pulsed-wave Doppler and color Doppler are extremely sensitive in detecting minimal PR in otherwise normal patients.[69,70] Functional PR is frequently present in pulmonary hypertension of any cause. Rarely, other disorders such as rheumatic heart disease, carcinoid, and endocarditis may cause PR. The extent and width of the jet is directly proportioned to the severity of PR and is best appreciated in the parasternal short axis view.[9]

PERCUTANEOUS BALLOON VALVULOPLASTY

PERCUTANEOUS BALLOON AORTIC VALVULOPLASTY

Percutaneous balloon aortic valvuloplasty was performed for the first time by Lababidi and coworkers[71] in 1984 in young children with congenital aortic stenosis.

Prior to aortic balloon valvuloplasty, the following parameters can be assessed by Doppler echocardiography:

1. The maximum velocity of the transaortic systolic flow
2. The maximum and mean systolic Doppler-determined gradients, by application of the modified Bernoulli equation (Fig. 5–24)
3. The continuous-wave Doppler echocardiographic systolic ejection time (DOPET) and the time from onset of systolic Doppler spectral envelope to maximal velocity (TTP)
4. The ratio of TTP/DOPET, to determine the severity of aortic stenosis[24]
5. The left ventricular ejection time

During aortic valvuloplasty, the following parameters can be monitored using Doppler echocardiography:

1. The degree of left ventricular outflow obstruction as indicated by the peak flow velocity across the aortic valve, as well as left ventricular ejection time
2. Changes in aortic regurgitant flow
3. Mitral valve inflow velocity profiles, which can indicate the acute changes in left ventricular diastolic function[72,73]

During the inflation of the balloon across the aortic valve, there is a noticeable decrease in the velocity of the aortic regurgitant jet. This reflects an increase in left ventricular diastolic pressure and a decrease in aortic pressure.

After aortic valvuloplasty, Doppler echocardiography is extremely helpful in evaluation of:

1. Changes in aortic valve area as calculated by the continuity equation, aortic valve gradient, and valve excursion (see Fig. 5–24)
2. The development of AR
3. Changes in diastolic function as determined by mitral valve velocity profile

Aortic regurgitation has been reported to occur in about 10% to 15% of patients; however, it is hemodynamically significant in <2% of the patients.[74,75] Clinical outcome of aortic valvuloplasty both in short-term (24 to 36 h) and long-term followup (6 months) has shown a 30% to 50% improvement in the aortic valve gradient and aortic valve area.[72,74,76] However, in 50% to 60% of patients, restenosis occurs within 6 months.[74,77]

Doppler echocardiographic evaluation of elderly patients with severe aortic stenosis before, during, and after percutaneous balloon aortic valvuloplasty is very important not only in the assessment of the success rate of the procedure itself, but also in providing prognostic information with regard to the followup evaluation (Table 5–2).[79–84] From the prognostic standpoint, aortic valve area is not the major parameter that determines outcome.[78] Rather, the echocardiographic left ventric-

Table 5–2. Results of Balloon Aortic Valvuloplasty

| Author | Year | No. Pts. | Age | Gradient (mm Hg) | | | AV Area (cm²) | | | Survival |
				Pre	Post	FU	Pre	Post	FU	
Lababidi et al[71]	1984	23	<30	113	32	NA	NA	NA	NA	NA
Nishimura et al[81]	1988	55	NA	48	33	46	0.54	0.85	0.62	NA
Kuntz et al[82]	1990	211	78	54	30	NA	0.6	0.9	NA	78%–1 yr
										70%–2 yr
Come[83]	1989	240	79	49 D	35 D	NA	0.6 D	0.8 D	NA	70%
				58 C	30 C		0.5 C	0.8 C		6 mo
Cribier et al[84]	1989	328	NA	NA	26–29	NA	NA	0.9–1.05		86%
										8 mo
O'Neill[80]	1991	492	79	54	28–30		0.47–0.52	0.78–0.85		63%–1 yr

Post = 24–72 hours after valvuloplasty; FU = follow-up study 6 months after valvuloplasty; D = Doppler echo-cardiogram; C = cardiac catheterization; NA = not applicable.

ular mass index, changes in left ventricular diastolic performance, and left ventricular volumes provide more important prognostic criteria that can be followed regularly by serial 2-D and Doppler echocardiography.[79] The most important variables in determining long-term survival in patients undergoing balloon aortic valvuloplasty are left ventricular dysfunction, the presence of coronary artery disease, and the use of multiple balloon inflations.[80]

PERCUTANEOUS BALLOON MITRAL VALVULOPLASTY

Two-dimensional and Doppler echocardiography play a major role in evaluating patients with mitral stenosis who are considered for percutaneous balloon mitral valvuloplasty. The magnitude of mitral stenosis and MR can be assessed very accurately with the use of pulsed Doppler (Fig. 5–25). In addition, the extent of pathologic involvement of the mitral valve by the rheumatic process can be appreciated by 2-D echocardiography. If severe fibrosis, calcification, and subvalvular commissural fusion are present, the results of balloon valvuloplasty can be disappointing. However, if a pliable, noncalcified valve without subvalvular involvement is documented by echocardiography, excellent results can be obtained from either balloon or surgical valvuloplasty. An echocardiographic score can be derived from 2-D echocardiography, which is helpful in the decision making regarding mitral valvuloplasty (Table 5–3).[85,86] The echocardiographic score is based on four parameters:

1. Leaflet mobility
2. Leaflet thickness
3. Degree of subvalvular involvement
4. Degree of calcification

Each of these parameters has a score of 1 to 4, with 4 having the greatest involvement. Patients with a score of <8 are usually good candidates for balloon valvuloplasty, and patients with a score of >10 have a higher complication rate and lower success rate.[86] Undoubtedly, with the advent and improvement of

Table 5–3. Components of Echocardiographic Score (see text for details)

LEAFLET MOBILITY
Grade 1. Highly mobile valve with restriction of only the leaflet tips
Grade 2. Midportion and base of leaflets have reduced mobility
Grade 3. Valve leaflets move forward in diastole mainly at the base
Grade 4. No or minimal forward movement of the leaflets in diastole
VALVULAR THICKENING
Grade 1. Leaflets near normal (4–5 mm)
Grade 2. Midleaflet thickening; marked thickening of the margins
Grade 3. Thickening extends through the entire leaflets (5–8 mm)
Grade 4. Marked thickening of all leaflet tissue (>8–10 mm)
SUBVALVULAR THICKENING
Grade 1. Minimal thickening of chordal structures just below the valve
Grade 2. Thickening of chordae extending up to one third of chordal length
Grade 3. Thickening extending to the distal third of the chordae length
Grade 4. Extensive thickening and shortening of all chordae extending down to the papillary muscle
VALVULAR CALCIFICATION
Grade 1. A single area of increased echo brightness
Grade 2. Scattered areas of brightness confined to leaflet margins
Grade 3. Brightness extending into the midportion of leaflets
Grade 4. Extensive brightness through most of the leaflet tissue

Adapted from Abascal et al.[85]

biplane transesophageal echocardiography, the aforementioned scoring system may be modified so that more accurate parameters regarding the prognosis of patients undergoing balloon valvuloplasty can be employed.

Several studies have addressed the question of the optimal echocardiographic score to determine the outcome of mitral valvuloplasty.[85–87] Early observations[88,90] showed that the presence of rigid, calcified valves and subvalvular disease as well as the fusion of chordae tendineae did not preclude a satisfactory result after balloon mitral valvuloplasty. However, other studies[87,89,92] as well as our own experience indicated that a total echocardiographic score of >8 correlates negatively with immediate outcome of balloon valvuloplasty (Fig. 5–26). Followup results also demonstrate that echocardiographic score is the single most important factor predictive of restenosis (Table 5–4).[93–97]

Short-term followup (up to 13 months) shows that patients with pliable noncalcified valves have a 5% to 7% recurrence of severe symptoms, but no significant stenosis. In patients with heavily calcified, nonpliable valves, the incidence of recurrent symptoms has been reported to range between 30% and 40% with a restenosis rate of 42%.[91]

In patients who undergo percutaneous balloon mitral valvuloplasty, the long-term follow-up can be undertaken by 2-D and Doppler echocardiography. Two-dimensional echocardiographic determination of MVA has correlated well with MVA calculated by cardiac catheterization.[87] However, immediately after valvuloplasty the correlation between Doppler estimate of the MVA and that obtained by cardiac catheterization is poor.[85,88] The discrepancy may be related to nonsimultaneous catheterization and Doppler measurements,[88] lack of left atrial and ventricular compliance measurements,[100] inaccuracies of the Gorlin equation in estimating MVA at catheterization in the presence of MR,[101] and as a result of small

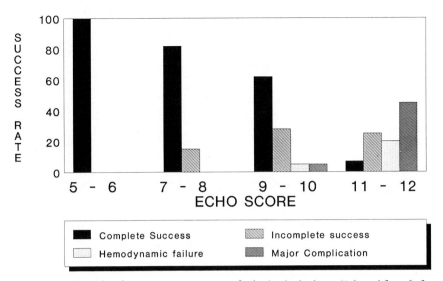

Figure 5–26. Relationship of echo score to outcome of mitral valvuloplasty. (Adapted from Lefevre, et al.[89])

left-to-right shunts not detected by oximetry. The correlation between valve area calculated by the pressure half-time method and the Gorlin formula improved at follow-up. At present, caution should be exercised when estimating the MVA by Doppler techniques immediately after balloon mitral valvuloplasty. Closure of the atrial septal defect after valvuloplasty also can be adequately assessed by Doppler echocardiography.

The progression or regression of MR that commonly occurs after mitral valvuloplasty is best evaluated by echocardiographic studies as well. After mitral valvuloplasty, no change in the severity of MR is encountered in 53% to 55% of

Table 5–4. Results of Balloon Mitral Valvuloplasty

Author	Year	No. Pts.	Age	Mean ES	MV area (cm²) Pre	MV area (cm²) Post	Gradient (mm Hg) Pre	Gradient (mm Hg) Post	Survival
McKay et al[93]	1989	737	54	7.9	1.0	2.0	14	6	97% 30 day
Palacios et al[94]	1989	320 T	NA	NA	NA	NA	NA	NA	
		210	64	≤8	1.0	2.2	15	5	99%–4 yr
		110	48	>8	0.8	1.7			75%–4 yr
Serra et al[95,96]	1989	146	NA	NA	1.1	2.3	16	5	NA
				≤8					94%–3 yr
				>8					72%–3 yr
Berland et al[97]	1990	183 T	NA	NA	NA	NA	NA	NA	NA
		109	54		1.04	2.12			
		74	28		1.03	2.18			

T = total number of patients; ES = echo score; MV = mitral valve.

patients, whereas an increase in MR by one grade occurs in 33% to 40%, and by two grades in 8% to 13%.[85,99] The most important mechanism for developing significant MR after mitral valvuloplasty appears to be a torn leaflet or ruptured chordae tendineae. Lesser degrees of mitral valve regurgitation are caused by excessive commissural split or anterior mitral prolapse and irregularities at the sites of coaptation that could be related to a dilated mitral anulus.[95,96,98] Another explanation for an apparent increase in the severity of MR is a marked decrease in the left atrial pressure, which produces an increase in the left ventricular to left atrial pressure gradient.[99]

CATHETERIZATION VS. ECHO DOPPLER MANAGEMENT OF VALVULAR HEART DISEASE

Although many studies have shown excellent correlation between Doppler echocardiography and cardiac catheterization in evaluating the severity of aortic and mitral valve disease,[16-19,21-26] few studies have addressed the comparison of management decisions reached after Doppler echocardiography or catheterization.[102,103]

Slater and associates[103] prospectively evaluated 189 consecutive patients with valvular heart disease who were being considered for surgical treatment on the basis of clinical information. All the patients underwent a complete Doppler echocardiographic examination and cardiac catheterization. The combination of Doppler echocardiographic and clinical evaluation was inadequate for clinical decision to operate in 21% of patients with aortic and 5% of patients with mitral valve disease. In contrast, the combination of cardiac catheterization and clinical evaluation was considered inadequate in 2% of patients with aortic and 2% of patients with mitral valve disease. There was overall agreement on whether to operate for 76% of patients when the two technologies were compared.[103] When individual valvular lesions were compared, there was agreement between both techniques in 92% for aortic regurgitation, 90% for mitral stenosis, and 83% for aortic stenosis but a disappointing 69% for MR.[103] However, when comparing each technology with clinical evaluation in deciding whether to operate, caution should be advised. Many physicians currently are not adequately trained in clinical skills when evaluating patients with valvular heart disease and have relied extensively on the Doppler echocardiographic examination.[104] With a careful Doppler echocardiographic examination making one measurement of distance and two velocity measurements, aortic valve area can be accurately determined.[105] According to one investigator,[105] "We no longer need to subject the majority of patients with aortic stenosis to invasive measurements of hemodynamics." This statement taken at face value may not apply to all patients because:

1. A technically perfect Doppler echocardiographic examination is not possible on all patients. However, transesophageal echocardiography may overcome this problem.
2. In older patients, coronary arteriography is frequently required to exclude associated coronary artery disease.
3. In patients with combined valvular disease (e.g., aortic stenosis and MR) Doppler echocardiography may not always provide precise quantification of the degree of MR, and although transesophageal echocardiography may

be more accurate,[106] cardiac catheterization may still be indicated in equivocal instances.

Therefore, in the majority of patients, especially elderly patients, both technologies (Doppler echocardiography and cardiac catheterization) are needed to arrive at the appropriate decision about surgery despite the added increases in costs.

SUMMARY

Although Doppler echocardiography plays an important role in evaluating patients with suspected valvular heart disease, it should not replace a careful history, a meticulous physical examination, an electrocardiogram, and well-performed posteroanterior and lateral chest x-rays. Two-dimensional echocardiography can reliably evaluate anatomic valvular lesions, estimate left and right ventricular function, and exclude associated pericardial disease. Doppler echocardiography provides accurate hemodynamic parameters of the severity of aortic and mitral stenosis and the degree of pulmonary hypertension. In addition, color-flow Doppler is helpful in providing semiquantitative information with regard to the degree of MR, AR, or TR. Doppler echocardiography is very useful in evaluating patients before and after valvuloplasty but may be inaccurate when compared with cardiac catheterization immediately following mitral balloon valvuloplasty. However, in the long-term followup, after valvuloplasty, Doppler echocardiography is ideally suited to predict restenosis. A properly performed echo-Doppler study may allow the clinician to send a young patient for surgery when warranted by the clinical symptoms. However, in older patients, especially those with suspected coronary artery disease, and in multivalvular disease, cardiac catheterization may still be required.

REFERENCES

1. Kotler, MN, Mintz, GS, Segal, BL, et al: Clinical uses of two-dimensional echocardiography. Am J Cardiol 45:1061, 1980.
2. Zonolla, L, Marino, P, Nicolosi, GL, et al: Two-dimensional echocardiographic evaluation of mitral valve calcification; sensitivity and specificity. Chest 82:154, 1982.
3. Depace, N, Kotler, MN, Soulen, R, et al: Two-dimensional echocardiographic detection of intra-atrial masses. Am J Cardiol 48:954, 1981.
4. Seward, JB, Khandheira, BK, Oh, JK, et al: Transesophageal echocardiography; technique, anatomic correlations, implementation, and clinical applications. Mayo Clin Proc 63:649, 1988.
5. Glover, MU, Warren, SE, Vieweg, WVR, et al: M-mode and two-dimensional echocardiography correlation with findings at catheterization and surgery in patients with mitral stenosis. Am Heart J 105:98, 1983.
6. Martin, RP, Rakowski, H, Kleiman, JH, et al: Reliability and reproducibility of two-dimensional echocardiographic measurements of the stenotic mitral valve orifice area. Am J Cardiol 43:560, 1979.
7. Wann, LS, Weyman, AE, Feigenbaum, H, et al: Determination of mitral valve area by cross-sectional echocardiography. Ann Intern Med 88:337, 1978.
8. Henry, WL, Griffith, JM, Michaelis, LL, et al: Measurement of mitral orifice area in patients with mitral valve disease by real-time two-dimensional echocardiography. Circulation 51:827, 1975.
9. Olson, LJ and Tajik, AJ: Echocardiography evaluation of valvular heart disease. In Marcus, Schelbert, Skorton, et al (eds): Cardiac Imaging: A Companion to Braunwald's Heart Disease. WB Saunders, Philadelphia, 1991, pp 419–448.

10. Ruckman, RN and Van Praagh: Anatomic types of congenital mitral stenosis. Report of 49 autopsy cases with consideration of diagnosis and surgical implications. Am J Cardiol 42:592, 1978.

11. Snider, AR, Roge, CL, Schiller, NB, et al: Congenital left ventricular inflow obstruction evaluated by two-dimensional echocardiography. Circulation 61:848, 1980.

12. Shone, JD, Sellers, RD, Anderson, RC, et al: The developmental complex of "parachute mitral valve," supravalvular ring of left atrium, subaortic stenosis and coarctation of aorta. Am J Cardiol 11:714, 1963.

13. Hatle, L, Brubakk, A, Tromsdal, A, et al: Noninvasive assessment of pressure drop in mitral stenosis by Doppler ultrasound. Br Heart J 40:131, 1978.

14. Holen, J and Simonsen, S: Determination of pressure gradient in mitral stenosis with Doppler echocardiography. Br Heart J 41:529, 1979.

15. Khandheira, BK, Tajik, AJ, Reeder, GS, et al: Doppler color flow imaging; a new technique for visualization and characterization of the blood flow jet in mitral stenosis. Mayo Clin Proc 61:623, 1986.

16. Stamm, RB and Martin, RP: Quantification of pressure gradients across stenotic valves by Doppler ultrasound. J Am Coll Cardiol 2:707, 1983.

17. Hatle, L, Angelsen, B, and Tromsdal, A: Noninvasive assessment of atrioventricular pressure half-time by Doppler ultrasound. Circulation 60:1096, 1979.

18. Holen, J, Aaslid, R, Landmark, K, et al: Determination of effective orifice area in mitral stenosis from noninvasive ultrasound Doppler data and mitral flow rate. Acta Med Scand 201:83, 1977.

19. Nakatani, S, Masuyama, T, Kodama, K, et al: Value and limitations of stenotic mitral valve area: Comparison of the pressure half-time and the continuity equation methods. Circulation 77:78, 1988.

20. Brandenburg, RO, Jr, Tajik, AJ, Edwards, WD, et al: Accuracy of two-dimensional echocardiographic diagnosis of congenitally bicuspid aortic valve: Echocardiographic anatomic correlation in 115 patients. Am J Cardiol 51:1469, 1983.

21. Currie, PJ, Seward, JB, Reeder, GS, et al: Continuous wave Doppler echocardiographic assessment of severity of calcific aortic stenosis; a simultaneous Doppler catheter correlative study in 100 adult patients. Circulation 71:1162, 1985.

22. Fan, PH, Kapur, KK, and Nanda, NC: Color guided Doppler echocardiographic assessment of aortic valve stenosis. J Am Coll Cardiol 12:441, 1988.

23. Hegrames, L and Hatle, L: Aortic stenosis in adults; noninvasive estimation of pressure differences by continuous wave Doppler echocardiography. Br Heart J 54:396, 1985.

24. Hatle, L, Angelsen, BA, and Tromsdal, A: Noninvasive assessment of aortic stenosis by Doppler ultrasound. Br Heart J 43:284, 1980.

25. Oh, JK, Taliercio, CP, Holmes, DR, Jr, et al: Prediction of the severity of aortic stenosis by Doppler aortic valve area determination; prospective Doppler catheterization correlation in 100 patients. J Am Coll Cardiol 11:1227, 1988.

26. Mann, DL, Usher, BW, Hammerman, S, et al: The fractional shortening velocity ratio: Validation of a new echocardiographic Doppler method for identifying patients with significant aortic stenosis. J Am Coll Cardiol 15:1578, 1990.

27. Daniels, SJ, Mintz, GS, and Kotler, MN: Rheumatic tricuspid valve disease: Two-dimensional echocardiographic, hemodynamic and angiographic correlations. Am J Cardiol 51:492, 1983.

28. Hauck, AJ, Freeman, DP, Ackermann, DM, et al: Surgical pathology of the tricuspid valve: A study of 363 cases spanning 25 years. Mayo Clin Proc 63:851, 1988.

29. Weyman, AE, Rankin, R, and King, H: Loeffler's endocarditis presenting as mitral and tricuspid stenosis. Am J Cardiol 40:438, 1977.

30. Callahan, JA, Wroblewski, EM, Reeder, GS, et al: Echocardiographic features of carcinoid heart disease. Am J Cardiol 50:762, 1982.

31. Denning, K, Henneke, KH, and Rudolph, W: Assessment of tricuspid stenosis by Doppler echocardiography (Abstract). J Am Coll Cardiol (Suppl A):237A, 1987.

32. Weyman, AE, Dillon, JC, Feigenbaum, H, et al: Echocardiographic differentiation of infundibular from valvular pulmonary stenosis. Am J Cardiol 36:21, 1975.

33. Weyman, AE, Hurwitz, RA, Girad, DA, et al: Cross-sectional echocardiographic visualization of the stenotic pulmonary valve. Circulation 56:769, 1977.

34. Lima, CO, Sahn, DJ, Valdes-Cruz, LM, et al: Noninvasive prediction of transvalvular pressure gradient in patients with pulmonary stenosis by quantitative two-dimensional echocardiography Doppler studies. Circulation 67:866, 1983.

35. Bruss, J, Jacobs, LE, and Kotler, M: Mechanism of mitral regurgitation in dilated cardiomyopathy. Echocardiography 8:219, 1991.
36. Roberts, WC and Perloff, JK: Mitral valvular disease; a clinicopathologic survey of the conditions causing the mitral valve to function abnormally. Ann Intern Med 77:939,1972.
37. Boltwood, CM, Tei, C, Wong, M, et al: Quantitative echocardiography of the mitral complex in dilated cardiopathy: The mechanism of functional mitral regurgitation. Circulation 68:498, 1983.
38. Maze, SS, Kotler, MN, Parry, WR, et al: An echocardiographic and Doppler study of the mechanisms of mitral regurgitation in left ventricular dilation. Am J Noninvasive Cardiol 2:313, 1988.
39. Kaul, S, Pearlman, JD, Tochstone, DA, et al: Prevalence and mechanisms of mitral regurgitative in left ventricular dilation. Am Heart J 118:963, 1989.
40. Kochar, G, Jacobs, CE, Blondheim, DS, et al: Quantification of mitral annular calcification in octogenarian patients. Echocardiography 8:329, 1991.
41. Abbasi, AS, Allen, MW, DeCristofaro, D, et al: Detection and estimation of the degree of mitral regurgitation by range-gated pulsed Doppler echocardiography. Circulation 61:143, 1980.
42. Veyrat, C, Ameur, A, Bas, S, et al: Pulsed Doppler echocardiographic indices for assessing mitral regurgitation. Br Heart J 51:130, 1984.
43. Quinones, MA, Young, JB, Waggoner, AD, et al: Assessment of pulsed Doppler echocardiography in detection and quantification of aortic and mitral regurgitation. Br Heart J 44:612, 1980.
44. Helmcke, F, Nanda, NC, Hsiung, MC, et al: Color Doppler assessment of mitral regurgitation with orthogonal planes. Circulation 75:175, 1987.
45. Spain, MG, Smith, MD, Grayburn, PA, et al: Quantitative assessment of mitral regurgitation by Doppler color flow imaging: Angiographic and hemodynamic correlations. J Am Coll Cardiol 13:585.
46. Sahn, DJ: Instrumentation and physical factors related to visualization of stenotic and regurgitant jet by Doppler color flow mapping. J Am Coll Cardiol 12:593, 1988.
47. Kurokawa, S, Takahashi, M, Sugiyama, T, et al: Noninvasive evaluation of the magnitude of aortic and mitral regurgitation by means of Doppler two-dimensional echocardiography. Am Heart J 120:639, 1990.
48. Pearson, AC, St. Vrain, J, Mrosek, D, et al: Color Doppler echocardiographic evaluation of patients with a flail mitral leaflet. J Am Coll Cardiol 16:232, 1990.
49. Blumlein, S, Bouchard, A, Schiller, NB, et al: Quantitation of mitral regurgitation by Doppler echocardiography. Circulation 74:306, 1986.
50. Seder, JD, Burke, JF, and Pauletto, FJ: Prevalence of aortic regurgitation by color flow Doppler in relation to aortic root size. J Am Soc Echo 3:316, 1990.
51. Louie, EK, Mason, TJ, Shah, R, et al: Determinants of anterior mitral leaflet fluttering in pure aortic regurgitation from pulsed Doppler study of the early diastolic interaction between the regurgitant jet and mitral inflow. Am J Cardiol 61:1085, 1988.
52. Ciobanu, M, Abbasi, AS, Allen, M, et al: Pulsed Doppler echocardiography in the diagnosis and estimation of severity of aortic insufficiency. Am J Cardiol 49:339, 1982.
53. Perry, GJ, Helmcke, F, Nanda, NC, et al: Evaluation of aortic insufficiency by Doppler color flow mapping. J Am Coll Cardiol 9:952, 1987.
54. Grayburn, PA, Handshoe, R, Smith, MD, et al: Quantitative assessment of the hemodynamic consequences of aortic regurgitation by means of continuous wave Doppler recordings. J Am Coll Cardiol 10:135, 1987.
55. Teague, SM, Heinsimer, JA, Anderson, et al: Quantification of aortic insufficiency by Doppler color flow mapping. J Am Coll Cardiol 9:952, 1987.
56. Masuyama, T, Kodama, K, Kitabatake, A, et al: Noninvasive evaluation of aortic regurgitation by continuous-wave Doppler echocardiography. Circulation 73:460, 1986.
57. Beyer, RW, Ramirez, M, Josephson, MA, et al: Correlation of continuous-wave Doppler assessment of chronic aortic regurgitation with hemodynamics and angiography. Am J Cardiol 60:852, 1987.
58. Samstad, SO, Hegrenaes, L, Skjaerpe, T, et al: Half time of the diastolic aortoventricular pressure difference by continuous wave Doppler ultrasound: A measure of the severity of aortic regurgitation. Br Heart J 61:336, 1989.
59. Touche, T, Prasqlier, R, Nitenberg, A, et al: Assessment and follow-up of patients with aortic regurgitation by an updated Doppler echocardiographic measurement of the regurgitant fraction in the aortic arch. Circulation 72:819, 1985.

60. Takenaka, K, Dabestani, A, Gardin, JM, et al: A simple Doppler echocardiographic method for estimating severity of aortic regurgitation. Am J Cardiol 57:1340, 1986.

61. Waller, B, Moriarty, A, Eble, J, et al: Etiology of pure tricuspid regurgitation based on anular circumference and leaflet area: Analysis of 45 necropsy patients with clinical and morphologic evidence of pure tricuspid regurgitation. J Am Coll Cardiol 7:1063, 1986.

62. Chopra, HK, Nanda, NC, Fan, P, et al: Can two-dimensional echocardiography and Doppler color flow mapping identify the need for tricuspid valve repair? J Am Coll Cardiol 14:1266, 1989.

63. Fisher, EA and Goldman, ME: Simple, rapid method for quantification of tricuspid regurgitation by two-dimensional echocardiography. Am J Cardiol 63:1375, 1989.

64. Miyatake, K, Okamoto, M, Kinoshita, N, et al: Evaluation of tricuspid regurgitation by pulsed Doppler and two-dimensional echocardiography. Circulation 66:777, 1982.

65. Suzuki, Y, Kambara, H, Kadota, K, et al: Detection and evaluation of tricuspid regurgitation using a real-time, two-dimensional, color-coded, Doppler flow imaging system: Comparison with contrast two-dimensional echocardiography and right ventriculography. Am J Cardiol 57:811, 1986.

66. Pennestri, F, Loperfido, F, Salvatori, MP, et al: Assessment of tricuspid regurgitation by pulsed Doppler echocardiography. Circulation 76:262, 1987.

67. Currie, PJ, Seward, JB, Chan, KL, et al: Continous wave Doppler determination of right ventricular pressure. A simultaneous Doppler-catheterization study in 127 patients. J Am Coll Cardiol 6:750, 1985.

68. Yock, PG and Popp, RL: Noninvasive estimation of right ventricular systolic pressure by Doppler ultrasound in patients with tricuspid regurgitation. Circulation 70:657, 1984.

69. Kostucki, W, Vandenbossche, JL, Friart, A, et al: Pulsed Doppler regurgitant flow patterns of normal valves. Am J Cardiol 58:309, 1986.

70. Miyatake, K, Okamoto, M, Kinoshita, N, et al: Pulmonary regurgitation studied with the ultrasonic pulsed Doppler technique. Circulation 65:969, 1982.

71. Lababidi, Z, Wu, J-R, and Walls, JT: Percutaneous balloon aortic valvuloplasty. Results in 23 patients. Am J Cardiol 53:194, 1984.

72. Nishimura, RA, Holmes, DR, Jr, Reeder, GS, et al: Doppler echocardiographic observations during percutaneous aortic balloon valvuloplasty. J Am Coll Cardiol 11:1219, 1988.

73. Rohey, R, Kuo, LC, Zoghbi, WA, et al: Determination of parameters of left ventricular diastolic filling with pulsed Doppler echocardiography: Comparison with cineangiography. Circulation 71:543, 1985.

74. Safian, RD, Berman, AD, Diver, DJ, et al: Balloon aortic valvuloplasty in 170 consecutive patients. N Engl J Med 319:125, 1988.

75. Litvak, F, Jakubowski, AT, Buchbinder, NA, et al: Lack of sustained clinical improvement in an elderly population after percutaneous aortic valvuloplasty. Am J Cardiol 62:270, 1988.

76. McKay, RG, Safian, RD, Lock, JE, et al: Assessment of left ventricular and aortic valve function after aortic balloon valvuloplasty in adult patients with critical aortic stenosis. Circulation 75:192, 1987.

77. Nishimura, RA, Holmes, DR, Jr, and Reeder, GS: Percutaneous balloon valvuloplasty. Mayo Clin Proc 65:198, 1990.

78. Cribier, A, Savin, T, Berland, J, et al: Percutaneous transluminal balloon valvuloplasty of adult aortic stenosis: Report of 92 cases. J Am Coll Cardiol 9:381, 1987.

79. Sheikh, KH, Davidson, CJ, Honan, M, et al: Clinical status 6 months after aortic valvuloplasty relates to changes in left ventricular diastolic performance and mass (Abstract). Circulation 80:II-360, 1989.

80. O'Neill, WW: Predictors of long-term survival after percutaneous aortic valvuloplasty: Report of the Mansfield scientific balloon aortic valvuloplasty registry. J Am Coll Cardiol 17:193, 1991.

81. Nishimura, RA, Holmes, DR, Jr, Reeder, GS, et al: Doppler evaluation of results of percutaneous aortic balloon valvuloplasty in calcific aortic stenosis. Circulation 78:791, 1988.

82. Kuntz, RD, Berman, AD, Diver, DJ, et al: Balloon aortic valvuloplasty in perspective (Abstract). J Am Coll Cardiol 15:5A, 1990.

83. Come, PC: For the NHLBI Balloon Valvuloplasty Registry—Doppler-echo evaluation of aortic stenosis severity pre- and post-balloon aortic valvuloplasty (Abstract). J Am Coll Cardiol 13:114A, 1989.

84. Cribier, A, Grigera, F, Eltchaninoff, H, et al: New developments in aortic balloon valvuloplasty (Abstract). J Am Coll Cardiol 13:17A, 1989.

85. Abascal, VM, Wilkins, GT, Choong, CY, et al: Mitral regurgitation after percutaneous balloon

mitral valvuloplasty in adults: Evaluation by pulsed Doppler echocardiography. J Am Coll Cardiol 11:257, 1988.

86. Block, PC: Who is suitable for percutaneous balloon mitral valvotomy? (Editorial) Int J Cardiol 20:9, 1988.

87. Abascal, VM, Wilkins, GT, Choong, CY, et al: Echocardiographic evaluation of mitral valve structure and function in patients followed for at least 6 months after percutaneous balloon mitral valvuloplasty. J Am Coll Cardiol 12:606, 1988.

88. Reid, CL, McKay, CR, Chandraratna, PAN, et al: Mechanisms of increase in mitral valve area and influence of anatomic features in double-balloon, catheter balloon valvuloplasty in adults with rheumatic mitral stenosis: Doppler and two-dimensional echocardiographic study. Circulation 76:628, 1987.

89. Lefevre, T, Bonan, R, Serra, A, et al: Percutaneous mitral valvuloplasty in surgical high risk patients. J Am Coll Cardiol 17:348, 1991.

90. Dietz, WA, Water, JB, Ramaswamy, K, et al: Adverse echocardiographic score does not preclude successful outcome in patients undergoing mitral valvuloplasty with Inoue balloon (Abstract). J Am Coll Cardiol 17:782, 1989.

91. Palacios, IF, Block, PC, Wilkins, GI, et al: Follow-up of patients undergoing percutaneous mitral balloon valvotomy: Analysis of factors determining restenosis. Circulation 79:782, 1989.

92. Block, PC, Tuzcu, M, and Palacios, IF: Two-year follow-up of percutaneous mitral valvotomy: Cardiac catheterization, echocardiography, and clinical status (Abstract). J Am Coll Cardiol 17:340A, 1991.

93. McKay, CR, Otto, C, Block, P, et al: Immediate results of mitral balloon commissurotomy in 737 patients (Abstract). Circulation 82:III-545, 1990.

94. Palacios, IF, Tuzcu, EM, Hewell, JB, et al: Four-year clinical follow-up of patients undergoing percutaneous mitral balloon valvotomy (Abstract). Circulation 82:III-545, 1990.

95. Serra, A, Bonan, R, Lefevre, T, et al: Hemodynamic and clinical follow-up after percutaneous mitral valvuloplasty (Abstract). J Am Coll Cardiol 15:5A, 1990.

96. Serra, A, Bonan, R, Barraud, P, et al: Long-term clinical results of balloon mitral valvuloplasty (Abstract). Circulation 82:III-500, 1990.

97. Berland, J, Rath, PC, Rocha, P, et al: Balloon mitral valvotomy in patients above 40 years of age: Immediate and 2 years follow-up (Abstract). J Am Coll Cardiol 17:339A, 1991.

98. Wisenbaugh, T, Skoularigis, J, Durau, H, et al: Mitral regurgitation following balloon mitral valvotomy: Differing mechanisms for severe versus moderate lesions (Abstract). Circulation 82:III-500, 1990.

99. Parro, A, Jr, Helmcke, F, Mahan, EF, III, et al: Value and limitations of color Doppler echocardiography in the evaluation of percutaneous balloon mitral valvuloplasty for isolated mitral stenosis. Am J Cardiol 67:1261, 1991.

100. Thomas, JD, Wilkins, GT, Choong, CY, et al: Inaccuracy in mitral pressure half-tissue immediately after percutaneous mitral valvotomy: Dependence of transmitral gradient and left atrial and ventricular compliance. Circulation 78:980, 1988.

101. Feldman, CS, Pearson, AC, Labovitz, AJ, et al: Comparison of hemodynamic pressure half-time method and Gorlin formula with Doppler and echocardiographic determination of mitral valve area in patients with combined mitral stenosis and regurgitation. Am Heart J 119:121, 1990.

102. Jaffe, WM, Roche, AHG, Coverdale, HA, et al: Clinical evaluation versus Doppler echocardiography in the quantitative assessment of valvular heart disease. Circulation 78:267, 1988.

103. Slater, J, Gindea, AJ, Freedberg, RS, et al: Comparison of cardiac catheterization and Doppler echocardiography in the decision to operate in aortic and mitral valve disease. J Am Coll Cardiol 17:1026, 1991.

104. Frankl, WS: Valvular heart disease: The technologic dilemma (Editorial). J Am Coll Cardiol 17:1037, 1991.

105. Miller, FA: Aortic stenosis: Most cases no longer require invasive hemodynamic study. J Am Coll Cardiol 13:551, 1989.

106. Jacobs, LE, Wertheimer, JH, Kotler, MN, et al: Quantification of mitral regurgitation: A comparison of transesophageal echocardiography and contrast ventriculography (Abstract). J Am Coll Cardiol 15:75A, 1990.

CHAPTER 6

Transesophageal Echocardiography in Valvular Heart Disease

Dean G. Karalis, M.D.
John J. Ross, Jr., R.C.P.T.
Bruce M. Brown, M.D.
Krishnaswamy Chandrasekaran, M.D.

Transthoracic echocardiography is the procedure of choice in the evaluation of patients with valvular heart disease. Transthoracic two-dimensional (2-D) and Doppler echocardiography provide reliable anatomic and hemodynamic information in most patients with valvular heart disease. However, accuracy is limited in patients with poor acoustic windows, that is, patients with chest deformities, obesity, or pulmonary disease causing ultrasonic interference from the chest wall, ribs, adipose tissue, or lungs. In most older patients, lower frequency transducers are required to achieve far field penetration, often at the expense of resolution of valvular structures, particularly the posteriorly located mitral valve. Furthermore, when evaluating a prosthetic mitral valve, the transthoracic approach is limited owing to attenuation and acoustic shadowing of heart structures from the prosthetic valve material.

In transesophageal echocardiography, the close proximity of the esophagus to the heart, the lack of interfering structures, and the use of higher frequency transducers provide superior quality images of the heart and valvular structures. Recently introduced transesophageal biplane imaging and continuous-wave Doppler capability has further enhanced the role of transesophageal echocardiography in identifying valvular pathology. In this chapter, we review both the strengths and limitations of transesophageal echocardiography in the evaluation of native and prosthetic valvular disease.

NATIVE AORTIC VALVULAR DISEASE

AORTIC STENOSIS

Transthoracic 2-D and Doppler echocardiography can adequately assess the severity of aortic stenosis in most patients. The morphology and mobility of the aortic valve can be determined by visualizing the valve cusps in both the parasternal

short and long axis views.[1] Although 2-D echocardiographic imaging provides anatomic information about the valve, Doppler echocardiography is needed to accurately assess the severity of stenosis. With Doppler echocardiography, the transvalvular pressure gradient can be measured, and by using the continuity equation to
calculate the aortic valve area, the severity of aortic stenosis can be reliably determined.[2,3] The reliability of the Doppler echocardiographic data, however, is dependent on proper technique and aligning the ultrasound beam parallel to the direction
of the aortic jet. This is of particular importance in patients with reduced cusp
separation from low cardiac output in whom an accurate gradient must be obtained
to determine if significant aortic stenosis is present. In certain patients, despite an
exhaustive transthoracic echocardiographic study, the maximal aortic flow velocity
cannot be determined, and the degree of aortic stenosis cannot accurately be
assessed.[2] This may create a clinical dilemma regarding the severity of stenosis if
the aortic valve is sclerotic or calcified and the maximal aortic flow velocity cannot
accurately be determined. Visualization by transesophageal echocardiography of an
aortic valve that opens normally excludes the diagnosis of significant aortic stenosis
and avoids the need for cardiac catheterization (Fig. 6–1).

Transesophageal echocardiography allows high-resolution imaging of the aortic valve and aortic root.[4,5] Using single-plane transesophageal echocardiography,
the number of aortic valve cusps and the aortic valve area can be determined in up
to 80% of patients[5] (Fig. 6–2). With the introduction of biplane imaging, better

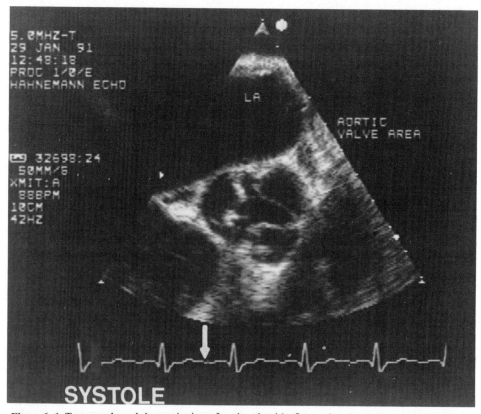

Figure 6–1. Transesophageal short axis view of a sclerotic tri-leaflet aortic valve. During systole, reduced
excursion of all three cusps are demonstrated. The planimetered aortic valve area is 1.5 cm². LA = left
atrium.

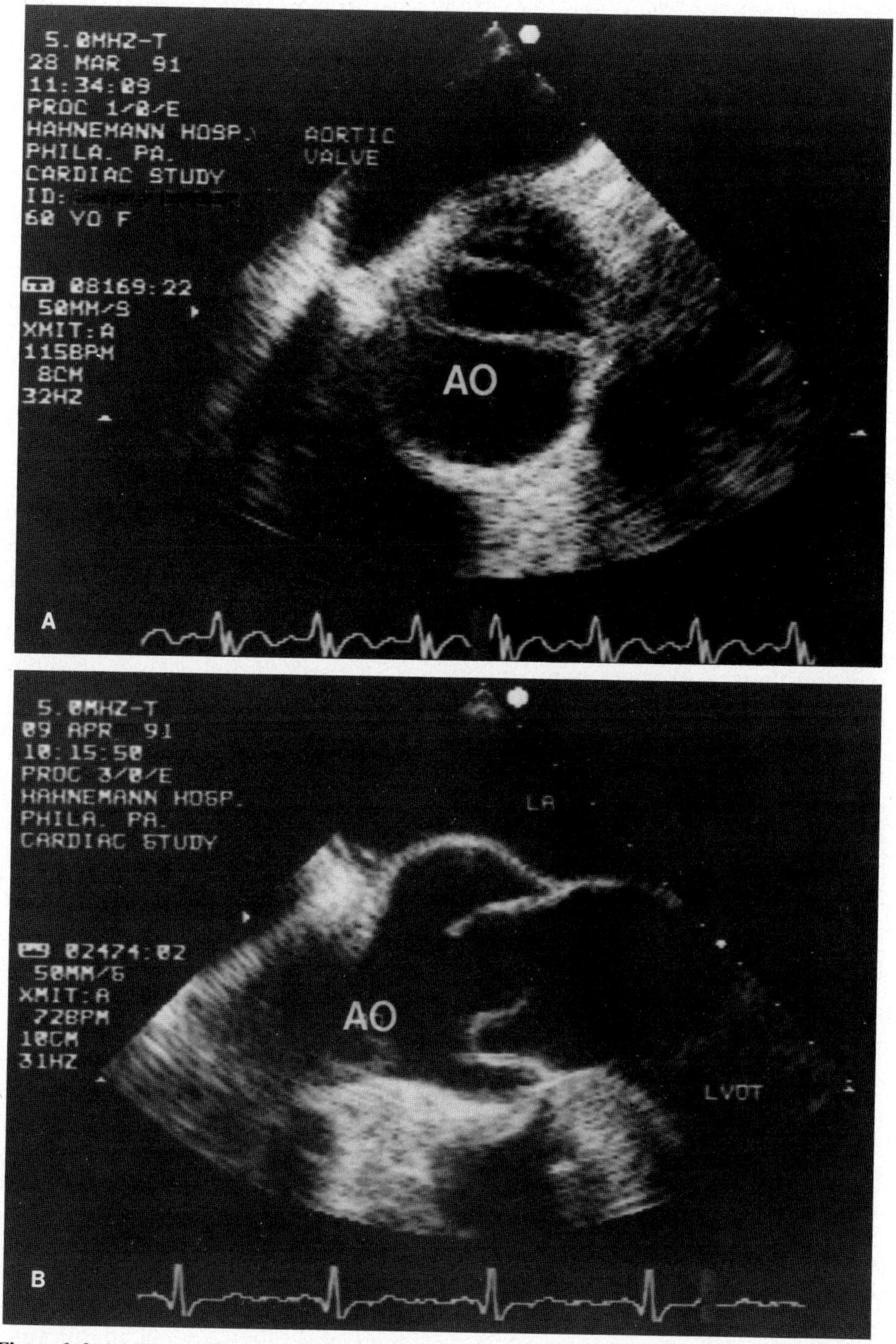

Figure 6–2. (*A*) Transesophageal basal short axis view of the aortic valve. Note the large anterior and smaller posterior cusp of the bicuspid aortic valve. (*B*) Long axis view of the bicuspid aortic valve shown in Figure (*A*). AO = aorta; LA = left atrium; LVOT = left ventricular outflow tract.

assessment of the aortic valve morphology is possible.[6] When the aortic valve is well visualized in its short axis, the planimetered area of the valve in systole correlates closely with the aortic valve area determined by the Gorlin formula by cardiac catheterization.[5] Furthermore, transesophageal echocardiography can reliably differentiate valvular aortic stenosis from supravalvular or subvalvular aortic stenosis.[7]

Continuous-wave Doppler, currently available from the transesophageal approach, allows Doppler gradients to be obtained across the left ventricular outflow tract and aortic valve.[8] Doppler gradients estimated from transesophageal echocardiography demonstrate good correlation with transvalvular gradients obtained from transthoracic echocardiography and cardiac catheterization.[9] However, continuous-wave Doppler from transesophageal echocardiography is limited by the fewer interrogating planes offered by the transesophageal approach.

AORTIC REGURGITATION

Color-flow Doppler echocardiography has significantly improved the ability to recognize and quantitate the degree of aortic regurgitation (AR) by the transthoracic approach.[10] In most patients, transesophageal echocardiography offers no advantage over the transthoracic approach in the recognition and quantification of AR.[11] Furthermore, in a patient with a mitral valve prosthesis, acoustic shadowing of the left ventricular outflow tract from the prosthesis may interfere with the evaluation of AR. Transesophageal echocardiography is of value if the image quality of the transthoracic study is poor. In addition, transesophageal echocardiography plays an important role in defining the etiology of AR by providing superior quality images of the aortic root, cusps, and left ventricular outflow tract. Transesophageal echocardiography is superior to transthoracic echocardiography in evaluating aortic root dilation,[12] type I aortic dissections[13,14] (Fig. 6–3), subaortic membrane,[11,15] and the complications of infective endocarditis, including valvular vegetations[16,17] (Fig. 6–4), perforation, flail leaflet, and perivalvular abscess,[11,20] all of which cause AR.

PROSTHETIC AORTIC VALVULAR DISEASE

As with native aortic valve regurgitation, transesophageal echocardiography offers no advantage in quantifying prosthetic aortic valve regurgitation unless the transthoracic study is suboptimal.[18] In patients who have a prosthesis in both the aortic and mitral positions, acoustic reverberations from the mitral prosthesis may shadow the left ventricular outflow tract, limiting the transesophageal evaluation of AR.[18] However, transesophageal echocardiography is important in demonstrating the underlying pathology responsible for the prosthetic valve malfunction and in discerning perivalvular from valvular regurgitation.[11] It is superior to transthoracic echocardiography in detecting torn cusps, valvular degeneration,[19] and the complications of infective endocarditis, specifically vegetations[17] and perivalvular abscess.[20]

Single-plane transesophageal echocardiography offers limited tomographic imaging planes of the aortic valve prosthesis. The leaflets of a bioprosthetic aortic valve can be adequately visualized in most cases; however, the opening and closing movements of the disc(s) or ball of a mechanical aortic valve prosthesis are difficult

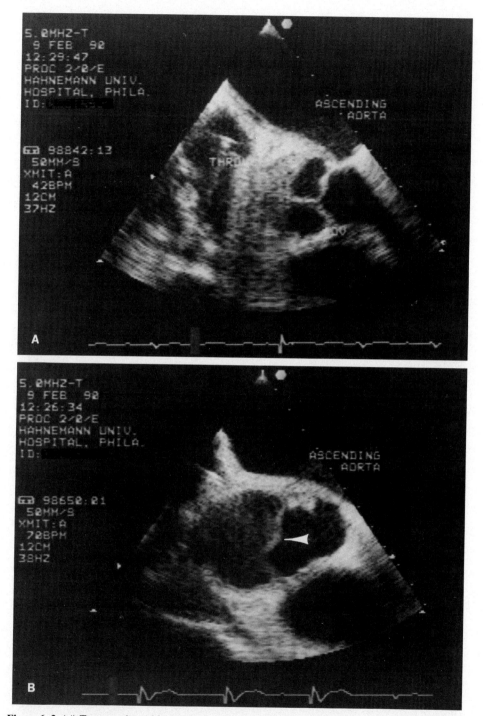

Figure 6–3. (*A*) Transesophageal long axis view of the aortic valve in a patient with a type I aortic dissection. Note the soft tissue echoes just above the aortic valve demonstrating a thrombus-filled false lumen. (*B*) In the same patient, a short axis view at the level of the ascending aorta clearly demonstrates the intimal flap *(arrow)* and the thrombosed false lumen.

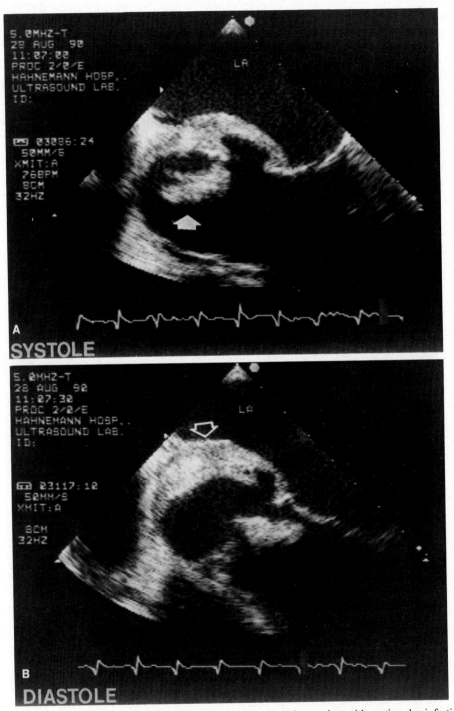

Figure 6–4. (*A*) Magnified view of the aortic valve during systole in a patient with aortic valve infective endocarditis. A large mobile vegetation *(arrow)* is seen on the posterior cusp of a bicuspid aortic valve. (*B*) In diastole the vegetation prolapses into the left ventricular outflow tract. Posterior to the aortic valve an echo dense abscess cavity is seen *(arrow)*. LA = left atrium.

to visualize consistently owing to attenuation by the surrounding prosthetic valve material.[21] This limits the role of transesophageal echocardiography in detecting stenosis of a mechanical aortic valve prosthesis. The introduction of biplane imaging and continuous-wave Doppler to the transesophageal exam may improve the assessment of prosthetic valve stenosis. Currently, transthoracic Doppler echocardiography, by estimating transvalvular pressure gradients across a prosthetic valve, remains the mainstay in evaluating prosthetic aortic valve stenosis.

NATIVE MITRAL VALVULAR DISEASE

MITRAL STENOSIS

Transesophageal echocardiography has added little in evaluating the severity of mitral stenosis but has added significantly in assessing the morphology of the stenotic valve. This is of particular importance if catheter balloon valvuloplasty is being considered.

Transthoracic 2-D echocardiography has been used to analyze the mitral valve morphology before performing catheter balloon valvuloplasty.[22,23] An echocardiographic scoring method, based on leaflet mobility and thickness, extent of subvalvular disease, and severity of valvular and commissural calcium has been used to evaluate patients before catheter balloon valvuloplasty. A less than optimal result would be expected with more extensive leaflet calcification and more restricted leaflet mobility.[22,23] Transthoracic echocardiography is often limited in distinguishing commissural calcium from calcium within the body of the leaflet and in assessing the extent of subvalvular disease.[24] These limitations become more apparent when the image quality of the transthoracic study is suboptimal. Transesophageal echocardiography allows better assessment of valve mobility and thickness, subvalvular involvement, and the extent of valvular and commissural calcification (Fig. 6–5).[25] This allows better screening of patients and appropriate triage to either catheter balloon valvuloplasty or mitral valve surgery.

The transthoracic approach is limited in adequately evaluating the left atrium and appendage for thrombus, which may complicate or preclude catheter balloon valvuloplasty. Transesophageal echocardiography is superior to transthoracic echocardiography in detecting thrombi in the body or appendage of the left atrium[26,27] as well as detecting spontaneous echo contrast within the left atrium (Fig. 6–6).[28,29] Transesophageal echocardiography is also of value in assisting the interventional cardiologist in the performance of balloon catheter valvuloplasty. By visualizing the fossa ovalis membrane, it can help guide the catheter during transseptal puncture; by visualizing the mitral valve, it can assure accurate placement of the dilating balloons thereby reducing the complications associated with catheter balloon valvuloplasty.[30,31] In addition, the transvalvular mitral gradient obtained using continuous-wave Doppler from the transesophageal approach correlates well with transmitral gradients obtained from transthoracic echocardiography and cardiac catheterization.[32] Therefore, transesophageal echocardiography performed during catheter balloon mitral valvuloplasty will allow the interventional cardiologist an immediate assessment of the postdilation transmitral gradient and the mitral valve area. In addition, it allows immediate recognition of the complications of the procedure, such as mitral regurgitation (MR) and atrial shunt.

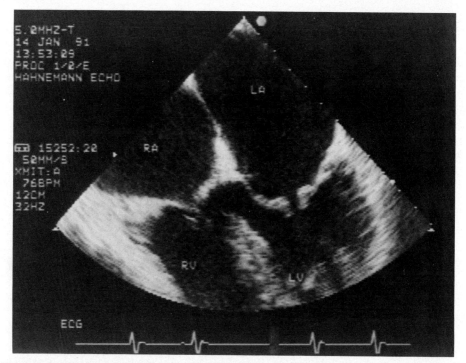

Figure 6–5. Transesophageal 4-chamber view demonstrating thickening and diastolic doming of the anterior and posterior mitral valve leaflets characteristic of rheumatic mitral valve disease. LA = left atrium; LV = left ventricle; RA = right atrium; RV = right ventricle.

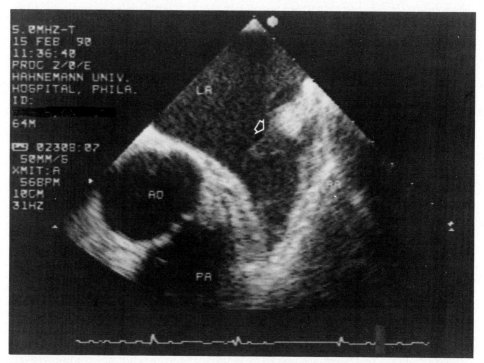

Figure 6–6. Transesophageal basal short axis view of the left atrial appendage demonstrating spontaneous echo contrast and laminated thrombus *(arrow)*. AO = aorta; LA = left atrium; PA = pulmonary artery.

112

MITRAL REGURGITATION

The retrocardiac approach of transesophageal echocardiography makes it ideal for evaluating pathology of the posteriorly located mitral valve. The use of a higher frequency transducer (5.0 mHz) and the close proximity of the left atrium to the esophageal transducer produces high-quality images of the mitral valve leaflets, annulus, and subvalvular apparatus.

Transesophageal echocardiography is superior to transthoracic echocardiography in evaluating the pathology responsible for MR (Fig. 6–7 and 6–8). It can better detect vegetations,[16,17] torn leaflets, torn chordae with a flail segment,[33,34] calcifications or inflammatory involvement. Single-plane transesophageal echocardiography may not allow the entire anulus or all segments of the mitral valve leaflets to be visualized in all patients. However, the additional tomographic plane offered by biplane imaging allows evaluation of the entire mitral valve in most patients.[35] This added anatomic information provided by transesophageal echocardiography is particularly useful in deciding whether or not an abnormal mitral valve can be surgically repaired or must be replaced. In addition, intraoperative transesophageal echocardiography plays a vital role during cardiac valve surgery in assessing the adequacy of mitral valve repair or reconstruction.[36]

Transesophageal echocardiography is more sensitive than transthoracic echocardiography in detecting MR.[37,38] This is best appreciated in patients with suboptimal transthoracic studies or in patients with mitral anular calcification or valvular calcification, which can interfere with interrogation of the left atrium for MR. From the transesophageal approach, the left atrium is foreshortened, and transthoracic color-flow Doppler criteria used to grade the severity of MR may not apply.[39] Therefore, the ratio of the regurgitant jet to left atrial area, the length of the jet into the left atrium, and the presence of systolic flow reversal in the pulmonary veins[40,41] must all be used to judge the severity of MR.

PROSTHETIC MITRAL VALVULAR DISEASE

Transthoracic Doppler echocardiography is of limited value in identifying prosthetic mitral valve regurgitation. However, it may provide indirect evidence that the mitral prosthesis is dysfunctional. An abnormally high transvalvular pressure gradient with a normal pressure half-time should suggest the presence of significant MR. However, ultrasound artifact cast into the left atrium from the prosthesis does not allow adequate visualization, localization, and quantification of the mitral regurgitant jet.[42]

Transesophageal echocardiography provides high quality images of the left atrium and atrial surface of the prosthesis. This allows easy recognition of the site and degree of MR. In patients with bioprosthetic valves, the problem of acoustic artifact may be less severe; however, when the valve leaflets become fibrosed or calcified, significant masking of flow in the left atrium may occur.

Transesophageal echocardiography has been shown to be more sensitive and accurate than transthoracic echocardiography in assessing the severity of MR for both mechanical and bioprosthetic mitral valves.[19,43,44] Transesophageal echocardiography can easily distinguish between physiologic prosthetic mitral valve regurgitation and pathologic perivalvular regurgitation. By transesophageal echocardiography, all normally functioning mechanical prosthetic mitral valves have some

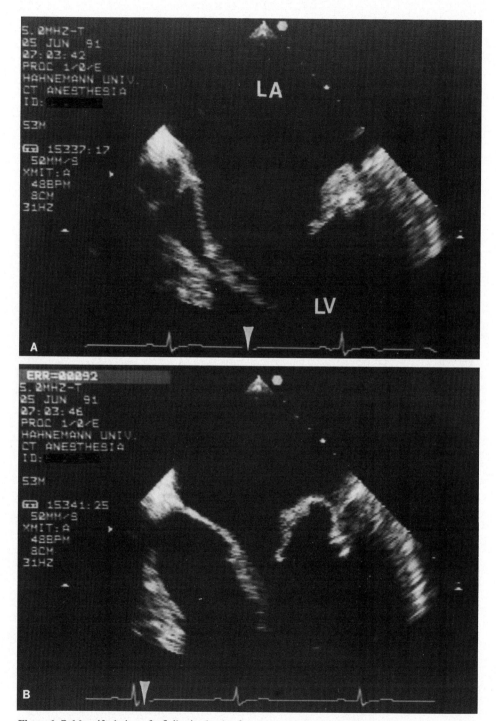

Figure 6–7. Magnified view of a flail mitral valve from the transesophageal 4-chamber view (*A*) through (*E*) are freeze-frames of the mitral valve from end-diastole to end-systole. The mitral valve is thickened consistent with myxomatous disease.

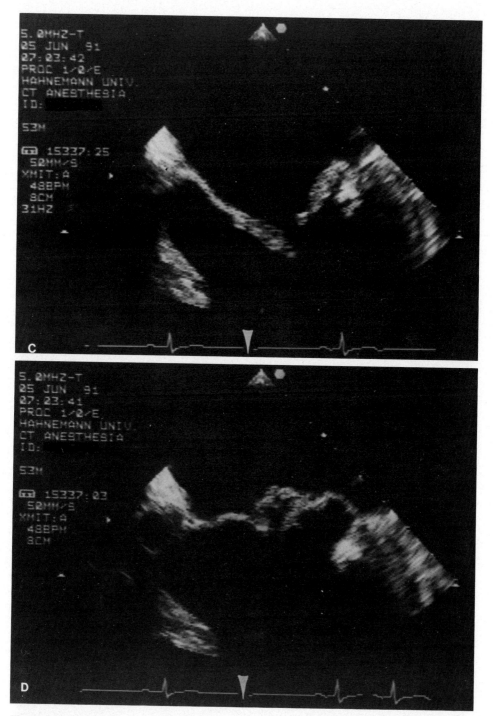

Figure 6–7. *Continued*

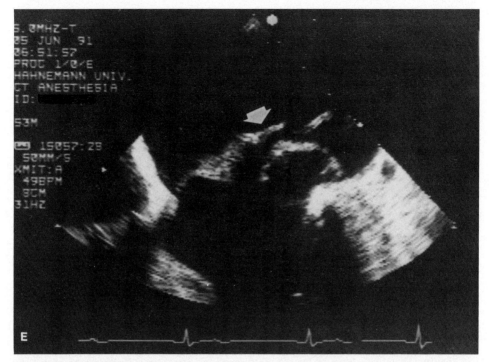

Figure 6–7. *Continued*

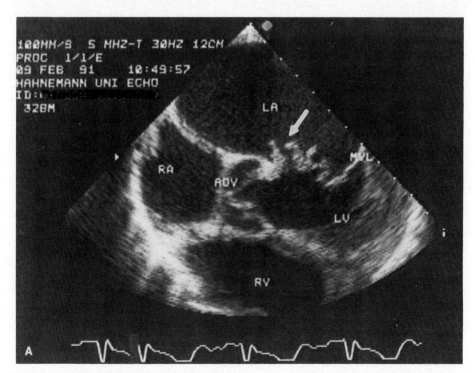

Figure 6–8. (*A*) Transesophageal 4-chamber view with aorta. Anterior mitral valve leaflet (MVL) perforation with overlaying vegetation is seen *(arrow).*

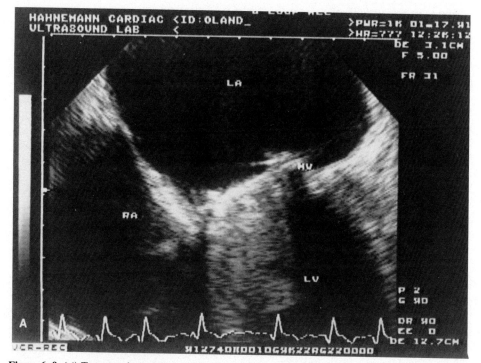

Figure 6–9. (*A*) Transesophageal 4-chamber view of a mechanical (St. Jude) mitral prosthesis. Characteristic acoustic shadowing of the left ventricle and left ventricular outflow tract from the prosthetic mitral valve is demonstrated.

degree of prosthetic MR.[45] This normally occurring regurgitation is always mild. By color-flow mapping, the regurgitant jet is small and of low velocity. Pathologic regurgitation is often more severe, and color-flow mapping demonstrates a regurgitant jet that is large and of high velocity with a mosaic pattern due to turbulence (Fig. 6–9). By imaging the prosthetic mitral valve in its short axis, the location of perivalvular dihiscence and the site of perivalvular regurgitation can be accurately determined. However, in some patients, owing to the position of the mitral prosthesis, a short axis view of the prosthetic valve cannot be obtained by single-plane transesophageal echocardiography. This limitation can be overcome by biplane transesophageal echocardiography.

In addition to better assessing the degree of MR, transesophageal echocardiography can better recognize the etiology of the prosthetic mitral valve malfunction. Transesophageal echocardiography has been shown to be superior to transthoracic echocardiography in detecting vegetations[17] (Fig. 6–10 and 6–11) and valve ring abscess.[20] This is particularly useful in culture negative endocarditis and allows earlier recognition of the complications of prosthetic valve endocarditis. Transesophageal echocardiography is superior to transthoracic echocardiography in detecting valve ring dehiscence and in visualizing the leaflets of a bioprosthetic mitral valve as well as recognizing valvular calcifications and torn and flail bioprosthetic cusps.[19,44]

In assessing suspected prosthetic mitral valve obstruction, transesophageal echocardiography provides important anatomic information. It can easily detect

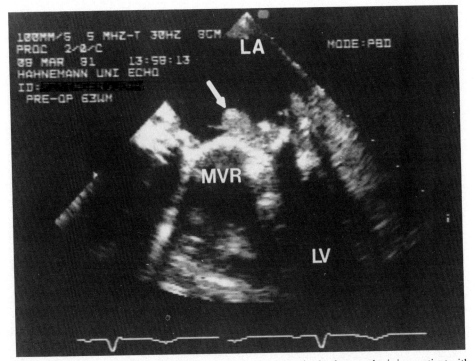

Figure 6–10. Transesophageal 4-chamber view of a mechanical mitral valve prosthesis in a patient with prosthetic valve endocarditis. A large vegetation *(arrow)* is seen on the atrial surface of the prosthesis, obstructing the lateral disc. LA = left atrium; LV = left ventricle; MVR = mitral valve replacement.

obstructing thrombi[12] or calcified, immobile bioprosthetic cusps. However, in some patients, the opening and closing movements of the prosthetic discs cannot be clearly appreciated. Biplane transesophageal echocardiography is helpful in these situations. Continuous-wave Doppler with transesophageal echocardiography can provide hemodynamic data by obtaining the antegrade peak velocity across the valve and by estimating the mitral valve area by the pressure half-time method.[32]

TRICUSPID VALVULAR DISEASE

The anterior location of the tricuspid valve makes it easily imaged by the transthoracic approach. Although the role of transesophageal echocardiography in evaluating tricuspid valvular disease is not well established, in most patients this approach offers improved visualization of the tricuspid valve leaflets and the inflow portion of the right ventricle. Similar to MR, tricuspid regurgitation (TR) can be easily detected and quantified by the transesophageal approach (Fig. 6–12).

Intraoperative transesophageal echocardiography is useful in assessing the severity of TR in patients with mitral valve disease. If severe TR persists after mitral valve surgery, then tricuspid valve repair may be warranted.

PULMONARY VALVULAR DISEASE

The pulmonic valve is visualized only in cross-section by single-plane transesophageal echocardiography. This precludes optimal evaluation. Biplane trans-

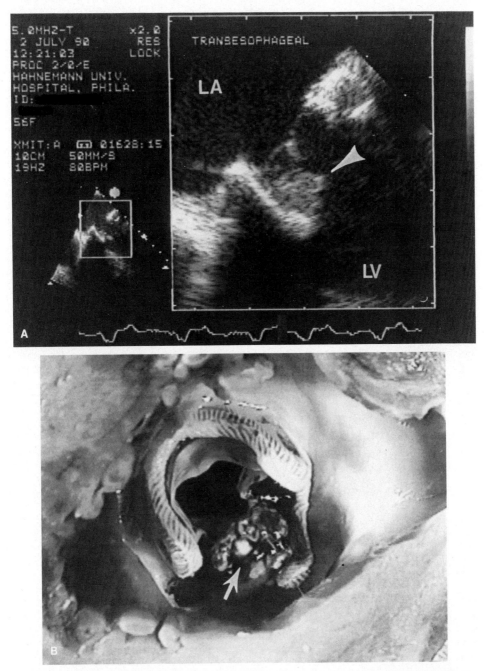

Figure 6–11. Transesophageal magnified view of a bioprosthetic mitral valve in a patient with infective endocarditis. (*A*) A large vegetation was present on the ventricular surface of the prosthesis *(arrow).* (*B*) At autopsy, the vegetation was confirmed.

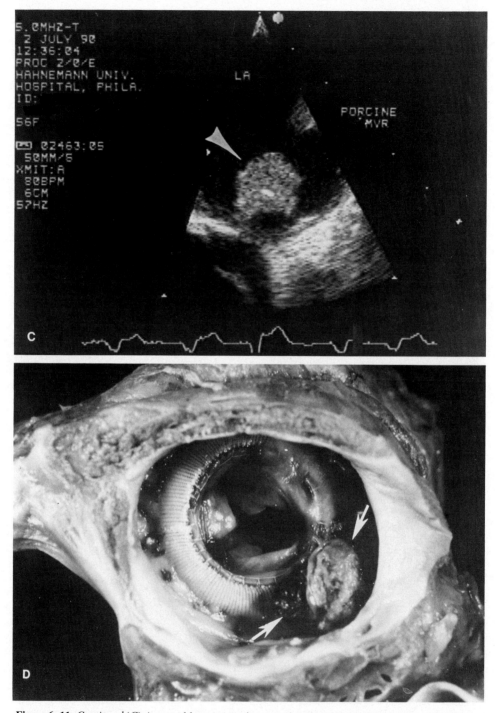

Figure 6–11. *Continued* (*C*) A second large vegetation was visualized on the atrial surface of the prosthesis *(arrow)*. (*D*) At autopsy the presence of the vegetation was confirmed *(arrow)*. LA = left atrium; LV = left ventricle.

esophageal echocardiography with the longitudinal scanning plane provides improved imaging of the pulmonary valve leaflets, its anulus, the main pulmonary artery, and the right ventricular outflow tract. Although transthoracic echocardiography can provide adequate information about the pulmonary valve in most patients, transesophageal echocardiography may be useful in patients with complex congenital heart disease.

CONCLUSION

Transesophageal echocardiography plays an important role in the assessment of patients with valvular heart disease. Although transesophageal echocardiography provides superior anatomic detail of the valvular pathology, both transthoracic and transesophageal echocardiography should be performed in patients with valvular heart disease. Transthoracic echocardiography can help determine the need for transesophageal echocardiography and provide data that may not easily be obtained from the transesophageal approach, particularly hemodynamic data in patients with stenotic valves. Newer developments, such as higher frequency and multiplane imaging transducers, will enhance the role of transesophageal echocardiography in valvular heart disease.

REFERENCES

1. Bansal, RC, Tajik, A, Seward, JB, et al: Feasibility of detailed two-dimensional echocardiographic examination in adults. Prospective study of 200 patients. Mayo Clin Proc 55:291, 1980.
2. Zoghbi, WA, Farmer, KL, Soto, JG, et al: Accurate noninvasive quantification of stenotic aortic valve area by Doppler echocardiography. Circulation 73:452, 1986.
3. Oh, JK, Taliercio, CP, Holmes, DR, et al: Prediction of the severity of aortic stenosis by Doppler aortic valve area determination: Prospective Doppler-catheterization correlation in 100 patients. J Am Coll Cardiol 11:1227, 1988.
4. Hofmann, T, Kasper, W, Meinertz, T, et al: Determination of aortic valve orifice area in aortic valve stenosis by two-dimensional transesophageal echocardiography. Am J Cardiol 59:330, 1987.
5. Chandrasekaran, K, Foley, R, Weintraub, A, et al: Evidence that transesophageal echocardiography can reliably and directly measure the aortic valve area in patients with aortic stenosis—a new application that is independent of LV function and does not require Doppler data. J Am Coll Cardiol 17:20A, 1991.
6. Bijoy, KK, Seward, JB, Edwards, WD, et al: Biplane transesophageal echocardiography: Anatomic correlation, new imaging planes, and clinical utility. Circulation 82(Suppl III):668, 1990.
7. Schwinger, ME and Kronzon, I: Improved evaluation of left ventricular outflow tract obstruction by transesophageal echocardiography. J Am Soc Echo 2:191, 1989.
8. Weintraub, A, Pandian, N, Simonetti, J, et al: CW Doppler in transesophageal echocardiography allows analysis of high velocity flows and enhances the utility of transesophageal echo. Circulation 82 (Suppl III):669, 1990.
9. Samdarshi, T, Fan, PH, Chouinard, M, et al: Intraoperative transesophageal color Doppler guided continuous wave Doppler assessment of aortic valve stenosis. Circulation 82(Suppl III):669, 1990.
10. Perry, GJ, Helmcke, F, Nanda, NC, et al: Evaluation of aortic insufficiency by Doppler color flow mapping. J Am Coll Cardiol 9:952, 1987.
11. Dittrich, HC, McCann, HA, Walsh, TP, et al: Transesophageal echocardiography in the evaluation of prosthetic and native aortic valves. Am J Cardiol 66:758, 1990.
12. Chandrasekaran, K, Bansal, RC, Mintz, GS, et al: Impact of transesophageal color flow Doppler echocardiography in current cardiology practice. Echocardiography 7:125, 1990.
13. Erbel, R, Daniel, W, Visser, C, et al and the European Cooperative Study Group for Echocardiography. Echocardiography in diagnosis of aortic dissection. Lancet 1:457, 1989.

14. Hashimoto, S, Kumada, T, Osakada, G, et al: Assessment of transesophageal Doppler echography in dissecting aortic aneurysm. J Am Coll Cardiol 14:1253, 1989.

15. Mugge, A, Daniel, WG, Wolpers, HG, et al: Improved visualization of discrete subvalvular aortic stenosis by transesophageal color-coded Doppler echocardiography. Am Heart J 117:474, 1989.

16. Erbel, R, Rohmann, S, Drexler, M, et al: Improved diagnostic value of echocardiography in patients with infective endocarditis by transesophageal approach: A prospective study. Eur Heart J 9:45, 1988.

17. Mugge, A, Daniel, WG, Frank, G, et al: Echocardiography in infective endocarditis: Reassessment of prognostic implications of vegetation size determined by the transthoracic and the transesophageal approach. J Am Coll Cardiol 14:631, 1989.

18. Brown, BM, Karalis, DG, Ross, JR, et al: Limited value of single plane transesophageal echocardiography in prosthetic aortic valve malfunction. J Am Soc Echo 4:284, 1991.

19. Alam, M, Serwin, JB, Rosman, HS, et al: Transesophageal echocardiographic features of normal and dysfunctioning bioprosthetic valves. Am Heart J 121:1149, 1991.

20. Daniel, WG, Mugge, A, Martin, RP, et al: Improvement in the diagnosis of abscesses associated with endocarditis by transesophageal echocardiography. N Engl J Med 324:795, 1991.

21. Nellessen, U, Schnittger, I, Appleton, CP, et al: Transesophageal two-dimensional echocardiography and color Doppler flow velocity mapping in the evaluation of cardiac valve prostheses. Circulation 78:848, 1988.

22. Reid, CL, McKay, CR, Chandraratna, PAN, et al: Mechanisms of increase in mitral valve area and influence of anatomic features in double-balloon, catheter balloon valvuloplasty in adults with rheumatic mitral stenosis: A Doppler and two-dimensional echocardiographic study. Circulation 76:628, 1987.

23. Herrmann, HC, Wilkins, GT, Abascal, VM, et al: Percutaneous balloon mitral valvotomy for patients with mitral stenosis. Analysis of factors influencing early results. J Thorac Cardiovasc Surg 96:33, 1988.

24. Reid, CL, Chandraratna, AN, Kawanishi, DT, et al: Influence of mitral valve morphology on double-balloon catheter balloon valvuloplasty in patients with mitral stenosis. Analysis of factors predicting immediate and 3-month results. Circulation 80:515, 1989.

25. Griffen, DL, Sheikh, KH, Harrison, JK, et al: Relationship of the echocardiographic score determined by transthoracic and transesophageal echocardiography to the success of balloon mitral valvuloplasty. Circulation 82(Suppl III):44, 1990.

26. Aschenberg, W, Schluter, M, Kremer, P, et al: Transesophageal two-dimensional echocardiography for the detection of left atrial appendage thrombus. J Am Coll Cardiol 7:163, 1986.

27. Kronzon, I, Tunick, PA, Glassman, E, et al: Transesophageal echocardiography to detect atrial clots in candidates for percutaneous transseptal balloon valvuloplasty. J Am Coll Cardiol 16:1320, 1990.

28. Daniel, WB, Nellessen, U, Schroder, E, et al: Left atrial spontaneous echo contrast in mitral valve disease: An indicator for an increased thromboembolic risk. J Am Coll Cardiol 11:1204, 1988.

29. Black, IW, Hopkins, AP, Lee, LCL, et al: Left atrial spontaneous echo contrast: A clinical and echocardiographic analysis. J Am Coll Cardiol 18:398, 1991.

30. Milner, MR, Goldstein, SA, Lindsay, J, et al: Transesophageal echocardiographic guidance for percutaneous balloon mitral valvuloplasty. Circulation 82(Suppl III):81, 1990.

31. Chirillo, F, Ramondo, A, Dan, M, et al: Transesophageal echocardiography during percutaneous balloon mitral valvuloplasty. Circulation 82(Suppl III):46, 1990.

32. Stewart, WJ, Loop, FD, Litowitz, H, et al: Intraoperative validation of Doppler-derived mitral gradients in patients with native mitral stenosis and prosthetic mitral valves. J Am Coll Cardiol 15:138A, 1990.

33. Schluter, M, Kremer, P, and Hanrath, P: Transesophageal 2-D echocardiographic feature of flail mitral leaflet due to ruptured chordae tendineae. Am Heart J 108:609, 1984.

34. Hozumi, T, Yoshikawa, J, Yoshida, K, et al: Direct visualization of ruptured chordae tendineae by transesophageal two-dimensional echocardiography. J Am Coll Cardiol 16:1315, 1990.

35. Fraser, AG, Stumper, OFW, VanHerwerden, LA, et al: Anatomy of imaging planes used to study the mitral valve: Advantages of biplane transesophageal echocardiography. Circulation 82(Suppl III):668, 1990.

36. Stewart, WJ, Currie, PJ, Salcedo, E, et al: Intraoperative Doppler color flow mapping for decision-making in valve repair for mitral regurgitation. Technique and results in 100 patients. Circulation 81:556, 1990.

37. Taams, MA, Gussenhoven, EJ, Cahalan, MK, et al: Transesophageal Doppler color flow imaging

in the detection of native and Bjork-Shiley mitral valve regurgitation. J Am Coll Cardiol 13:95, 1989.

38. Akamatsu, S, Kagawa, K, Terazawa, E, et al: Physiologic mitral regurgitation: A study with transesophageal Doppler echocardiography. Circulation 82(Suppl III):45, 1990.

39. Smith, MD, Harrison, MR, Pinton, R, et al: Regurgitant jet size by transesophageal compared with transthoracic Doppler color flow imaging. Circulation 83:79, 1991.

40. Klein, AL, Cohen, GI, Davison, MB, et al: Importance of sampling both pulmonary veins in the transesophageal assessment of severity of mitral regurgitation. J Am Coll Cardiol 17:199A, 1991.

41. Klein, AL, Obarski, TP, Stewart, WJ, et al: Transesophageal Doppler echocardiography of pulmonary venous flow: A new marker of mitral regurgitation severity. J Am Coll Cardiol 18:518–526, 1991.

42. Sprecter, DL, Adamick, R, Adams, D, et al: In vitro color flow, pulsed and continuous wave Doppler ultrasound masking of flow by prosthetic valves. J Am Coll Cardiol 9:1306, 1987.

43. Van den Brink, RBA, Visser, CA, Basart, DCG, et al: Comparison of transthoracic and transesophageal color Doppler flow imaging in patients with mechanical prostheses in the mitral valve position. Am J Cardiol 63:1471, 1989.

44. Khandheria, BK, Seward, JB, Oh, JK, et al: Value and limitations of transesophageal echocardiography in assessment of mitral valve prostheses. Circulation 83:1956, 1991.

45. Mohr-Kahaly, S, Kupferwasser, I, Erbel, R, et al: Regurgitant flow in apparently normal valve prostheses: Improved detection and semiquantitative analysis by transesophageal two-dimensional color-coded Doppler echocardiography. J Am Soc Echo 3:187, 1990.

CHAPTER 7

Cardiac Magnetic Resonance Imaging

Robert M. MacMillan, M.D., F.A.C.C.

Magnetic resonance imaging (MRI) acquires high-resolution tomographic images through the heart and great vessels.[1] Electrocardiographic gating is required.[2] Images can be obtained in any plane without manipulating the patient.[3] The technique is completely noninvasive. Subjects to be imaged must be in sinus rhythm, not subject to claustrophobia, and be free of metallic foreign bodies or implants with certain exceptions.[4] At present, three basic imaging modes are available: spin-echo, gradient-echo, and phase-velocity mapping.[5] Spin-echo imaging provides high-resolution static images of the heart, which are predominantly used for morphologic evaluation. The blood pool appears black owing to little or no signal return, resulting in high-contrast images of cardiac structures. Gradient-echo imaging (GRASS cine, cine MRI) results in the blood pool appearing bright white and cardiac tissues appearing less bright. This method allows sequential images to be obtained through the cardiac cycle, which can be viewed as a cine. Phase-velocity mapping encodes information about spatial movement and can be used to measure blood flow.[6]

Magnetic resonance imaging can be used to evaluate cardiac anatomy,[7] chamber dimensions,[8,9] ventricular volumes and ejection fraction,[10] left ventricular segmental wall motion,[11] left ventricular mass,[12] cardiac masses,[13] coronary bypass grafts,[14] pericardial disease,[15] congenital heart disease,[16] and great vessel disease.[17] The ability of MRI to assess cardiac valvular function is essential for complete evaluation of the heart. This chapter will review the current capability of MRI to evaluate the cardiac valves.

AORTIC REGURGITATION

Gradient-echo imaging can detect aortic regurgitation (AR) as a region of signal loss corresponding to the regurgitant blood that appears in early diastole at the base of the aortic valve and is seen to move down into the body of the left ventricle with successive images in later diastole[18,19] (Fig. 7–1). The mechanism for this signal loss is not completely understood. Signal loss is associated with turbulence or acceleration of flow through orifices.[20,21] A small degree of turbulent signal loss is nor-

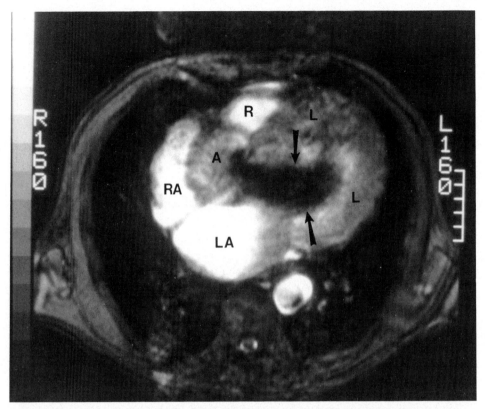

Figure 7–1. Axial gradient-echo image through the left ventricular cavity in early diastole. An area of signal loss *(arrows)* representing aortic regurgitation is seen filling the left ventricular cavity as it arises from the aorta through an incompetent aortic valve. A = aorta; L = left ventricle; LA = left atrium; R = right ventricle; RA = right atrium.

mally seen around the anterior mitral valve leaflet in early diastole and must be distinguished from signal loss secondary to mild AR. The optimal planes of imaging for AR are coronal, axial, and long axis. In evaluating the accuracy of diagnosis of AR on the basis of signal loss in the left ventricle, sensitivity and specificity were found to be 100% when compared with cineangiography at catheterization.[22]

Several methods have been employed to quantitate AR using cine MRI. Right and left ventricular volumes can be measured using a modified Simpson's formula. Regurgitant fraction is determined as left ventricular stroke volume minus right ventricular stroke volume divided by left ventricular stroke volume.[23] Pflugfelder and associates[25] studied 10 normal volunteers and 25 patients with AR documented and graded for severity by Doppler echocardiography. Regurgitant fraction calculated from analysis of cine magnetic resonance images was 4% to 7% for normal volunteers and 31% ± 8% in mild, 45% ± 11% in moderate, and 56% ± 9% in severe AR ($p < 0.05$ for moderate and severe vs. normal and mild).

Aortic regurgitation also may be quantitated by analyzing the characteristics of the regurgitant signal loss. Wagner and coworkers[24] measured the total volume of signal loss in 38 patients with mild, moderate, or severe AR classified by two-dimensional (2-D) echocardiography or angiography. The calculated signal loss was 27.3 ml (± 3.2 SEE; n = 24) in mild, 49.7 ml (± 2.9 SEE; n = 7) in moderate, and 75.8 ml (± 5.7 SEE; n = 6) in severe regurgitation. A good correlation was found between the volume of the signal loss and the regurgitant volume calculated for cine MRI volume measurements of the difference of right and left ventricular stroke volume (r = 0.84). Pflugfelder and associates[25] studied 10 normal volunteers and 25 patients with AR documented and graded by Doppler echocardiography. The total area of diastolic left ventricular signal loss by MRI was 0 cm^2 in normal volunteers, 24 ± 13 cm^2 in eight patients with mild AR, 49 ± 11 cm^2 in nine patients with moderate AR, and 62 ± 20 cm^2 in eight patients with severe AR. Nishamura and colleagues[22] measured the length and area of regurgitant signal loss in the left ventricle. The best correlation with angiography was the ratio of signal loss area to the area of the left ventricle for grading of AR. Variations in the echo time (TE) and display settings cause differences in the measured area of the regurgitant signal loss.[26] Quantification of valvular regurgitation by cine MRI requires strict standardization of display and imaging parameters.

AORTIC STENOSIS

Gradient-echo imaging is the preferred mode of MRI for diagnosis of aortic stenosis. The optimal imaging planes are axial, coronal, long axis, and modified

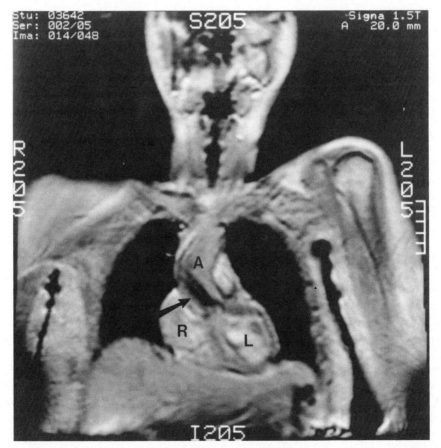

Figure 7–2. Coronal gradient-echo image through the left ventricle (L), right atrium (R), and aorta (A). Note the black "jet" in the ascending aorta *(arrow)* during early systole, indicative of turbulence in this patient with mild aortic stenosis.

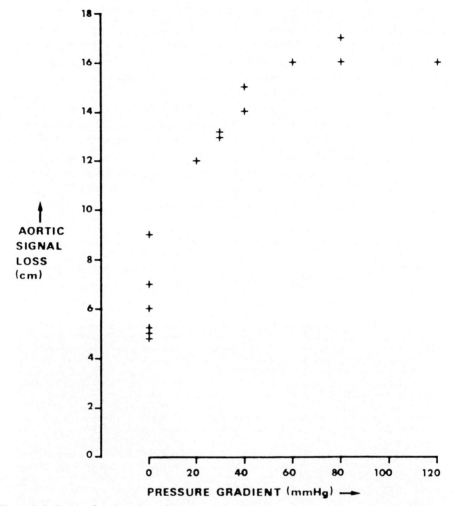

Figure 7–3. Graph of peak-peak aortic valve pressure gradient versus maximum length of signal loss distal to aortic valve on gradient-echo MRI. (From Mitchell et al.,[28] p. 188, with permission.)

short axis. Sufficient resolution exists to detect thickened leaflets, restricted opening excursion of leaflets, and signal loss at the valve plane owing to valvular calcification. Systolic turbulence seen as signal loss in the ascending aorta has been observed to be a major predictor of aortic valvular stenosis[27] (Fig. 7–2). Mitchell and coworkers[28] demonstrated a significant correlation (T = 0.86; $p < 0.002$) between severity of pressure gradient across the aortic valve and length of the signal loss in the ascending aorta by gradient-echo imaging (Fig. 7–3). The presence of signal loss in the ascending aorta up to 9 cm above the aortic valve without associated aortic valve gradient may be attributed to reduced aortic valve area (sclerosis) that has not reached critical level to generate a transaortic valve gradient ($<$50% cross-sectional area reduction). Increased transvalvular flow rates in AR can produce signal loss suggestive of aortic stenosis.[28] Other identifiers of significant aortic stenosis are the presence of a narrow high-velocity jet of signal loss just distal to the aortic valve plane and signal loss just proximal to the aortic valve plane reflecting prestenotic acceleration of blood flow.[29] Direct measurement of aortic valve orifice area remains theoretically possible using high-resolution thin (3 mm) slices through and parallel to the aortic valve plane; however, aortic valve area cannot be determined at present. Magnetic resonance imaging also can provide nonspecific supportive evidence of aortic stenosis by demonstration of dilated ascending aorta and increased left ventricular mass.

MITRAL REGURGITATION

Mitral valve regurgitation is detected by an area of signal loss appearing in the left atrium using gradient-echo imaging[18] (Fig. 7–4). This area of signal loss corresponds to the regurgitant volume of blood seen on angiography and the disturbance observed with pulsed Doppler echocardiography. The size and duration of the signal loss increases with the degree of mitral regurgitation (MR).[28] The optimal imaging planes for detecting MR are axial and long axis.

Magnetic resonance imaging compared with color-flow and pulsed-Doppler echocardiography for detection of MR produced no false positives (sensitivity 94%, specificity 100%).[30] Nishamura and coworkers[31] compared the extent and severity of the regurgitant jet by MRI and color-flow Doppler mapping when classified as 4+ (severe), 3+ (moderate), 2+ (mild), and 1+ (minimal). The results of the two methods were the same in 14 (70%) of 20 patients, with 5 patients differing by one grade and one patient by two grades. Pflugfelder and colleagues[32] studied 26 patients with MR using gradient-echo MRI and color Doppler echocardiography or contrast ventriculography. In patients with mild MR, signal loss was seen in 3.3 ± 1.2 anatomic slices (10 mm slice thickness) compared with 4.9 ± 1.4 levels in patients with moderate MR (p = ns) and in 7.0 ± 1.4 levels in severe MR (p <

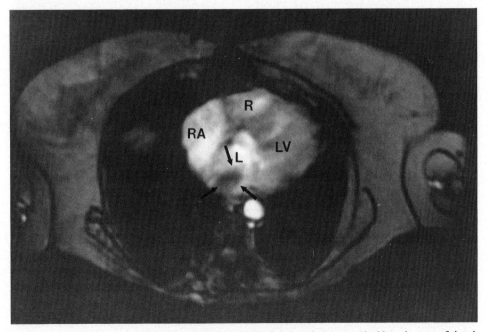

Figure 7–4. Axial gradient-echo image through the midleft atrium in late systole. Note the area of signal loss in the left atrium *(arrows)* representing blood regurgitated through the incompetent mitral valve. L = left atrium; LV = left ventricle; R = right ventricule; RA = right atrium.

0.001 vs. mild MR). The total area of maximal systolic left atrial signal loss observed in all levels was 10 ± 6 cm^2 in mild, 31 ± 17 cm^2 in moderate ($p <$ 0.001), and 96 ± 30 cm^2 in severe MR ($p < 0.001$). Glogar and associates[33] compared gradient-echo MRI with angiography, 2-D echocardiography, Doppler sonography, and color-flow mapping. The ratio of regurgitant jet area/left atrium area as determined by MRI showed good correlation with a comparable ratio from color Doppler sonography ($r = 0.87$; $p < 0.001$). The determination of left and right ventricular stroke volume in the same study allowed calculation of the volume of regurgitant fraction, which showed a correlation with invasively determined regurgitant fraction of $r = 0.87$ ($p < 0.001$).[33]

MITRAL VALVE PROLAPSE

Using gradient-echo imaging in the long axis planar view, the anterior and posterior mitral valve leaflets can be easily seen. Mitral valve prolapse can be detected by observing the anterior and/or posterior leaflets breaking the plane of the mitral anulus during systole and prolapsing into the left atrium (Fig. 7–5). No comparative studies have been reported as to the accuracy of MRI to diagnose mitral valve prolapse.

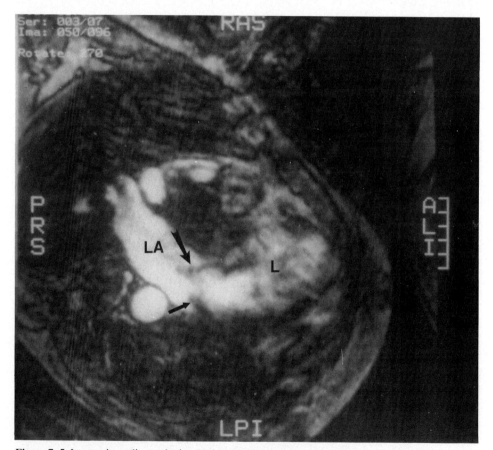

Figure 7–5. Long axis gradient-echo image through the mitral valve in ventricular systole. There is prolapse of the anterior mitral valve leaflet *(large arrow)* and of the posterior mitral valve leaflet *(small arrow)* into the left atrium. L = left ventricle; LA = left atrium.

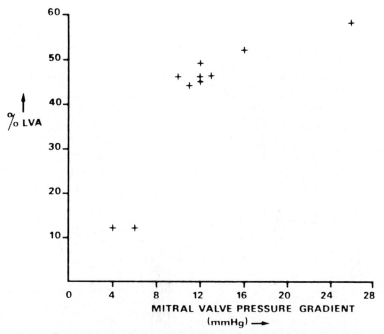

Figure 7–6. Graph of mean mitral valve pressure gradient against area of signal loss distal to the mitral valve as a percentage of left ventricular cross-sectional area on gradient-echo MRI. (From Mitchell et al.,[28] p. 193, with permission.)

MITRAL STENOSIS

Spin-echo imaging can be used to detect anatomic abnormalities associated with mitral stenosis such as left atrial enlargement,[34] thickened chordae tendineae and mitral valve leaflets, and focal areas of signal loss in the valve and anulus indicative of calcification. Gradient-echo imaging is the method of choice for evaluation of the mitral valve. The optimal plane of imaging is the long axis. Patients must be in sinus rhythm, which limits the applications of MRI because many patients with mitral stenosis are in atrial fibrillation. Gradient-echo imaging of the stenotic valve can detect thickened leaflets and chordae with restricted opening movement. A central jet of signal loss can be seen in early diastole entering the left ventricle through the mitral valve and moving into the body of the left ventricle. This signal loss corresponds to turbulent blood flow as it enters the left ventricle. Mitchell and colleagues[28] demonstrated a highly significant correlation ($T = 0.77$; $p < 0.01$) between the size of signal loss as a proportion to left ventricular cross-sectional area and catheter-measured gradient, with a leveling off at gradients greater than 16 mm Hg (Fig. 7–6). Difficulty with this method occurs when moderate or severe AR coexists, which contributes signal loss to the left ventricle.

THE TRICUSPID VALVE

TRICUSPID REGURGITATION

Gradient-echo imaging is the preferred mode of imaging for detection of tricuspid regurgitation (TR). The plane of the tricuspid valve is almost perpendicular to the axial plane, and usually two of the valve's leaflets are easily seen in represen-

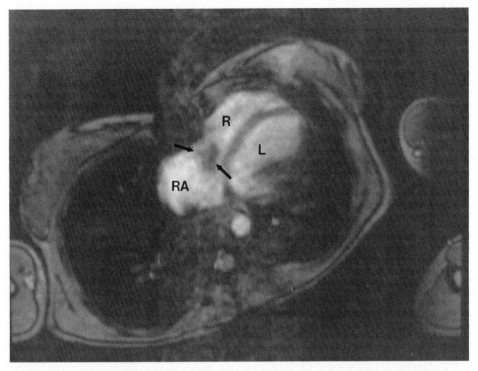

Figure 7-7. Long axis gradient-echo image through the tricuspid valve during systole. Note the dark area of signal loss *(arrows)* in the right atrium representing regurgitant blood from the right ventricle through an incompetent tricuspid valve. L = left ventricle; R = right ventricle; RA = right atrium.

tative sections through the central portions of the valve.[18] The optimal planes of imaging for detection of TR are axial and long axis. Tricuspid regurgitation is identified as a jet of signal loss extending from the valve into the right atrium[35] (Fig. 7-7). The sensitivity for detection of TR compared with cineangiography was 86%.[22] Quantitation of TR by MRI has not been reported.

TRICUSPID STENOSIS

Gradient-echo imaging is the preferred mode of imaging. Normal tricuspid valve flow of blood into the right ventricle produces only minimal signal loss along the leaflet edges. Excessive turbulence across the tricuspid valve and into the right ventricle as a jet of signal loss has been associated with hemodynamically documented tricuspid stenosis.[36] Quantitation of tricuspid stenosis has not been reported.

THE PULMONARY VALVE

The pulmonic valve is poorly imaged in the axial plane. It is seen reasonably well in the coronal plane. Excursion and subvalvular width are easily appreciated.[18] Gradient-echo imaging is the mode of choice. Pulmonary regurgitation (PR) is detected as a jet of signal loss passing into the right ventricular outflow tract in diastole. Pulmonic stenosis can be suspected by excessive turbulence as a jet of signal loss in systole in the pulmonary artery. Comparative studies for accuracy of detection and quantitation of pulmonary valve stenosis or regurgitation have not been reported.

VALVULAR PROSTHETICS

All artificial valves may be safely imaged at high-field strengths with the exception of the Starr-Edwards mitral pre-6000 series (used from 1960 to 1964), which should not be scanned at field strengths greater than 0.35 Tesla when valve dehiscence is suspected.[37] The valves are seen as an area of discrete signal loss with little or no detail being discernible. Unlike computed tomography, magnetic resonance images of the prosthetic valves cause minimal distortion or artifact formation of surrounding structures. Valvular dysfunction due to disc, hemidisc, or ball restriction cannot be seen. Valvular regurgitation (VR) can be detected as a jet of signal loss appearing in the more proximal chamber (Fig. 7-8). It is not possible to distinguish paravalvular from VR at present.

SUMMARY

All four cardiac valves can be imaged using MRI. Gradient-echo imaging is the preferred mode of imaging. Valvular regurgitation seen as an area of signal loss

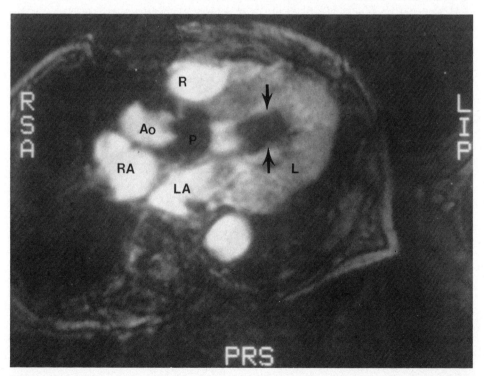

Figure 7-8. Long axis gradient-echo image through the left ventricle from a patient with a St. Jude aortic valve prosthesis (*P*). Aortic regurgitation is seen as an area of signal loss *(arrows)* in the left ventricular cavity during diastole. Ao = ascending aorta; L = left ventricle; LA = left atrium; R = right ventricle; RA = right atrium.

in the more proximal chamber can be diagnosed with a high degree of accuracy when compared with 2-D Doppler echocardiography and catheterization angiography. Aortic and mitral stenosis can be semiquantitatively diagnosed, but no method for determining valve areas is currently available. Cardiac prosthetic valves can be imaged but appear only as localized signal loss. Prosthetic valve regurgitation can be diagnosed in the same way as native valve regurgitation.

At present, MRI, though not a widely used modality, can contribute significantly to the diagnosis of cardiac valve disorders. With the addition of fast magnetic resonance scanning, which can eliminate the need for electrocardiographic gating, it will be possible for patients with cardiac rhythm irregularities to be scanned, thus broadening the base of patients with valve disease who can be diagnosed.

REFERENCES

1. Higgins, CB: Overview of MR of the heart—1986. AJR 146:907, 1986.
2. Dimick, RN, Hedlund, LW, Herfkens, RJ, et al: Optimizing electrocardiograph electrode placement for cardiac-gated magnetic resonance imaging. Invest Radiol 22:17, 1987.
3. Dinsmore, RE, Wismer, GL, Levine, RA, et al: Magnetic resonance imaging of the heart: Positioning and gradient angle election for optimal imaging plane. AJR 143:1135, 1984.
4. Shellock, FG, Kanal, E, and SMRI Safety Committee: Policies, Guidelines and Recommendations for MR imaging safety and patient management. JMRI 1:97, 1991.
5. Cranney, GB, Lotan, CS, and Pohost, GM: Evaluation of aortic regurgitation by nuclear magnetic resonance imaging. Curr Probl Cardiol 15(2):87, 1990.
6. Underwood, SR, Fermin, DN, Klipstein, RH, et al: Magnetic resonance velocity mapping: Clinical application of a new technique. Br Heart J 57:404, 1987.
7. Higgins, CB, Stark, D, McNamara, M, et al: Multiplane magnetic resonance imaging of the heart and major vessels: Studies in normal volunteers. AJR 142:661, 1984.
8. Markiewicz, W, Sechtem, U, and Higgins, CB: Evaluation of the right ventricle by magnetic resonance imaging. Am Heart J 113:8, 1978.
9. Kaul, S, Wismer, GL, Brady, TJ, et al: Measurement of normal left heart dimensions using optimally oriented MR images. AJR 146:75, 1986.
10. MacMillan, RM, Murphy, JH, Kresh, JY, et al: Left ventricular volume using cine-MRI: Validation by catheterization ventriculography. Am J Card Imag 4:79, 1990.
11. MacMillan, RM, Ivanoff, J, Tulchinsky, M, et al: Clinical applications of magnetic resonance imaging of the heart and great vessels. Angiology 1991 (in press).
12. Maddahi, J, Crues, J, Berman, DS, et al: Noninvasive quantification of left ventricular myocardial mass by gated proton nuclear magnetic resonance imaging. J Am Coll Cardiol 10:682, 1987.
13. Go, RT, O'Donnell, JK, Underwood, DA, et al: Comparison of gated cardiac MRI and 2-D echocardiography of intracardiac neoplasms. AJR 145:21, 1985.
14. Rubinstein, RI, Askenase, AD, Thickman, D, et al: Magnetic resonance imaging to evaluate patency of aortocoronary bypass grafts. Circulation 76:786, 1987.
15. Soulen, RL, Stark, DD, and Higgins, CB: Magnetic resonance imaging of constrictive pericarditis. Am J Cardiol 55:48, 1985.
16. Chung, KJ, Simpson, IA, Sohn, DJ, et al: Cine magnetic resonance imaging in congenital heart disease. Dynamic Cardiovascular Imaging 1:133, 1987.
17. Dinsmore, RE, Liberthson, RR, Wismer, GL, et al: Magnetic resonance imaging of thoracic aortic aneurysms: Comparison with other imaging methods. AJR 146:309, 1986.
18. Schieber, M, Axel, L, Reichek, N, et al: Correlation of cine MR with two-dimensional pulsed Doppler echocardiography in valvular insufficiency. J Comput Assist Tomogr 11:627, 1987.
19. Utz, JA, Herfkens, RJ, Heinsimer, JA, et al: Valvular regurgitation: Dynamic MR imaging. Radiology 168:91, 1988.
20. Evans, AJ, Blinder, RA, Herfkens, RJ, et al: Effects of turbulence on signal intensity in gradient-echo images. Invest Radiol 23:512, 1988.
21. Cook, SL, Maurer, G, Berman, DS, et al: Effect of flow rate and orifice size on flow jets visualized by fast NMR imaging: A phantom study (Abstract). J Am Coll Cardiol 11(Suppl A):156, 1988.

22. Nishamura, F, Yoshimo, Y, Mihara, J, et al: Advantage of cine-MR imaging for evaluation of valvular regurgitation. Japanese Circulation Journal 54:288, 1990.

23. Sechtem, U, Pflugfelder, PW, Cassidy, MM, et al: Mitral or aortic regurgitation: Quantification of regurgitant volumes with cine MR imaging. Radiology 167:425, 1988.

24. Wagner, S, Aufferman, W, Buser, P, et al: Diagnostic accuracy and estimation of the severity of valvular regurgitation from the signal void on cine magnetic resonance images. Am Heart J 118:760, 1989.

25. Pflugfelder, PW, Landzberg, JS, Cassidy, MM, et al: Comparison of cine MR imaging with Doppler echocardiography for evaluation of aortic regurgitation. AJR 152:729, 1989.

26. Suzuki, J, Caputo, GR, Kondo, C, et al: Cine MR imaging of valvular heart disease: Display and imaging parameters affect the size of the signal void caused by valvular regurgitation. AJR 155:723, 1990.

27. Metcalfe, M, Jones, RA, Redpath, TW, et al: Low-field cine magnetic resonance imaging in aortic valve disease. Br J Radiol 62:1063, 1989.

28. Mitchell, L, Jenkins, JPR, Watson, Y, et al: Diagnosis and assessment of mitral and aortic disease by cine-flow magnetic resonance imaging. Magnetic Resonance in Medicine 12:181, 1989.

29. deRoos, A, Reichek, N, Axel, L, et al: Cine MR imaging in aortic stenosis. J Comput Assist Tomogr 13:421, 1989.

30. Aurigemma, G, Reichek, N, Scheibler, M, et al: Evaluation of mitral regurgitation by cine magnetic resonance imaging. Am J Cardiol 66:621, 1990.

31. Nishamura, T, Yamada, N, Itoh, AA, et al: Cine MR imaging in mitral regurgitation. Comparison with color Doppler flow imaging. AJR 153:721, 1989.

32. Pflugfelder, PW, Sechtem, UP, White, RD, et al: Noninvasive evaluation of mitral regurgitation by analysis of left atrial signal loss in cine magnetic resonance. Am Heart J 117:1113, 1989.

33. Glogar, D, Globits, S, Neuhold, A, et al: Assessment of mitral regurgitation by magnetic resonance imaging. Magnetic Resonance Imaging 7:611, 1989.

34. Hill, JA, Akins, EW, Fitzsimmons, JR, et al: Mitral stenosis: Imaging by nuclear magnetic resonance. Am J Cardiol 57:351, 1985.

35. Higgins, CB, Sechtem, UP, and Pflugfelder, P: Cine MR: Evaluation of cardiac ventricular function and valvular function. Int J Cardiac Imag 3:21, 1988.

36. Cohen, ML, Spray, T, Gutierrez, F, et al: Congenital tricuspid valve stenosis with atrial septal defect and left anterior fascicular block. Clin Cardiol 13:497, 1990.

37. Williams, KD and Drazer, BP: Magnets, metal and medical devices: The good, the bad and the ugly. BNI Quarterly 5:46, 1989.

38. Randall, PA, Kohman, LJ, Scalzetti, EM, et al: Magnetic resonance imaging of prosthetic cardiac valves in vitro and in vivo. Am J Cardiol 62:973, 1988.

PART 4

Clinical Considerations

CHAPTER 8

Endocarditis: Recognition, Management, and Prophylaxis

Abdolghader Molavi, M.D.

During the past 2 decades, infective endocarditis has undergone a striking evolution, with changes in the age of patients, the recognized underlying cardiac conditions, the etiologic organisms, and the approach to therapy.[1] The mean age of patients with this disease has gradually increased, and the proportion of those who have rheumatic valvular disease as an underlying lesion has decreased. Mitral valve prolapse has been recognized as the leading cardiac condition in adults with subacute bacterial endocarditis. Prosthetic valves and degenerative valvular disease have become frequent underlying conditions in patients with endocarditis. The increasing use of intravascular devices has provided a nosocomial source for development of this infection.[2] Surgical therapy has become an essential part of the management in a significant proportion of patients with endocarditis.

DIAGNOSIS

The clinical features of infective endocarditis also have undergone remarkable changes. The classic peripheral manifestations, including Osler nodes, Janeway lesions, and Roth spots, have become uncommon. An increasing proportion of patients have no detectable murmur when they first come to medical attention. A change in the character of heart murmur, common in patients with acute endocarditis, is rarely noted in those with subacute valvular infection.

The diagnosis of endocarditis is based on the clinical findings and demonstration of a continuous bacteremia. New developments in echocardiography have greatly advanced the value of this procedure for the detection of both valvular vegetations and the intracardiac complications associated with this infection.

BLOOD CULTURES

The bacteriologic diagnosis of infective endocarditis is facilitated by the relative constancy of bacteremia originating from the vegetations.[3] Quantitative studies of blood cultures have shown that bacteria are discharged from endocardial vegetations at a relatively constant rate, rather than haphazardly as a result of the breaking off of infected particles,[4] and that arterial blood cultures have no demonstrable advantage over venous blood cultures for detecting bacteremia in patients with endocarditis.[4,5]

The relative constancy of bacteremia in infective endocarditis accounts for the fact that, in the absence of previous antimicrobial therapy, nearly all blood cultures are positive in the vast majority of patients.[6] Administration of antibiotics within 2 weeks before blood cultures are obtained substantially reduces the proportion of positive cultures, particularly in patients with endocarditis caused by streptococci or HACEK organisms. The acronym HACEK describes a group of fastidious gram-negative bacilli that include Haemophilus species, *Actinobacillus actinomycetemcomitans, Cardiobacterium hominis,* and Eikenella and Kingella species. All of these organisms require incubation in atmospheres of 5% to 10% CO_2 for optimal growth and have a predilection for infecting the heart valves when causing human disease.

The volume of blood obtained for culture is an important factor in the detection of bacteremia.[7,8] Quantitative blood cultures in patients with infective endocarditis have shown that in most cases bacteremia is low grade. Werner and associates[6] found that 24% of blood cultures from patients with streptococcal endocarditis contained between 1 and 10 colony-forming units per milliliter of blood. In adults with suspected endocarditis, no less than 10 ml of blood should be drawn for each culture set in order to furnish an inoculum adequate to initiate bacterial growth.

In a patient with suspected endocarditis, at least three sets of blood cultures should be obtained at no less than hourly intervals within the first 24 hours. Collection of additional blood cultures may be necessary in patients who have received antibiotics in the preceding 2 weeks and in those with endocarditis due to HACEK organisms. The vast majority of organisms causing endocarditis are detected within 7 days of incubation.[7] If blood cultures reveal no growth after a period of 7 days, an additional 2 weeks of incubation is recommended.

The presence of bacteremia in a patient with a prosthetic valve does not necessarily imply an associated endocarditis. Prosthetic valves are relatively resistant to colonization by most gram-negative bacilli. If there is an identifiable focus for gram-negative bacteremia and the bacteremia clears promptly with antimicrobial therapy, the patient can usually be treated for bacteremia alone. However, if bacteremia persists or the source of infection is not apparent, the patient should be assumed to have prosthetic valve endocarditis. Because gram-positive bacteria adhere readily to prostheses, their presence in blood cultures is more frequently associated with prosthetic valve infection.

Polymicrobial endocarditis occurs most commonly in intravenous drug users.[9] Detection of all the infecting organisms is essential for the selection of appropriate antimicrobial therapy. If these include a fastidious slow-growing organism, positive blood cultures may be discarded before the fastidious pathogen can be isolated.

Culture-Negative Endocarditis

Blood cultures are negative in 2% to 5% of patients with infective endocarditis. The higher rates reported in some series are probably related to the low volume of blood sampled, previous antimicrobial therapy, and inadequate laboratory techniques.[7] Culture-negative endocarditis is usually due to organisms that do not grow readily in blood cultures, such as *Coxiella burnetii* (Q fever) and the genera Chlamydia spp., Mycoplasma spp., Legionella spp., Mycobacterium spp., Brucella spp., *Histoplasma capsulatum,* and Aspergillus spp.

Q fever endocarditis may develop on native as well as prosthetic heart valves.[10,11] The course is chronic, and the aortic valve is involved in more than 80% of the cases. Elevated liver enzymes (aspartate aminotransferase and alkaline phosphatase), thrombocytopenia, and hypergammaglobulinemia are commonly present. Diagnosis is usually made by finding an elevated complement fixing antibody to phase I *Coxiella burnetii* antigen.[10] A phase I antibody titer greater than 1:200 is considered virtually diagnostic of Q fever endocarditis.

Legionella endocarditis may develop on either native or prosthetic valves.[12] The course is chronic, and high titers of antibody to *Legionella pneumophila* are usually present. Cultures of lysed concentrate of blood (lysis-centrifugation system) or blind subcultures of culture bottles onto buffered charcoal yeast extract agar can result in the isolation of the organism.

Endocarditis is a rare complication of brucellosis. The aortic valve is most commonly involved.[13] Because brucellae require special media for optimal growth, blood cultures may be negative if the infection is not suspected and the microbiology laboratory is not notified. Brucella antibody, present in high titers in all cases, is useful to rule out this infection in a patient with culture-negative endocarditis.

Endocarditis due to *Chlamydia psittaci* occurs usually in association with psittacine bird exposure.[14] The course is subacute, and the diagnosis is established by serologic means or by histologic findings in the heart valves. Valvular infections due to *Chlamydia trachomatis* and *Chlamydia pneumoniae* also have been reported.[15]

Endocarditis due to *Mycoplasma pneumoniae* and *Mycoplasma hominis*[16] has been reported. Diagnosis was made by serologic means without culture confirmation.

Endocarditis due to Aspergillus spp. may develop on normal, damaged, or prosthetic heart valves.[17,18] Large obstructing vegetations and embolization to major arteries may occur. Blood cultures are positive in only 15% of the cases. Diagnosis is usually made by histopathology or culture of the valve tissue.

Histoplasma capsulatum is the third most common cause of fungal endocarditis.[19,20] Endocardial involvement occurs in the setting of subacute or chronic disseminated histoplasmosis. Blood cultures are frequently negative. Diagnosis is established by demonstration of the organism in bone marrow or liver biopsy, the excised valve, or an embolus removed from a peripheral artery.

ECHOCARDIOGRAPHY

Since the initial observations in 1973,[21,22] ultrasound examination of the heart has provided increasingly better images and is currently the diagnostic imaging procedure of choice in patients with suspected endocarditis. A series of three major technical advances has greatly enhanced the value of this noninvasive technique in the diagnosis of infective endocarditis—the advent of two-dimensional (2-D) echocardiography, the introduction of color-flow Doppler technology, and the introduction of transesophageal imaging.[23,24]

Transthoracic 2-D echocardiography is of limited diagnostic value in approximately 30% of patients with endocarditis due to such factors as obesity, emphysema, and chest wall deformity. With the transesophageal approach, the chest wall interference and intrathoracic attenuation are eliminated. Furthermore, the ability to move the transducer closer to the heart allows the use of high-frequency (5 mHz), high-resolution transducers that provide improved image quality, better sensitivity for color-flow Doppler studies, and improved visualization of all left-sided structures and prosthetic valves.

Echocardiography can assist in the recognition of endocarditis primarily by visualizing vegetations, and secondarily, by detecting the intracardiac complications of infection, such as paravalvular abscesses and valvular destruction leading to regurgitation.[25]

Vegetations

In contrast to M-mode echocardiography, 2-D imaging provides information about the size, shape, and mobility of vegetations. Vegetations in the 1- to 2-mm range approach the limits of resolution of the system and are difficult to detect. As the size or the echogenicity of the lesion increases, the sensitivity of the technique improves. The sensitivity of transthoracic 2-D echocardiography for detecting vegetations is approximately 60%, with a range of 38% to 78% in reported series.[26-32] The actual sensitivity is subject to debate because most studies have been based on the clinical diagnosis of infective endocarditis as opposed to histopathologic findings. The specificity, which is an indicator of how often a positive test correctly identifies the presence of vegetations, is more than 95% in skilled hands.

The identification of the vegetations has been considerably improved by the use of transesophageal echocardiography. Mugge and coworkers[30] compared the sensitivities of transthoracic and transesophageal imaging in 80 patients with 91 infected valves proved by surgery or autopsy. Transthoracic echocardiography revealed "definite" vegetations on 53 (58%) of 91 valves and a "possible vegetation" on 17 valves (19%). In contrast, transesophageal echocardiography visualized a "definite" vegetation on 82 (90%) of 91 valves and a "possible" vegetation on 6 valves (6%). The difference was especially striking for prosthetic valves; only 8 (36%) of 22 transthoracic echocardiograms showed definite or possible vegetations whereas 19 (86%) of 22 transesophageal images had positive findings. Echocardiography could not distinguish between vegetations and ruptured leaflets or chordae tendineae—conditions that may or may not be associated with infective endocarditis. The absence of echocardiographically visualized vegetations, even by the transesophageal approach, does not exclude the possibility of infective endocarditis.

Erbel and colleagues[29] compared the clinical values of transesophageal and transthoracic echocardiography in 96 consecutive patients with infective endocarditis. All vegetations larger than 10 mm were detected by both transesophageal and transthoracic echocardiograms. However, transthoracic echocardiography detected only 69% of moderately sized vegetations (6 to 10 mm) and 25% of small vegetations (less than 5 mm) that were detected by transesophageal approach.

Serial echocardiograms are not indicated in a patient who is doing well clinically. Even after successful therapy, many of the vegetations observed on echocardiographic studies persist for months, and some have been detected 3 years following an episode of endocarditis.[28]

Intracardiac Complications

In addition to vegetations, echocardiography can detect cardiac complications of endocarditis such as valve disruption, perivalvular abscess, septal abscess, mycotic aneurysm formation, and prosthetic valve dehiscence. This information is extremely valuable to both the physician managing the patient and to the surgeon who must plan the operative approach.

Transthoracic 2-D echocardiography may detect abscesses associated with endocarditis, particularly those located in the aortic root.[33-36] Transesophageal echocardiography, however, is substantially more sensitive than the transthoracic approach. Daniel and associates[37] reported a prospective study of 118 consecutive patients in whom infective endocarditis was documented by either direct inspection during surgery or histologic examination at autopsy. A total of 137 valves, including 103 native and 34 prosthetic valves, were infected. The anatomic evaluation during surgery or at autopsy revealed 46 definite regions of abscess in 44 (37%) of the 118 patients. The abscesses were found in the aortic root of native valve (14 abscesses), the ring of an infected aortic prosthetic valve (12 abscesses) or mitral prosthetic valve (4 abscesses), the interventricular septum (9 abscesses), the apparatus of native mitral valve (6 abscesses), and the papillary muscle (1 abscess). With *abscess* defined as a definite region of reduced echodensity or echolucency on the echocardiogram, transthoracic echocardiography identified only 13 (28%) of 46 abscesses, as compared with 40 (87%) of 46 detected by transesophageal approach. Although the specificity and the positive predictive value of the two techniques were similar, the sensitivity and the negative predictive value of the transesophageal method were substantially higher. Three of four false-positive diagnoses on transesophageal echocardiography were in patients with prosthetic valves or annular calcification.

Doppler echocardiography provides definition of the direction and velocity of blood flow and thus allows characterization of intracardiac complications of endocardial infection, including valvular insufficiency, cusp perforation, or functional valvular stenosis. In patients with ruptured sinus of Valsalva's aneurysm, the site of rupture and the chamber into which rupture occurs can be demonstrated[38]; this information may be an important determinant of the surgical approach. Aortic valve endocarditis may be complicated by infection of the mitral-aortic intervalvular fibrosa with formation of a pseudoaneurysm or a subaortic abscess that can rupture into the left atrium.[39] Precise preoperative diagnosis is important; this lesion should be differentiated from a ruptured aneursym of the sinus of Valsalva or perforation of the anterior mitral leaflet, also a complication of aortic valve endocarditis. Transthoracic echocardiography using color-flow imaging can demonstrate the jet location and orientation but may not provide definitive diagnosis. Transesophageal echocardiography provides an accurate diagnosis in such cases.[39,40]

The metal and plastic components of prosthetic valves generate shadows and artifacts that preclude a complete Doppler color-flow examination of suspected mitral prosthetic regurgitation by the transthoracic approach. Transesophageal echocardiography allows unobstructed visualization of the mitral prosthesis and the entire left atrium. It permits estimation of regurgitation through the prosthesis, visualization of the site of regurgitation, and identification of masses that may be adherent to the prosthesis itself or present in the left atrium. The sensitivity and specificity of transesophageal echocardiography for detection and characterization of mitral prosthetic dysfunction ranges from 90% to 95%.[41] With aortic prostheses, transesophageal echocardiography can differentiate valvular from paravalvular regurgitation.[42] However, the quantitation of regurgitation may be difficult because the left ventricular outflow tract can be obscured by the "shadowing" of nonbiologic prostheses.

Transesophageal echocardiography should be performed when the site, extent, and functional importance of cardiac infection have not been clearly defined by conventional echocardiographic studies. Specific indications include persistent fever or bacteremia, which suggest ongoing infection and the possible formation of abscess, and the presence of a prosthetic heart valve that may limit the accuracy of transthoracic echocardiography.[43]

ANTIMICROBIAL THERAPY

A number of widely accepted principles provide the framework for antimicrobial therapy of infective endocarditis. These principles relate to the selection of drugs, the dose, the route of administration, and the duration of therapy.

In most infections, once bacterial replication is inhibited, phagocytic cells eradicate the causative organism. In endocarditis, however, bacteria are located within vegetations, a meshwork of platelet-fibrin strands into which phagocytic cells cannot penetrate. Because eradication of infection depends solely on the activity of antimicrobials, unaided by host defenses, the use of bactericidal agents is necessary to achieve cure. Clinical experience has shown that treatment of endocarditis with bacteriostatic agents is associated with a high incidence of relapse or failure to control the infection. Reliable and consistent achievement of serum bactericidal concentrations mandates parenteral administration of antibiotics that are commonly used to treat endocarditis.

Antimicrobial treatment should begin promptly but does not usually need to be immediate in a patient with suspected subacute endocarditis. Most of these patients have been ill for a few weeks before the diagnosis is established. Therefore, a 1- to 2-day delay in treatment until cultures are collected and preliminary microbiologic data are available is of no significance. If death occurs before therapy is begun in such cases, it is usually due to unpredictable complications that are not prevented by antimicrobial therapy, such as rupture of a mycotic aneurysm or embolic occlusion of a coronary artery. In contrast, it is imperative that treatment of acute endocarditis is not delayed, especially when it is caused by *Staphylococcus aureus,* because of the rapidity with which valve leaflets, papillary muscles, or chordae tendineae may rupture or myocardial or septal abscesses can develop. Despite the urgent need for treatment in such cases, administration of antimicrobials should be withheld until sufficient blood cultures have been obtained, usually no more than 2 to 3 hours.

In contrast to most infections, effective treatment of infective endocarditis requires a prolonged course of therapy. In the absence of phagocytic cells, the organisms within vegetations multiply freely and reach very high population densities (10^9 to 10^{10} colony-forming units per gram of tissue). At such densities, microorganisms exist in a state of reduced metabolic activity, multiplying very slowly,[44] and consequently are less susceptible to the bactericidal action of antibiotics. This phenomenon and the total reliance on antimicrobials to eradicate infection account for the requirement of prolonged therapy. With rare exceptions, infective endocarditis should be treated for no less than 4 weeks. The exceptions are endocarditis caused by "penicillin-susceptible" *Streptococcus viridans* and selected cases of right-sided *S. aureus* endocarditis associated with intravenous drug abuse, which may be treated with a 2-week course of two-drug regimens.

Home therapy with parenteral antibiotics should be considered only in the patient who has responded well to initial treatment in the hospital, whose condition is stable, and for whom medical supervision can be maintained.

Gram-positive cocci (e.g., Staphylococcus spp., Streptococcus spp., and Enterococcus spp.) are the etiologic organisms in most cases of infective endocarditis. In an attempt to standardize acceptable regimens for endocarditis due to these organisms, the American Heart Association (AHA) sponsored a writing group from the Committee on Rheumatic Fever, Endocarditis, and Kawasaki disease to review the subject and make recommendations. This committee has published their conclusions, citing specific treatment regimens.[45] Since there are numerous species of gram-positive cocci, with varying susceptibilities to antibiotics, the recommended regimens are numerous and complex.

Viridans Streptococci and *Streptococcus bovis*

The viridans streptococci include a diverse group of Streptococcus species, for example, *S. sanguis, S. mitis, S. intermedius, S. anginosus, S. mutans,* and *S. salivarius,* that produce either green (alpha) or no (gamma) hemolysis when cultured on blood agar. Though some strains may possess Lancefield group antigens, most clinical isolates within each species lack group antigens and are, therefore, nongroupable.

Approximately 5% of cases of viridans streptococcal endocarditis are caused by nutritionally variant strains (mostly *S. mitis*). These organisms grow poorly in blood culture media and fail to grow on subculture onto routine blood agar. Media must be supplemented with thiol compounds, such as cysteine, or the active forms of vitamin B_6 (pyridoxal or pyridoxamine but *not* pyridoxine) for the isolation, identification, and subsequent antimicrobial susceptibility testing of these organisms.[46]

Viridans streptococci are usually highly sensitive to penicillin G. For therapeutic purposes, these organisms are classified, based upon minimum inhibitory concentrations (MIC) of penicillin G, into three groups: penicillin-susceptible (defined arbitrarily by MIC ≤ 0.1 μg/ml), relatively resistant to penicillin (MIC > 0.1 μg/ml and < 0.5 μg/ml), and penicillin-resistant (MIC ≤ 0.5 μg/ml).[45]

Streptococcus bovis, a group D streptococcus, is a normal inhabitant of the gastrointestinal tract. Endocarditis due to this organism occurs primarily in elderly men and is often associated with carcinoma of the colon. Endocarditis due to *S. bovis* is treated with the same regimens as that caused by viridans streptococci.

Viridans Streptococci Susceptible to Penicillin G (MIC ≥ 0.1 μg/ml)

Native valve endocarditis due to viridans streptococci and *S. bovis* that are "susceptible" to penicillin may be treated with either a 4-week regimen of penicillin G[47,48] or a 2-week regimen of penicillin G combined with either gentamicin or streptomycin (Table 8–1).[49,50]

Penicillin G alone, administered intravenously for 4 weeks, is highly effective for the treatment of penicillin-susceptible streptococcal endocarditis. The relapse

Table 8–1. Suggested Therapeutic Regimens for Endocarditis due to Penicillin-Susceptible Viridans Streptococci or *Streptococcus bovis* (Minimum Inhibitory Concentration ≤0.1 µg/ml)

Antibiotic	Adult Dose and Route	Pediatric Dose and Route	Duration of Therapy, wk
Regimens for Patients not Allergic to Penicillin			
1. **Aqueous crystalline penicillin G**	10–20 million U/24 h IV either continuously or in 6 equally divided doses	150,000–200,000 U/kg per 24 h IV (not to exceed 20 million U/24 h) either continuously or in 6 equally divided doses	4
2. **Aqueous crystalline penicillin G**	10–20 million U/24 h IV either continuously or in 6 equally divided doses	150,000–200,000 U/kg per 24 h IV (not to exceed 20 million U/24 h) either continuously or in 6 equally divided doses	2
With **gentamicin** or	1 mg/kg IM or IV (not to exceed 80 mg) every 8 h	2.0–2.5 mg/kg IV (not to exceed 80 mg) every 8 h	2
With **streptomycin**	7.5 mg/kg IM (not to exceed 500 mg) every 12 h	15 mg/kg IM (not to exceed 500 mg) every 12 h	2
Regimens for Penicillin-Allergic Patients			
1. **Cephalothin** or	2 g IV every 4 h	100–150 mg/kg per 24 h IV (not to exceed 12 g/24 h) in equally divided doses every 4–6 h	4
Cefazolin	1 g IM or IV every 8 h	80–100 mg/kg per 24 h IM or IV (not to exceed 3 g/24 h) in equally divided doses every 8 h	4
2. **Vancomycin**	30 mg/kg per 24 h IV in 2 or 4 equally divided doses, not to exceed 2 g/24 h unless serum levels are monitored	40 mg/kg per 24 h IV in 2 or 4 equally divided doses, not to exceed 2 g/24 h unless serum levels are monitored	4

Source: Adapted from Bisno et al.[45]
Key: IM = intramuscularly; IV = intravenously.

rate among patients treated with this regimen is 0.6%. Therapy must be continued for 4 weeks. In one trial, treatment for 10 to 14 days resulted in an unacceptably high relapse rate of 15%.[51]

The combination of penicillin G with either gentamicin or streptomycin exerts a synergistic bactericidal action against viridans streptococci and *S. bovis* both *in vitro* and in experimental endocarditis.[52] Penicillin G combined with either gentamicin or streptomycin administered parenterally for 2 weeks is an alternative to the 4-week regimen of penicillin G. In a study of 277 cases treated with the 2-week regimen, the overall relapse rate was 2%, which is not significantly different from that associated with the 4-week regimen of penicillin G.[49] The 2-week regimen is considered appropriate for uncomplicated endocarditis due to penicillin-susceptible viridans streptococci in patients at low risk for aminoglycoside toxicity. This regimen is not recommended for patients with impaired renal function, those particularly susceptible to the risk of aminoglycoside-induced ototoxicity (the elderly), or those with complications such as myocardial abscess or extracardiac foci of infection.

At present, gentamicin is more commonly used than streptomycin in the two-drug regimen. Determinations of gentamicin serum levels are more readily available, and in contrast to streptomycin, gentamicin can be administered either intravenously or intramuscularly. Some strains of viridans streptococci exhibit high-level resistance to streptomycin, defined as MIC >1000 μg/ml. There is no synergy between penicillin and streptomycin against these organisms both *in vitro* and in experimental animal models.[53] For endocarditis caused by these strains, gentamicin rather than streptomycin must be used when the two-drug regimen is employed.

Penicillin G administered parenterally for 4 weeks combined with either gentamicin or streptomycin for the first 2 weeks has been used to treat endocarditis due to penicillin-susceptible viridans streptococci.[54] This regimen, which is also recommended by the AHA Committee,[45] provides the greatest bactericidal activity. The cure rate, however, is not superior to that achieved by penicillin G alone administered for 4 weeks.

In patients with a history of immediate hypersensitivity reactions to penicillin, vancomycin administered intravenously for 4 weeks is the drug of choice. If the penicillin allergy is not of the immediate type, a first-generation cephalosporin (usually cefazolin or cephalothin) administered intravenously for 4 weeks may be used. Although the prolonged elimination half-lives of some second- and third-generation cephalosporins (such as cefonicid and ceftriaxone) may facilitate outpatient therapy, the use of these compounds for the treatment of streptococcal endocarditis is not recommended.

For patients with prosthetic valve endocarditis caused by penicillin-susceptible viridans streptococci or *S. bovis,* a 6-week regimen of penicillin G combined with gentamicin or streptomycin for at least the first 2 weeks is recommended.

Viridans Streptococci Relatively Resistant to Penicillin G (MIC >0.1 μg/ml and <0.5 μg/ml) and Nutritionally Variant Streptococci

For native-valve endocarditis due to viridans streptococci or *S. bovis* relatively resistant to penicillin G, a 4-week course of penicillin G, combined with an aminoglycoside (gentamicin or streptomycin) for the first 2 weeks, is recommended (Table 8–2).[45] The data to support this recommendation, however, are limited, and penicillin G alone administered for 4 weeks may be adequate.[55] In patients with a history of immediate hypersensitivity reactions to penicillin, vancomycin alone for 4 weeks is the substitute of choice. If the pencillin allergy is not of the immediate type, a 4-week course of a first-generation cephalosporin combined with an aminoglycoside for the first 2 weeks may be used.

Endocarditis due to nutritionally variant streptococci is associated with a higher incidence of bacteriologic failure, a higher frequency of relapse after therapy, and a higher mortality rate than that caused by other viridans streptococci.[56] It is treated, therefore, with regimens that are recommended for strains relatively resistant to penicillin G, even if the isolate is penicillin susceptible.

For patients with prosthetic valve endocarditis caused by viridans streptococci or *S. bovis* with penicillin MIC >0.1 μg/ml, a 6-week regimen of combined therapy with penicillin G and gentamicin is recommended.

Table 8–2. Suggested Therapeutic Regimens for Endocarditis due to Viridans Streptococci or *Streptococcus bovis* Relatively Resistant to Penicillin G (MIC >0.1 μg/ml and <0.5 μg/ml)

Antibiotic	Adult Dose and Route	Pediatric Dose and Route	Duration of Therapy, wk
1. **Aqueous crystalline penicillin G**	20 million U/24 h IV either continuously or in 6 equally divided doses	150,000–200,000 U/kg per 24 h IV (not to exceed 20 million U/24 h) either continuously or in 6 equally divided doses	4
With **gentamicin** or	1 mg/kg IM or IV (not to exceed 80 mg) every 8 h	2.0–2.5 mg/kg IV (not to exceed 80 mg) every 8 h	2
With **streptomycin**	7.5 mg/kg IM (not to exceed 500 mg) every 12 h	15 mg/kg IM (not to exceed 500 mg) every 12 h	2

Source: Adapted from Bisno et al.[45]
Key: IM = intramuscularly; IV = intravenously.

Viridans Streptococci Resistant to Penicillin G (MIC ≤0.5 μg/ml)

Endocarditis due to viridans streptococci or *S. bovis* requiring ≥0.5 μg/ml of penicillin for inhibition is treated with the same regimens as those for enterococcal endocarditis (Table 8–3).

OTHER STREPTOCOCCI

Group B streptococcal endocarditis is relatively uncommon.[57] Large friable vegetations are a frequent feature, and embolization may occur early in the course. Combined therapy with penicillin and an aminoglycoside is more effective *in vitro* and in experimental group B streptococcal endocarditis than is penicillin G alone. Patients with group B streptococcal endocarditis should be treated with penicillin G administered for 4 weeks combined with gentamicin or streptomycin for the first 2 weeks of therapy.

Endocarditis due to group C and G streptococci is usually marked by valve destruction with resultant congestive heart failure and recurrent systemic embolization.[58] Abscesses of major organs including brain, spleen, and kidneys have been described. Because of the acute and destructive nature of this infection, combination therapy with penicillin G and an aminoglycoside for 4 weeks is recommended.

Pneumococcal endocarditis has declined sharply in incidence since the advent of penicillin.[59] Concomitant meningitis is present in 60% to 70% of cases. Penicillin G administered for 4 weeks is the treatment regimen of choice.

ENTEROCOCCI

Enterococci are the third most common cause of native valve endocarditis, accounting for 10% to 15% of all cases. These organisms, previously included in the group D Streptococcus, are now considered to represent a separate genus, *Enterococcus,* which is comprised of several of species including *E. faecalis* and *E. faecium. Enterococcus faecalis* is the predominant species, with a tendency to infect older men more frequently than women. Most patients with enterococcal bacteremia do not have endocarditis. Clinical features that suggest an associated endocarditis include the absence of an identifiable extracardiac focus of infection, the

Table 8–3. Suggested Therapeutic Regimens for Endocarditis due to Enterococci (or to Viridans Streptococci Resistant to Penicillin G [MIC $\geq$0.5 μg/ml])

Antibiotic	Adult Dose and Route	Pediatric Dose and Route	Duration of Therapy, wk
Regimens for Patients not Allergic to Penicillin			
1. **Aqueous crystalline penicillin G**	20–30 million U/24 h IV either continuously or in 6 equally divided doses	200,000–300,000 U/kg per 24 h IV (not to exceed 30 million U/24 h) given continuously or in 6 equally divided doses	4–6
With **gentamicin**	1 mg/kg IM or IV (not to exceed 80 mg) every 8 h	2.0–2.5 mg/kg IM or IV (not to exceed 80 mg) every 8 h	4–6
or With **streptomycin**	7.5 mg/kg IM (not to exceed 500 mg) every 12 h	15 mg/kg IM (not to exceed 500 mg) every 12 h	4–6
2. **Ampicillin**	12 g/24 h IV given continuously or in 6 equally divided doses	300 mg/kg per 24 h IV (not to exceed 12 g/24 h) in 4 to 6 equally divided doses	4–6
With **gentamacin**	1 mg/kg IM or IV (not to exceed 80 mg) every 8 h	2.0–2.5 mg/kg IM or IV (not to exceed 80 mg) every 8 h	4–6
or With **streptomycin**	7.5 mg/kg IM (not to exceed 500 mg) every 12 h	15 mg/kg IM (not to exceed 500 mg) every 12 h	4–6
Regimen for Penicillin-Allergic Patients			
1. **Vancomycin**	30 mg/kg per 24 h IV in 2 or 4 equally divided doses, not to exceed 2 g/24 h unless serum levels are monitored	40 mg/kg per 24 h IV in 2 or 4 equally divided doses, not to exceed 2 g/24 h unless serum levels are monitored	4–6
With **gentamicin**	1 mg/kg IM or IV (not to exceed 80 mg) every 8 h	2.0–2.5 mg/kg IM or IV (not to exceed 80 mg) every 8 h	4–6
or With **streptomycin**	7.5 mg/kg IM (not to exceed 500 mg) every 12 h	15 mg/kg IM (not to exceed 500 mg) every 12 h	4–6

Source: Adapted from Bisno et al.[45]
Key: IM = intramuscularly; IV = intravenously.

presence of underlying valvular heart disease or heart murmur, and acquisition in the community.[60]

Enterococci are intrinsically resistant to most antibiotics. Whereas the great majority of viridans streptococci are inhibited by ≤ 0.1 μg/ml of penicillin G, enterococci require 0.4 to 25 μg/ml for inhibition (median MIC = 2.0 μg/ml). Ampicillin is nearly twice as active as penicillin G against these organisms. Strains of enterococci that produce penicillinase and are resistant to penicillin and ampicillin have been isolated.[61] High-level resistance to penicillin/ampicillin (MIC > 200 μg/ml) without penicillinase production has also been described, particularly among *E. faecium*.[62] Enterococci are uniformly resistant to cephalosporins but, with rare exceptions,[63] are sensitive to vancomycin.

Enterococci are characteristically tolerant to the bactericidal action of antibiotics that inhibit cell-wall synthesis; the minimum bactericidal concentrations (MBC) of penicillin G, ampicillin, and vancomycin (> 100 μg/ml) greatly exceed the corresponding MICs. This lack of bactericidal activity is due to unique features of the enterococcal cell wall and a defective autolytic enzyme system.[64,65]

Enterococci are usually resistant to aminoglycosides.[66] Strains with low-level resistance (defined by MIC ≤ 1000 μg/ml) to an aminoglycoside are killed synergistically when the drug is combined with penicillin G, ampicillin, or vancomycin. Synergistic killing does not occur if a strain exhibits high-level aminoglycoside resistance (MIC > 1000 μg/ml). Currently, 40% of clinical isolates of enterococci exhibit high-level resistance to streptomycin. Only rare enterococcal strains, however, are highly resistant to gentamicin.

Treatment of enterococcal endocarditis (see Table 8–3) is begun with either penicillin G or ampicillin combined with gentamicin. For patients allergic to penicillin, vancomycin is substituted for ampicillin. If the infecting strain exhibits only low-level resistance (MIC ≤ 1000 μg/ml) to both gentamicin and streptomycin, either drug may be used as they are equally effective.[67] If the isolate has low-level resistance to only one of the two aminoglycosides, that agent should be used. If high-level resistance is demonstrated for both streptomycin and gentamicin, other aminoglycosides should be tested to find an alternative with MIC ≤ 1000 μg/ml. If none is found, it is unlikely that the addition of an aminoglycoside would be beneficial. Optimal therapy of endocarditis caused by such a strain has not been established, and valve replacement may be necessary for cure. Pending further data, long-term therapy (8 to 12 weeks) with large doses of penicillin (40 million U/d) is recommended.

For endocarditis due to beta-lactamase-producing strains of enterococci, either ampicillin-sulbactam or vancomycin combined with an aminoglycoside may be used. For strains with high-level penicillin resistance without penicillinase production (usually *E. faecium*), vancomycin plus an aminoglycoside is employed.

Combination therapy for enterococcal endocarditis should continue for a minimum of 4 weeks. A 6-week course of combined therapy is recommended for patients whose symptoms of infection have existed for more than 3 months before institution of appropriate therapy,[67] patients with prosthetic valve endocarditis, and patients with relapse following 4 weeks of therapy.

The serum concentrations of aminoglycosides should be monitored to avoid ototoxicity or nephrotoxicity, which may occur with prolonged therapy. Because the rationale for use of these agents in enterococcal endocarditis is to provide a synergistic bactericidal effect with penicillin G, ampicillin, or vancomycin, the serum levels need not be as high as those required for the treatment of gram-negative bacillary infections. The dosages of gentamicin and streptomycin should be adjusted to achieve peak serum levels of 3 to 4 μg/ml and 15 to 20 μg/ml, respectively.

STAPHYLOCOCCI

Staphylococcus aureus is the second most common cause of infective endocarditis, accounting for 25% to 35% of all cases, and is the most frequent organism in endocarditis associated with intravenous drug abuse.[65] Coagulase-negative staphylococci are the most common cause of prosthetic valve endocarditis, occurring within 12 months of valve replacement. In contrast, these organisms rarely cause native valve endocarditis, accounting for only 1% to 3% of cases.[69,70] In the absence of an intravascular catheter, the isolation of a coagulase-negative Staphylococcus species from multiple blood cultures suggests endocardial infection if the patient has a predisposing cardiac condition. This presumption is further strengthened if the isolates from separate cultures are shown to represent a unique strain.

Native Valve Endocarditis

The great majority of *S. aureus* isolates, whether community or hospital acquired, are resistant to penicillin G. The drug of choice, therefore, is nafcillin or oxacillin, administered intravenously for 4 to 6 weeks[45] (Table 8–4). Killing of staphylococci *in vitro* and in experimental endocarditis is enhanced by adding an aminoglycoside to nafcillin or oxacillin. In a multicenter study of *S. aureus* endocarditis, addition of gentamicin for the first 2 weeks of a 6-week course of nafcillin, although associated with more rapid clearing of bacteremia, failed to improve the cure rates and resulted in an increased incidence of nephrotoxicity.[71] The AHA Committee recommendations include an optional addition of gentamicin to either nafcillin or oxacillin for the first 3 to 5 days of therapy in the hope of minimizing damage to the heart valve while avoiding adverse reactions associated with more prolonged courses of aminoglycosides.[45] In patients with endocarditis caused by a penicillin-sensitive *S. aureus,* penicillin G with or without a brief course of gentamicin may be used.

Vancomycin, administered intravenously for 4 to 6 weeks, is the drug of choice in patients with a history of immediate hypersensitivity reactions to penicillin. Cefazolin or cephalothin, with or without an initial 3 to 5 days of gentamicin, may be used with caution in patients with other manifestations of penicillin allergy.

Endocarditis due to methicillin-resistant *S. aureus* must be treated with vancomycin. The addition of gentamicin for the initial 3 to 5 days of therapy may be considered only if the infection is caused by a gentamicin-susceptible strain.

The adjunctive role of rifampin in the therapy of *S. aureus* endocarditis is controversial. The *in vitro* effects of this agent in combination with nafcillin or vancomycin against *S. aureus* are highly variable. Addition of rifampin (300 mg orally every 8 hours) to the therapeutic regimen may be considered in patients with complicating meningitis[72] or those with low serum bactericidal activity during therapy if the organism is susceptible.

Uncomplicated right-sided *S. aureus* endocarditis associated with intravenous drug abuse has been treated successfully with a 2-week course of nafcillin combined with an aminoglycoside. In a group of 50 patients who had no extrapulmonary

Table 8–4. Suggested Therapeutic Regimens for Endocarditis
due to Staphylococci in the Absence of Prosthetic Material

Antibiotic	Adult Dose and Route	Pediatric Dose and Route	Duration of Therapy
Methicillin-Susceptible Staphylococci			
A. Regimens for patients not allergic to penicillin			
1. **Nafcillin** or **oxacillin**	2 g IV every 4 h	150–200 mg/kg per 24 h IV (not to exceed 12 g/24 h) in 4 to 6 equally divided doses	4–6 wk
With optional addition of **gentamicin**	1 mg/kg IM or IV (not to exceed 80 mg) every 8 h	2.0–2.5 mg/kg IV (not to exceed 80 mg) every 8 h	3–5 d
B. Regimens for penicillin-allergic patients			
1. **Cephalothin**	2 g IV every 4 h	100–150 mg/kg per 24 h IV (not to exceed 12 g/24 h) in equally divided doses every 4 to 6 h	4–6 wk
or **Cefazolin**	2 g IV every 8 h	80–100 mg/kg per 24 h IV (not to exceed 6 g/24 h) in equally divided doses every 8 h	4–6 wk
With optional addition of **gentamicin**	1 mg/kg IM or IV (not to exceed 80 mg) every 8 h	2.0–2.5 mg/kg IV (not to exceed 80 mg) every 8 h	3–5 d
2. **Vancomycin**	30 mg/kg per 24 h IV in 2 or 4 equally divided doses, not to exceed 2 g/24 h unless serum levels are monitored	40 mg/kg per 24 h IV in 2 or 4 equally divided doses, not to exceed 2 g/24 h unless serum levels are monitored	4–6 wk
Methicillin-Resistant Staphylococci			
Vancomycin	30 mg/kg per 24 h IV in 2 or 4 equally divided doses, not to exceed 2 g/24 h unless serum levels are monitored	40 mg/kg per 24 h IV in 2 or 4 equally divided doses, not to exceed 2 g/24 h unless serum levels are monitored	4–6 wk

Source: Adapted from Bisno et al.[45]
Key: IM = intramuscularly; IV = intravenously.

metastatic infectious complications, a cure rate of 94% was achieved with this regimen.[73] However, vancomycin combined with an aminoglycoside was not effective
when administered for 2 weeks. There are data to suggest that vancomycin may
not be as effective as nafcillin or oxacillin in the treatment of *S. aureus* endocarditis.[74]

Native valve endocarditis due to coagulase-negative staphylococci is treated
with either nafcillin (or oxacillin) or vancomycin, depending upon the sensitivity
of the infecting strain, with the optional addition of gentamicin for the initial 3 to
5 days of therapy.

Prosthetic Valve Endocarditis

COAGULASE-NEGATIVE STAPHYLOCOCCI. Prosthetic valve endocarditis due to coagulase-negative staphylococci occurs commonly within 12 months of valve replacement, and the infecting organisms are usually methicillin resistant.

The optimal antibiotic therapy for prosthetic valve endocarditis caused by methicillin-resistant coagulase-negative staphylococci is provided by vancomycin plus rifampin administered for a minimum of 6 weeks combined with gentamicin for the initial 2 weeks of therapy[45] (Table 8-5). If the infecting strain is resistant to gentamicin, another aminoglycoside to which it is sensitive should be used. If none is found, the aminoglycoside treatment should be omitted. Resistance to rifampin may develop during therapy; therefore, organisms isolated from surgical specimens or from blood cultures at relapse should be retested for antimicrobial sensitivity.

Prosthetic valve endocarditis due to methicillin-susceptible coagulase-negative

Table 8-5. Suggested Therapeutic Regimens for Staphylococcal Endocarditis in the Presence of a Prosthetic Valve or Other Prosthetic Material

Antibiotic	Adult Dose and Route	Pediatric Dose and Route	Duration of Therapy, wk
Regimen for Methicillin-Resistant Staphylococci			
Vancomycin	30 mg/kg per 24 h IV in 2 or 4 equally divided doses, not to exceed 2 g/24 h unless serum levels are monitored	40 mg/kg per 24 h IV in 2 or 4 equally divided doses, not to exceed 2 g/24 h unless serum levels are monitored	≥6
With **rifampin**	300 mg PO every 8 h	20 mg/kg per 24 h PO (not to exceed 900 mg/24 h) in 2 equally divided doses	≥6
and With **gentamicin**	1.0 mg/kg IM or IV (not to exceed 80 mg) every 8 h	2.0–2.5 mg/kg IV (not to exceed 80 mg) every 8 h	≥2
Regimen for Methicillin-Susceptible Staphylococci			
Nafcillin or **oxacillin**	2 g IV every 4 h	150–200 mg/kg per 24 h IV (not to exceed 12 g/24 h) in in 4 to 6 equally divided doses	≥6
With **rifampin**	300 mg PO every 8 h	20 mg/kg per 24 h PO (not to exceed 900 mg/24 h) in 2 equally divided doses	≥6
and With **gentamicin**	1.0 mg/kg IM or IV (not to exceed 80 mg) every 8 h	2.0–2.5 mg/kg IV (not to exceed 80 mg) every 8 h	≥2

Source: Adapted from Bisno et al.[45]
Key: IM = intramuscularly; IV = intravenously; PO = orally.

staphylococci is treated with either nafcillin or oxacillin plus rifampin for a minimum of 6 weeks combined with gentamicin for the initial 2 weeks of therapy. In
penicillin-allergic patients, vancomycin (or a first-generation cephalosporin if
allergy is minor) is substituted for the penicillinase-resistant penicillin.

COAGULASE-POSITIVE STAPHYLOCOCCI (*S. AUREUS*). Prosthetic valve endocarditis caused by methicillin-sensitive *S. aureus* is treated with nafcillin or oxacillin
for a minimum of 6 weeks plus gentamicin given for the initial 2 weeks of therapy.
If infection is caused by a methicillin-resistant strain, vancomycin should be substituted for penicillinase-resistant penicillin, and an aminoglycoside to which the
infecting organism is sensitive should be used. The therapeutic advantage of adding
rifampin is not established.

GRAM-NEGATIVE BACILLI

Gram-negative bacilli account for about 5% of cases of native valve endocarditis, 13% of cases of prosthetic valve endocarditis (mostly early prosthetic valve
infections), and 30% of cases of endocarditis associated with intravenous drug
abuse.[75-79]

Treatment of endocarditis due to enteric gram-negative bacilli, such as *Esch-
erichia coli, Klebsiella, Enterobacter,* and *Serratia marcescens,* must be individualized on the basis of the *in vitro* susceptibility data. The drug of choice in most
cases is a third-generation cephalosporin (such as ceftriaxone) or aztreonam administered parenterally in full doses. Imipenem may be used if the isolate is resistant
to cephalosporins. These antibiotics are highly active against Enterobacteriaceae
and produce high serum bactericidal titers. The therapeutic advantage of adding an
aminoglycoside (usually gentamicin) is not established but should be considered,
particularly in patients with prosthetic valve endocarditis. Treatment is continued
for a minimum of 6 weeks. Quinolones (e.g., ciprofloxacin, ofloxacin) are bactericidal and highly active against gram-negative bacilli. They are an alternative to
beta-lactam antibiotics for the treatment of endocarditis caused by gram-negative
bacilli.

Pseudomonas aeruginosa endocarditis occurs most commonly in association
with intravenous drug abuse.[80] Optimal therapy is provided by an extended-spec-
trum penicillin (e.g., piperacillin or azlocillin 3.0 g IV every 4 hours) or ceftazidime
(2 g IV every 8 hours) combined with high-dose tobramycin (8 mg/kg per day IV
in divided doses every 8 hours) or netilmicin. Serum tobramycin levels should be
monitored to maintain peak levels in the range of 12 to 20 μg/ml and at least 10
times the MBC of the infecting blood isolate. Treatment should be continued for
at least 6 weeks. Medical therapy may be successful in *P. aeruginosa* endocarditis
involving the right side of the heart. In left-sided Pseudomonas endocarditis the
medical cure rate may be as low as 11%.[81] Early valve replacement is currently
recommended once the diagnosis is confirmed.[81,82]

Endocarditis due to Haemophilus species, including *H. parainfluenzae, H.
aphrophilus,* and *H. paraphrophilus,* is not uncommon. Combined therapy with
ampicillin and gentamicin is effective if the infecting organism is sensitive to ampicillin.[83] Alternative regimens, which should be used if the organism is resistant to
ampicillin, include a third-generation cephalosporin with or without an aminoglycoside, aztreonam with or without an aminoglycoside, and ciprofloxacin. Therapy
should be continued for 4 weeks.

DIPHTHEROIDS

Diphtheroid endocarditis occurs primarily in patients with valvular prostheses. The drug of choice is vancomycin. Combination therapy with penicillin and gentamicin is also effective if the infecting strain is susceptible to gentamicin.[84] Treatment should be continued for 6 weeks.

FUNGI

Candida spp. are the most common cause of fungal endocarditis, followed by Aspergillus spp. and *Histoplasma capsulatum.* Candida endocarditis usually occurs in association with intravenous drug abuse and in patients with prosthetic valves and those receiving prolonged intravenous antibiotics or hyperalimentation. Amphotericin B is the drug of choice, but medical therapy alone is seldom successful in achieving a cure. Surgery (valvulectomy for tricuspid endocarditis, valve replacement for left-sided endocarditis) should be performed soon after the diagnosis is established. Following surgery, amphotericin B is continued for 6 to 8 weeks. The therapeutic advantage of adding 5-fluorocytosine to amphotericin B in Candida endocarditis is not established.

EMPIRIC THERAPY

Initial empiric therapy for native valve endocarditis presenting subacutely, before results of blood cultures are known, is directed against viridans streptococci and enterococci (i.e., penicillin combined with gentamicin). If the onset is acute, antistaphylococcal coverage is added. In patients with prosthetic valve endocarditis or endocarditis associated with intravenous drug abuse, combined therapy with vancomycin and gentamicin is given for the initial empiric therapy. When the infecting organism is identified and its antibiotic susceptibilities are known, specific therapy can be instituted.

CULTURE-NEGATIVE ENDOCARDITIS

Patients with subacute endocarditis and negative blood cultures are usually treated with ampicillin and gentamicin to cover streptococci and HACEK organisms. Careful follow-up and continued search for an etiologic agent is mandatory. If there is no clinical response, other organisms, such as *Coxiella burnetii,* Legionella, Chlamydia, and filamentous fungi, should be considered.

Q fever endocarditis is treated with doxycycline (100 mg PO every 12 hours) in combination with trimethoprim-sulfamethoxazole (160 mg trimethoprim and 800 mg sulfamethoxazole PO every 8 hours). Treatment is continued for 1 to 2 years or longer. The prognosis with medical therapy is poor, and valve replacement is often necessary for cure. Perivalvular abscess complicating Q fever endocarditis has been reported.[85]

MONITORING ADEQUACY OF THERAPY

The serum bactericidal test (SBT) is a direct method for measuring, during antimicrobial therapy, the bactericidal activity of a patient's serum against the organism causing infection. It is the highest dilution of the patient's serum that kills a standard inoculum of the infecting organism *in vitro.* There are many variables in the performance of the test, including the composition of the diluent, the preparation of the inoculum, and the bactericidal endpoint, that affect the results.[86-89] Using a standard SBT, a multicenter study was undertaken to determine the value of the test to predict the outcome of infection among patients with bacterial endocarditis.[90] When all the infecting organisms were considered together, a peak SBT level of ≥1:32 had a predictive value of 98.9% for bacteriologic cure whereas a level of <1:32 had a predictive value for failure of only 28.6%. Thus, although bacteriologic cure could be accurately predicted, the test was a poor predictor of bacteriologic failure. Unless precluded by drug toxicity, it is desirable to achieve a peak SBT of ≥1:32 during treatment of bacterial endocarditis.

Determinations of serum bactericidal titers are not necessary in most cases of infective endocarditis, particularly those caused by streptococci or staphylococci. The serum bactericidal titer is useful when response to therapy is suboptimal or when endocarditis is caused by unusual organisms, such as gram-negative bacilli. The test may result in misleading information in assessing regimens that rely on combinations of antibiotics to produce synergistic bactericidal activity, such as those used in enterococcal endocarditis.

Anticoagulation during active endocarditis, on a theoretical basis to decrease vegetation size, is contraindicated because of the risk of bleeding from an unrecognized mycotic aneurysm or intracranial emboli. In a series of patients with endocarditis, a major intracranial hemorrhage occurred in 3 of 7 patients (43%) treated with anticoagulants compared with only 10 of 211 patients (4.7%) not anticoagulated.[91] However, anticoagulation should be maintained in patients with prosthetic valves that would normally require anticoagulation.

Blood cultures should be obtained daily in the first week after initiating therapy to document clearance of bacteremia. Blood cultures also should be obtained once or twice in the 8 weeks after completion of antibiotic therapy. Relapses, should they occur, manifest themselves by clinical and bacteriologic means and usually respond to retreatment.

Most patients with infective endocarditis become afebrile after 7 to 10 days of appropriate antimicrobial therapy. The common causes of persistent or recurrent fever include (1) perivalvular or myocardial abscesses, (2) splenic abscesses, (3) pulmonary or systemic emboli, (4) drug fever, and (5) thrombophlebitis.

SURGICAL THERAPY

Valve replacement during active infection, first described in 1965,[92] has become an increasingly important adjunct to antimicrobial treatment in the management of infective endocarditis. Many of the complications of endocarditis that contribute to mortality and are not responsive to medical therapy are amenable to aggressive, prompt surgical intervention.

LEFT-SIDED ENDOCARDITIS

The generally accepted indications for cardiac surgery in patients with ongoing native valve endocarditis are congestive heart failure and refractory infection unresponsive to antimicrobial therapy.[93,94]

Congestive Heart Failure

Refractory congestive heart failure, due to incompetence of the aortic or mitral valve or both, is the most frequent cause of death in patients with infective endocarditis and is the prime indication for valve replacement in left-sided endocarditis. The pathoanatomy of valvular dysfunction includes leaflet perforation, erosion of leaflet edges, destruction of leaflets at their commissural attachment, ruptured chordae, and flail leaflets. The virulence of the infecting organism and the size of the vegetation, although statistically correlated with the development of heart failure, are not valuable in predicting whether hemodynamic failure will occur in an individual patient. Among patients with native valve endocarditis treated surgically, heart failure is cited as the indication for operation in more than 85%.[95]

Aortic valve endocarditis is more commonly associated with hemodynamic decompensation than is mitral valve infection. The hemodynamic instability resulting from acute aortic regurgitation progresses rapidly and unpredictably. Therefore, when acute aortic regurgitation is complicated by congestive heart failure, prompt surgery is indicated. In a series of 28 patients with endocarditis who developed acute aortic regurgitation, 4 without heart failure were treated medically and all survived.[96] In contrast, 7 of 11 patients with mild congestive heart failure and 7 of 8 with moderate-to-severe congestive heart failure died during medical therapy. However, 4 of 5 patients with moderately severe heart failure who underwent surgery survived.

In a patient with aortic valve endocarditis, early recognition of valvular dysfunction that will proceed to significant heart failure is essential for appropriate management. The hyperdynamic left ventricle, large stroke volume, wide pulse pressure, and long decrescendo diastolic murmur, which are typical of chronic AR, are not found in acute aortic insufficiency. The left ventricle is often not notably enlarged; stroke volume and pulse pressure are small, and the diastolic murmur is usually soft and brief. The rapid backflow of blood across the aortic valve into a noncompliant small left ventricle results in a prompt rise in left ventricular end-diastolic pressure and closure of the mitral valve before the left ventricle contracts. If closure of the mitral valve, as determined by echocardiography, occurs before the Q wave, the left ventricular end-diastolic pressure is very high, and surgical intervention is urgently required.

Although mitral valve dysfunction due to infective endocarditis is usually manifested as regurgitation, occasionally patients develop mitral stenosis caused by large obstructing vegetations. If low cardiac output and pulmonary edema in this setting are misinterpreted as myocardial depression, the corrective potential for valve replacement will be missed. Echocardiography would clarify the underlying lesion and facilitate the selection of appropriate treatment.

Unresponsive Infection

Infective endocarditis that is unresponsive to antimicrobial therapy is another important and generally accepted indication for surgery. Persistent bacteremia despite appropriate antimicrobial therapy is a prime example of uncontrolled infection. Endocarditis complicated by paravalvular invasion and endocarditis caused by fungi and certain gram-negative bacilli are usually refractory to medical therapy.

PERSISTENT BACTEREMIA. Bacteremia persisting after a variable number of days of appropriate antimicrobial therapy, depending upon the clinical setting, is an indication for surgery on the infected valve. Computed tomography of the abdomen should be performed before surgery, and splenectomy should precede valve replacement if splenic abscesses are present.

PARAVALVULAR INFECTION AND ABSCESS. Infection that has extended beyond the valve leaflet into the valve annulus and adjacent myocardial structures is rarely eradicated by antibiotics. This complication occurs more commonly in the setting of aortic valve endocarditis[97] and is usually associated with *S. aureus* and other virulent organisms, although it may be caused by relatively avirulent organisms such as viridans streptococci (particularly *S. mitis*). Early detection of paravalvular infection and abscess with prompt surgery will minimize tissue destruction and simplify the task of surgical reconstruction.

Clinical clues that suggest paravalvular invasion include fever that persists despite appropriate antimicrobial therapy,[98] new electrocardiographic conduction abnormalities,[99] and purulent pericarditis, which indicates extension of infection from an annular abscess to the pericardial surface. The conduction system runs particularly close to the aortic valve annulus in the region of the right coronary and noncoronary cusps. The development of a new and persistent conduction abnormality, which is not otherwise explained, particularly in a patient with infected aortic valve, usually indicates the presence of a septal abscess.[99] Transesophageal echocardiography is the most sensitive technique for detecting paravalvular abscesses and should be performed if clinical findings suggest that they may be present.

FUNGAL ENDOCARDITIS. Fungal endocarditis is almost always unresponsive to medical therapy. Only a few cases have been treated successfully with antimicrobial therapy.[20,100,101] Optimal management includes early valve replacement followed by a prolonged course of antifungal therapy. There is no evidence to suggest that a few days or weeks of amphotericin B therapy decreases any of the surgical problems and, in fact, this approach may allow embolic events from the friable bulky vegetations that are commonly present.

GRAM-NEGATIVE BACILLARY ENDOCARDITIS. Endocarditis caused by certain gram-negative bacilli, particularly *P. aeruginosa,* is often refractory to antimicrobial therapy.[82] Patients who, in the absence of extracardiac infection, remain bacteremic or persistently febrile after 7 to 10 days of antibiotic therapy should be considered for cardiac surgery. Owing to the high mortality of left-sided *P. aeruginosa* endocarditis treated medically, early valve replacement is recommended.[81,82]

Relative Indications

Cardiac valve replacement in patients with infective endocarditis entails both immediate and long-term risks. These include early operative mortality, recurrent endocarditis involving the prosthesis, periprosthetic leakage and the need for reoperation, thromboembolic complications, and, in patients receiving a mechanical valve, the risk of long-term anticoagulant therapy. In the clinical settings already discussed and accepted widely as indications for surgery, the morbidity and mortality associated with antibiotic therapy alone dramatically outweigh those surgery-related risks. However, in a number of clinical settings, the risk-to-benefit ratio of surgery versus continued medical therapy is less clear, and the physician must weigh the alternatives carefully. These include the presence of a large vegetation, systemic emboli, and relapse following appropriate antimicrobial therapy.

Systemic emboli occur in approximately one third of patients with left-sided infective endocarditis. Because these events may result in irreversible organ dysfunction or death, prevention is a desirable goal. This rationale has led to the recommendation that elective valve replacement be considered if a large echocardiographically detected vegetation, defined as greater than 10 mm at its longest diameter, is present.[94] Studies that correlate vegetation size to the risk of embolism show that although embolization occurs more frequently in patients with large vegetations than in those with smaller lesions, the differences are not statistically significant.[102] Location of vegetation may be an important factor in this regard. Mugge and colleagues[30] found that large vegetations only when located on native mitral valve were associated with an increased risk for embolic events. However, Steckelberg and colleagues[103] found that there was not a significant increase in the risk for emboli among patients with large vegetations, including the subgroup of patients with mitral valve involvement.

The presence of large vegetations is associated with an increased risk of developing heart failure and, therefore, the need for surgery.[26,28,32] However, in the absence of hemodynamic compromise, the presence of a large vegetation by itself is not an indication for valve replacement.[104]

Another controversial recommendation has been that elective valve replacement be considered in patients who have two systemic emboli. There are, however, no data to indicate that a patient with two major emboli is at an increased risk for another embolic event. Furthermore, the rate of embolic events declines steadily after initiation of antimicrobial therapy.[103] Surgery to prevent subsequent emboli might be justified if after one or more systemic emboli there is a residual echocardiographically demonstrable, large highly mobile vegetation. Until there is additional data, emboli remain a controversial indication for surgery.

Relapse of native valve endocarditis is not by itself an indication for cardiac surgery. Patients with relapse of uncomplicated endocarditis due to streptococci or the HACEK organisms are often cured with a second course of antimicrobial therapy. Relapsed endocarditis caused by organisms resistant to multiple drugs, however, may warrant surgery.

RIGHT-SIDED ENDOCARDITIS

In contrast to left-sided endocarditis, in which congestive heart failure is the usual indication for surgical intervention, in right-sided endocarditis refractory infection is the most frequent indication for surgery.[105,106] Most patients with right-sided endocarditis are intravenous drug users in whom the infecting organisms (gram-negative aerobic bacilli, fungi) are difficult to eradicate with antimicrobial therapy.

Right-sided heart failure secondary to tricuspid insufficiency is not usually associated with major hemodynamic instability and does not justify surgery during active infection. Persistent fever and toxicity during therapy in addicts with right-sided endocarditis are usually due to metastatic foci of infection or recurrent pulmonary emboli rather than uncontrolled valvular infection and should not be considered sole indications for surgical intervention. Pulmonary emboli, septic or bland may occur in right-sided endocarditis and produce pulmonary infarction or lung abscess with or without empyema. However, neither recurrent pulmonary emboli nor the presence of large tricuspid vegetations (>10 mm) are by themselves indications for surgical intervention in addicts with tricuspid valve endocarditis.[105]

Tricuspid valve replacement in intravenous drug users is complicated by the high frequency with which these patients resume intravenous drug use and acquire endocarditis on the inserted prosthetic valve. Unless prohibited by significant pulmonary hypertension, valve excision without replacement is the preferred procedure in addiction-related tricuspid valve endocarditis.[107,108] Mild-to-moderate right-sided heart failure may develop, but this is easily tolerated. Subsequent valve replacement is advised only when medical management fails to control the right heart failure. In a group of 55 patients who underwent tricuspid valve excision without replacement, only 6 required the insertion of a prosthesis to control medically refractory right heart failure.[109]

Another surgical approach for tricuspid valve endocarditis is vegetectomy, debridement of infected tissues, and valvuloplasty.[110–114] This procedure, which can be performed if the infection is sufficiently localized, has the advantage of preserving valvular competency.

PROSTHETIC VALVE ENDOCARDITIS

The indications for cardiac surgery in patients with prosthetic valve endocarditis are similar to those for native valve infection. Surgical intervention is mandated by hemodynamic instability resulting from prosthesis dysfunction, paravalvular invasion infection, persistent bacteremia, and fungal endocarditis. Nearly one half of patients with prosthetic valve endocarditis will require cardiac surgery during active infection. The risk of recurrent endocarditis after the surgical removal of an infected prosthesis is approximately 5%.

The pathology of prosthetic valve endocarditis explains the frequent necessity of surgical intervention. Local spread of the infectious process into the valve anulus is commonly present. Unusually large vegetations may obstruct blood flow and cause functional valvular stenosis or a combination of stenosis and regurgitation. The pathologic findings in porcine bioprostheses that become infected within 1 year after placement are similar to those in mechanical valves. However, when infection occurs more than 1 year after surgery, it is more likely to be confined to the leaflets. Valve replacement may still be required because of leaflet destruction and acute valve incompetence or because of damage that subsequently results in the development of leaflet rigidity and valve stenosis.

Patients with prosthetic valve endocarditis and moderate-to-severe heart failure secondary to prosthesis dysfunction require emergency valve replacement.[115,116] The mortality rate for those treated medically is 100%[116,117]; valve replacement combined with antimicrobial therapy reduces mortality to approximately 50%. Emergency valve replacement also is required in patients who develop acute prosthetic obstruction due to large vegetations.

Invasion of paravalvular or anular tissue, with abscess formation and valve dehiscence, mandates surgical intervention. This complication occurs most frequently in patients with aortic valve endocarditis. The clinical finding of a paravalvular leak in a patient with prosthetic valve endocarditis is presumptive evidence of a valve ring abscess. Prosthetic valve endocarditis caused by coagulase-negative staphylococci or S. aureus is frequently complicated by invasive infection and valve dysfunction; consequently most patients will require surgical treatment if the infection is to be cured. The risk of death or periprosthetic leakage requiring repeat cardiac surgery is greater when surgery is performed for paravalvular abscess than for congestive heart failure.

Because of the high frequency of major emboli and lack of response to medical therapy, early valve replacement is recommended for fungal prosthetic valve endocarditis. Persistent bacteremia for more than a few days after the initiation of appropriate antimicrobial therapy and in the absence of an extracardiac focus of infection mandates surgical intervention.

Infections of prosthetic valves due to organisms other than viridans streptococci and the HACEK organisms[118] are difficult to eradicate with antibiotics alone; most patients will require surgery. Relapsed prosthetic valve endocarditis after a course of appropriate antimicrobial therapy is often associated with paravalvular invasive infection; consequently most patients will require surgical treatment if the infection is to be cured.

The role of systemic emboli as an indication for surgery in patients with prosthetic valve endocarditis is similar to that described for native valve endocarditis.

TIMING OF SURGERY

The mortality rate for patients treated surgically for endocarditis is directly related to the hemodynamic dysfunction at the time of surgery. For optimal outcome, patients that will ultimately require surgery should be identified before the development of overwhelming hemodynamic instability or extensive perivalvular tissue destruction. Endocarditis complicated by intractable heart failure due to valve dysfunction is an indication for urgent cardiac surgery regardless of the duration of previous antibiotic therapy. Similarly, a patient with prosthetic valve endocarditis and valve dysfunction due to invasive perivalvular infection should undergo emergency cardiac surgery.

PROPHYLAXIS

The rationale for antimicrobial prophylaxis in infective endocarditis is based on three well-recognized facts. First, persons with certain structural abnormalities of the heart or great vessels are at greatly increased risk for developing infective endocarditis. Second, 15% to 20% of cases of infective endocarditis occur as a consequence of transient bacteremia caused by dental and surgical procedures and instrumentation involving mucosal surfaces colonized with bacteria.[119,120] Third, infective endocarditis occurring after these procedures is usually caused by streptococci and enterococci, which have predictable antibiotic susceptibility patterns.

A key element in the development of endocarditis is the occurrence of a transient bacteremia.[120] Transient bacteremia arises when a mucosal surface colonized with bacteria is traumatized.[121] It is usually a benign, self-limited event with no symptoms and no sequelae, except in patients who are at risk for developing infective endocarditis. Transient bacteremias occur commonly in everyday life in association with activities such as mastication and brushing or flossing of the teeth. However, when associated with dental or surgical procedures, the magnitude of bacteremia is greater and the corresponding risk of endocarditis is substantially higher.

Controlled clinical trials to evaluate the efficacy of antimicrobials in preventing endocarditis associated with dental and surgical procedures have not been done and may never be because of the large number of subjects required.[122] It is, however, possible to demonstrate the efficacy of prophylaxis by case-control studies[123] or by selecting a subgroup of patients at highest risk for endocarditis. In a retrospective study of patients with prosthetic heart valves, no cases of endocarditis occurred after 287 procedures for which antimicrobial prophylaxis was given, whereas 6 cases followed 390 procedures for which it was omitted.[124] Indirect evidence of the prophylactic efficacy of antibiotics is the paucity of reported cases of endocarditis in persons who have received adequate prophylaxis.

Even if prophylaxis for endocarditis were completely effective, less than 10% of all cases could be prevented. Viridans streptococci and enterococci, organisms against which prophylaxis is targeted, account for 50% of all endocarditis cases. However, only 25% of patients with endocarditis due to viridans streptococci and 40% of those with endocarditis caused by enterococci develop their infection in association with procedures for which prophylaxis could be given.[119,125] Furthermore, only one half of patients with endocarditis have a recognized or recognizable predisposing cardiac condition that would qualify them for prophylaxis.

Antimicrobial agents administered prophylactically before dental or surgical procedures do not prevent the transient bacteremias that may occur. They may, however, interfere with the adherence of bacteria to cardiac lesions, eradicate organisms that adhere to the lesions, or prevent their multiplication long enough for the host defenses to eradicate them.

Patients in whom endocarditis developed despite administration of prophylactic antibiotics have been reported.[126] Most of these infections occurred after dental procedures, and 75% were caused by viridans streptococci. In two thirds of the cases, the infecting organisms were sensitive to the antibiotic(s) that had been given for prophylaxis.

The AHA first published guidelines for preventing endocarditis in 1965. A fourth revision was published in December 1990.[127] Like the previous revisions, the current recommendations are based upon a review of the available data on the relationship of endocarditis to underlying cardiac lesions and to procedures that may cause transient bacteremia, the frequency and magnitude of transient bacteremia following particular procedures, and the efficacy of prophylactic antibiotics in experimental endocarditis. The updated guidelines offer improved practicality and close agreement with advice offered by the Endocarditis Working Party of the British Society for Antimicrobial Chemotherapy,[128] and recommendations published in *The Medical Letter of Drug Therapy.*[129]

CARDIAC LESIONS

The risk of developing infective endocarditis depends upon the underlying cardiac lesion. An essential step in deciding whether to use prophylaxis is to assess the relative risk presented by the patient's preexisting heart disease. Although few quantitative data are available, clinical experience shows that certain lesions are associated with a higher risk of endocarditis than others. Antimicrobial prophylaxis is recommended only for patients with high-risk cardiac lesions (Table 8–6).[127] Patients who have prosthetic heart valves, a previous history of endocarditis, or surgically constructed systemic-pulmonary shunts are at highest risk for endocarditis. Other conditions that present a high risk of endocarditis include rheumatic and other acquired valvular dysfunction, hypertrophic cardiomyopathy, and many congenital cardiac malformations, including bicuspid aortic valve, ventricular septal defect, patent ductus arteriosus, and cyanotic congenital heart disease.

Table 8–6. Cardiac Conditions

Endocarditis prophylaxis recommended:
- Prosthetic cardiac valves, including bioprosthetic and homograft valves
- Previous bacterial endocarditis, even in the absence of heart disease
- Most congenital cardiac malformations
- Rheumatic and other acquired valvular dysfunction, even after valvular surgery
- Hypertrophic cardiomyopathy
- Mitral valve prolapse with valvular regurgitation

Endocarditis prophylaxis not recommended:
- Isolated secundum atrial septal defect
- Surgical repair without residua beyond 6 months of secundum atrial septal defect, ventricular septal defect, or patent ductus arteriosus
- Previous coronary artery bypass graft surgery
- Mitral valve prolapse without valvular regurgitation
- Physiologic, functional, or innocent heart murmurs
- Previous Kawasaki disease without valvular dysfunction
- Previous rheumatic fever without valvular dysfunction
- Cardiac pacemakers and implanted defibrillators

Source: Adapted from Dajani et al.[127]

Mitral Valve Prolapse

Among adults with subacute native valve endocarditis, mitral valve prolapse is the underlying lesion in 20% to 30% of cases.[130–133] Mitral valve prolapse is estimated to occur in 4% to 7% of the population. However, only individuals with mitral-regurgitant murmurs are at substantially high risk for endocarditis.[134] In a case-control study, the risk of developing infective endocarditis was 35 times greater among those with a murmur than those who did not have a murmur.[135] Individuals who have a mitral valve prolapse associated with thickening or redundancy of the valve leaflets may also be at increased risk for endocarditis,[136] particularly men who are 45 years of age or older.

The AHA recommends prophylaxis for individuals with mitral valve prolapse who have *valvular regurgitation* (VR). This definition would rule out prophylaxis for those with mitral valve prolapse manifested only by a systolic click. However, what is meant by VR is not specified. Clearly, prophylaxis is indicated for individuals who have a holosystolic murmur. Whether the presence of a late systolic murmur, either spontaneous or evoked, or echocardiographic evidence of regurgitation without auscultatory findings warrants prophylaxis remains to be clarified.

Degenerative Valve Lesions

Infective endocarditis associated with degenerative (sclerotic or calcific) forms of valvular disease is being recognized with increasing frequency.[132] Murmurs originating from such aortic or mitral valvular lesions are common in elderly patients; however, the existent data do not allow accurate estimations of the risk-benefit ratio of prophylaxis for these patients. The current AHA recommendations are relatively silent on this issue. Some clinicians advocate prophylaxis for those patients who have clinical and echocardiographic evidence of significant valvular dysfunction. It is not practical, nor in all likelihood risk-beneficial, to mandate prophylaxis for all elderly patients with nondescript systolic murmurs.

Procedures Requiring Prophylaxis

Three variables must be taken into consideration to determine which procedures do (Table 8–7) or do not require antimicrobial prophylaxis: (1) the frequency with which a particular procedure has been epidemiologically associated with endocarditis, (2) the frequency with which the procedure gives rise to transient bacteremia, and (3) whether the organisms entering the blood are those commonly associated with endocarditis. Viridans streptococci and enterococci adhere much more readily to platelet-fibrin deposits on valvular endothelium than do gram-negative bacilli and are more likely to cause endocarditis after transient bacteremias. Antimicrobial prophylaxis is recommended for procedures that are likely to produce bacteremia due to viridans streptococci or enterococci.

Dental and Upper Respiratory Tract Procedures

Transient bacteremia occurs frequently after a wide range of dental and oropharyngeal procedures known to induce gingival or mucosal bleeding. In one study, transient bacteremia was detected in 59% of adults following dental extraction under general anesthesia.[137] Bacteremia usually occurs within 1 to 5 minutes of the extraction, lasts only a few minutes, and is low grade (10 to 15 colony-forming units per ml of blood). Viridans streptococci are the most frequent isolates. Without prophylaxis, the risk of developing endocarditis after dental extraction in a person with preexisting valvular heart disease is probably less than 1 in 500.[138]

Antimicrobial prophylaxis for endocarditis is indicated for all dental proce-

Table 8–7. Procedures for Which Endocarditis Prophylaxis Is Recommended

Dental procedures:
    Dental extraction
    Professional dental cleaning
    Periodontal surgery
Oropharyngeal and respiratory tract procedures:
    Tonsillectomy
    Adenoidectomy
    Surgical procedures involving respiratory mucosa
    Bronchoscopy with a rigid bronchoscope
Genitourinary procedures:
    Cystoscopy
    Prostatic surgery
    Urethral dilation
    Urethral catheterization if urinary tract infection is present
    Urinary tract surgery if urinary tract infection is present
Gastrointestinal procedures
    Gallbladder surgery
    Esophageal dilation
    Sclerotherapy for esophageal varices
    Intestinal surgery
Gynecologic and obstetric procedures
    Vaginal hysterectomy
    Vaginal delivery in the presence of infection
Incision and drainage of infected tissue

Source: Adapted from Dajani et al.[127]

dures likely to induce gingival or mucosal bleeding, including dental extractions, periodontal surgery, and professional dental cleaning. If a series of dental procedures is required, it may be prudent to maintain an interval of 7 days between procedures to reduce potential for the emergence of microbial resistance in the oral flora. Injection of local intraoral anesthetic (except intraligamentary injections), filling of cavities along the gum line, simple adjustment of orthodontic appliances, and spontaneous shedding of primary teeth do not require antimicrobial prophylaxis.

Nonpreventable, non–procedure-associated endocarditis due to viridans streptococci is largely related to transient bacteremias that occur in everyday life. Poor dental hygiene and periodontal infection enhance the frequency and intensity of these bacteremias and the associated risk of endocarditis in individuals with predisposing cardiac lesions. Such individuals should establish and maintain the best possible oral health to reduce potential sources of transient bacteremia. Topical chlorhexidine applied to gingiva 3 to 5 minutes before tooth extraction reduces the frequency and the magnitude of any resulting bacteremia and may be used as an adjunct to antibiotic prophylaxis, particularly in patients who are at high risk or have poor dental hygiene.

Antimicrobial prophylaxis is also recommended for nondental procedures that allow migration of bacteria from the oropharynx and respiratory tract into the bloodstream. These include tonsillectomy, adenoidectomy, surgical procedures involving respiratory mucosa, and bronchoscopy with a rigid bronchoscope. Prophylaxis is not recommended for endotracheal intubation and bronchoscopy with a flexible bronchoscope (with or without biopsy), except in patients who have prosthetic heart valves, a previous history of endocarditis, or surgically constructed systemic-pulmonary shunts, where it is considered optional. Endocarditis has not been reported in association with insertion of tympanostomy tubes.

Genitourinary and Gastrointestinal Procedures

Surgery or instrumentation of the genitourinary or gastrointestinal tract may be associated with transient bacteremia that can cause endocarditis in persons with predisposing cardiac lesions. The genitourinary tract is the portal of entry for enterococci in 20% to 50% of patients with endocarditis due to this organism. The frequency of bacteremia following urinary tract procedures is particularly high if urinary tract infection is present. Possible sources of bacteremia when the urine is sterile include normal urethral flora and bacteria in the prostate, if present.

Antimicrobial prophylaxis is recommended for cystoscopy, prostatic surgery, urethral dilation, urethral catheterization or urinary tract surgery in the presence of infected urine, vaginal hysterectomy, and vaginal delivery in the persence of infection. The current AHA recommendations also include prophylaxis for gallbladder surgery, intestinal surgery, esophageal dilation, and sclerotherapy for esophageal varices.

Very few cases of bacterial endocarditis related to gastrointestinal diagnostic procedures have been reported, and most of those are inadequately documented.[139] The mean incidence of transient bacteremia associated with these procedures, including esophagogastroduodenoscopy, proctosigmoidoscopy, colonoscopy, endoscopic retrograde cholangiopancreatography, barium enema, and liver biopsy, ranges from 3% to 6%.[140,141] Although some of these bacteremias are caused by

Table 8–8. Procedures for Which Endocarditis Prophylaxis Is
Not Recommended

Dental/oral procedures:
    Filling of cavities above the gum line
    Simple adjustment of orthodontic appliances
    Shedding of primary teeth
    Injection of local intraoral anesthetic (except intraligamentary injections)
Lower respiratory tract procedures*
    Endotracheal intubation
    Bronchoscopy with a flexible bronchoscope, with or without biopsy
Genitourinary procedures*
    Urethral catheterization in the absence of infection
Gastrointestinal procedures*
    Gastrointestinal endoscopies with or without biopsy
Gynecologic and obstetric procedures*
    Cesarean section
    In the absence of infection:
      Uncomplicated vaginal delivery
      Dilation and curettage
      Therapeutic abortion
      Sterilization procedures
      Insertion or removal of intrauterine devices
Cardiac catheterization

Source: Adapted from Dajani et al.[127]
*In patients who have prosthetic heart valves, a previous history of endocarditis, or surgically constructed systemic-pulmonary shunts or conduits, physicians may choose to administer prophylactic antibiotics.

enterococci, the majority are due to anaerobes or gram-negative enteric bacilli that are unlikely to cause endocarditis.

Prophylaxis is not recommended for gastrointestinal endoscopies with or without biopsy, barium enema, percutaneous liver biopsy, cesarean section, and in the absence of infection for urethral catheterization, uncomplicated vaginal delivery, dilation and curettage, therapeutic abortion, sterilization procedures, and insertion or removal of intrauterine devices (Table 8–8). However, in patients with prosthetic heart valves, surgically constructed systemic-pulmonary shunts, or a previous history of endocarditis, administration of prophylactic antibiotics for these low-risk procedures is considered optional.

PROPHYLACTIC REGIMENS

Prophylaxis is most effective when it is given perioperatively in doses that are sufficient to provide adequate serum concentrations at the time the procedure is performed. To reduce emergence of microbial resistance, prophylactic antibiotics should be started shortly before the procedure and continued for no more than 6 to 8 hours.

Dental and Upper Respiratory Tract Procedures

Endocarditis following dental and upper respiratory procedures is usually caused by viridans streptococci. Antimicrobial prophylaxis, therefore, is specifically directed against these organisms (Table 8–9).

In the new AHA recommendations, amoxicillin has replaced penicillin V as

Table 8–9. Recommended Prophylactic Regimen for Dental,
Oral, or Upper Respiratory Tract Procedures

Standard Regimen

Patients not allergic to penicillins:
　　Amoxicillin, 3.0 g orally 1 h before procedure; then 1.5 g 6 h after initial dose
Penicillin-allergic patients:
　　Erythromycin ethylsuccinate, 800 mg, or **erythromycin stearate,** 1.0 g, orally 2 h before proce-
　　dure; then half the dose 6 h after initial dose

or

　　Clindamycin, 300 mg orally 1 h before procedure, then 150 mg 6 h after initial dose

Parenteral Regimen for Patients Unable to Take Oral Medications

Patients not allergic to penicillins:
　　Ampicillin, 2.0 g IV or IM, 30 minutes before procedure, followed by ampicillin, 1.0 g IV or IM,
　　or amoxicillin, 1.5 g PO, 6 h after initial dose
Penicillin-allergic patients:
　　Clindamycin, 300 mg IV, 30 minutes before procedure, followed by 150 mg IV or PO, 6 h after
　　initial dose

Source: Adapted from Dajani et al.[127]
Initial pediatric doses are as follows: amoxicillin, 50 mg/kg; erythromycin ethylsuccinate or erythromycin stearate,
20 mg/kg; clindamycin, 10 mg/kg, and ampicillin 50 mg/kg. Follow-up doses should be one half the initial dose. **Total
pediatric dose should not exceed total adult dose.** The following weight ranges also may be used for the initial pediatric
dose of amoxicillin: <15 kg, 750 mg; 15–30 kg, 1500 mg; and >30 kg, 3000 mg (full adult dose).

the standard oral agent for prophylaxis in patients undergoing dental, oral, or upper
respiratory procedures. Importantly, the oral regimen is also recommended for the
highest-risk patients (e.g., those with prosthetic valves). The in vitro activity of
amoxicillin against viridans streptococci is comparable with that of penicillin V.
However, amoxicillin is better absorbed from the gastrointestinal tract and has a
longer elimination half-life, resulting in higher and more prolonged blood levels.

For penicillin-allergic individuals, erythromycin or clindamycin is recommended. In choosing an erythromycin preparation, the rate of absorption is a critical variable in determining when the initial dose is given. After oral administration, erythromycin stearate and erythromycin ethylsuccinate achieve peak serum
levels at 1 to 3 hours; however, enteric-coated tablets do not provide peak levels
until 3 to 5 hours after ingestion. Because of more reliable absorption, the new
AHA recommendations specify erythromycin ethylsuccinate or erythromycin stearate for penicillin-allergic individuals. For those who cannot tolerate either penicillins or erythromycin, clindamycin is the recommended alternative.

For individuals at risk who are unable to take oral medication, parenteral
ampicillin is recommended. In the presence of penicillin allergy, intravenous clindamycin may be used.

Patients who have received a recent therapeutic course of penicillin, or who
are on oral penicillin V for prevention of rheumatic fever, may harbor in their oral
cavity viridans streptococci that are relatively resistant to penicillin. For those who
have just completed a course of penicillin and whose dental problems are not
urgent, it may be prudent to delay dental procedures for 2 to 3 weeks to allow
reconstitution of normal oral flora. For patients whose problems require more
immediate attention and those who are on penicillin V for prevention of rheumatic

fever, an alternative agent (i.e., erythromycin or clindamycin) should be selected for endocarditis prophylaxis. This problem does not arise in patients who are receiving monthly intramuscular benzathine penicillin G prophylaxis for rheumatic fever.

Antibiotic regimens used to prevent recurrences of acute rheumatic fever are not adequate for the prevention of infective endocarditis. Therefore, patients who are already on a prophylactic regimen for rheumatic fever must receive endocarditis prophylaxis at the time of dental or surgical procedures.

Genitourinary and Gastrointestinal Tract Procedures

Infective endocarditis following genitourinary or gastrointestinal tract surgery or instrumentation is usually caused by enterococci. Although transient gram-negative bacteremia may occur in association with these procedures, gram-negative bacilli are only rarely responsible for endocarditis. Thus, antimicrobial prophylaxis is directed primarily against enterococci (Table 8–10).

The recommended regimen for prevention of bacterial endocarditis in patients undergoing genitourinary or gastrointestinal procedures is ampicillin plus gentamicin, both administered parenterally, followed by one dose of oral amoxicillin or a second dose of both parenteral agents. In penicillin-allergic individuals, parenterally administered vancomycin plus gentamicin, which may be repeated once, should be used. These parenteral regimens are recommended for all patients with high-risk cardiac lesions, particularly those at highest risk, that is, patients with prosthetic heart valves, a previous history of endocarditis, or surgically constructed systemic-pulmonary shunts. For low-risk patients, an alternative oral regimen (amoxicillin) is provided.

CARDIAC SURGERY

Patients undergoing open heart surgery with placement of mechanical or bioprosthetic valves are at high risk for postoperative infective endocarditis. Endocarditis in these patients is most often due to coagulase-negative staphylococci or *S. aureus*. Although a first-generation cephalosporin is most commonly used, vanco-

Table 8–10. Regimens for Genitourinary/Gastrointestinal Procedures

---

Patients not allergic to penicillin (standard regimen):
   Ampicillin, 2.0 g IM or IV plus **gentamicin,** 1.5 mg/kg (not to exceed 80 mg) IM or IV 30 minutes before procedure; followed by **amoxicillin,** 1.5 g orally 6 h after initial dose; alternatively, the parenteral regimen may be repeated once 8 h after initial dose
Penicillin-allergic patients:
   Vancomycin, 1.0 g IV slowly over 1 h plus **gentamicin,** 1.5 mg/kg (not to exceed 80 mg) IM or IV, 1 h before procedure; may be repeated once 8 h after initial dose
Alternate low-risk patient regimen:
   Amoxicillin, 3.0 g orally 1 h before procedure; then 1.5 g 6 h after initial dose

---

Source: Adapted from Dajani et al.[127]
   Initial pediatric doses are as follows: ampicillin, 50 mg/kg; amoxicillin, 50 mg/kg; gentamicin, 2.0 mg/kg; and vancomycin, 20 mg/kg. Follow-up doses should be half the initial dose. **Total pediatric dose should not exceed total adult dose.**

mycin is the most logical choice because the majority of coagulase-negative staphylococci are methicillin-resistant and therefore resistant to cephalosporins. High prevalence of infections caused by methicillin-resistant *S. aureus* in a particular institution should prompt usage of vancomycin for perioperative prophylaxis.

Antimicrobial prophylaxis for cardiac surgery should be started immediately before the operative procedure and continued for 24 hours. The effects of cardiopulmonary bypass and compromised postoperative renal function on the clearance of antibiotics should be considered in dosing schedules during the procedure.

Prophylactic antibiotics are not required for cardiac catheterization and angiography because with adequate aseptic techniques the occurrence of endocarditis following these procedures is extremely low.

REFERENCES

1. Kaye, D: Changing pattern of infective endocarditis. Am J Med 78(Suppl 6B):157, 1985.
2. Terpenning, MS, Buggy, BP, and Kauffman, CA: Infective endocarditis: Clinical features in young and elderly patients. Am J Med 83:626, 1987.
3. Weiss, H and Ottenberg, R: Relation between bacteria and temperature in subacute bacterial endocarditis. J Infect Dis 50:61, 1932.
4. Beeson, PB, Brannon, ES, and Warren, JV: Observations on the sites of removal of bacteria from the blood in patients with bacterial endocarditis. J Exp Med 81:9, 1945.
5. Mallen, MS, Hube, EL, and Brenes, M: Comparative study of blood cultures made from artery, vein, and bone marrow in patients with subacute bacterial endocarditis. Am Heart J 33:692, 1947.
6. Werner, AS, Cobbs, CG, Kaye, D, et al: Studies on the bacteremia of bacterial endocarditis. JAMA 202:199, 1967.
7. Washington, JA: Blood cultures: An overview. Eur J Clin Microbiol Infect Dis 8:803, 1989.
8. Arpi, M, Bentzon, MW, Jensen, J, et al: Importance of blood volume cultured in the detection of bacteremia. Eur J Clin Microbiol Infect Dis 8:838, 1989.
9. Raucher, B, Dobkin, J, Mandel, L, et al: Occult polymicrobial endocarditis with *Haemophilus parainfluenzae* in intravenous drug abusers. Am J Med 86:169, 1989.
10. Tobin, MJ, Cahill, N, Gearty, G, et al: Q fever endocarditis. Am J Med 72:396, 1982.
11. Fernandez-Guerrero, ML, Muelas, JM, and Aquado, JM: Q fever endocarditis on porcine bioprosthetic valves. Ann Intern Med 108:209, 1988.
12. Tompkins, LS, Roessler, BJ, Redd, SC, et al: Legionella prosthetic-valve endocarditis. N Engl J Med 318:530, 1988.
13. Jacobs, F, Abramowicz, D, Vereerstraeten, P, et al: Brucella endocarditis: The role of combined medical and surgical treatment. Rev Infect Dis 12:740, 1990.
14. Jones, RB, Priest, JB, and Kuo, GC: Subacute chlamydoal endocarditis. JAMA 247:655, 1982.
15. Marrie, TJ, Harczy, M, Mann, OE, et al: Culture-negative endocarditis probably due to *Chlamydia pneumoniae.* J Infect Dis 161:127, 1990.
16. Cohen, JI, Sloss, LJ, Kundsin, R, et al: Prosthetic valve endocarditis caused by *Mycoplasma hominis.* Am J Med 86:819, 1989.
17. Carrizosa, J, Levison, ME, Lawrence, T, et al: Cure of *Aspergillus ustus* endocarditis of prosthetic valve. Arch Intern Med 133:486, 1974.
18. Rinaldi, MG: Invasive aspergillosis. Rev Infect Dis 5:1061, 1983.
19. Goodwin, RA, Jr, Shapiro, JL, Thurman, GH, et al: Disseminated histoplasmosis: Clinical and pathologic correlations. Medicine 51:1, 1980.
20. Kanawaty, D, Stalker, JB, and Munt, PW: Nonsurgical treatment of Histoplasma endocarditis involving a bioprosthetic valve. Chest 99:253, 1991.
21. Dillon, JC, Feigenbaum, H, Konecke, LL, et al: Echocardiographic manifestations of valvular vegetations. Am Heart J 86:698, 1973.
22. Spangler, RD, Johnson, MC, Holmes, J, et al: Echocardiographic demonstration of bacterial vegetations in active infective endocarditis. J Clin Ultrasound 1:126, 1973.
23. Matsuzaki, M, Toma, Y, and Kusukawa, R: Clinical applications of transesophageal echocardiography. Circulation 82:709, 1990.

24. Taams, MA, Gussenhoven, EJ, Bos, E, et al: Enhanced morphological diagnosis in infective endo-
    carditis by transesophageal echocardiography. Br Heart J 63:109, 1990.
25. Martin, RP: The diagnostic and prognostic role of cardiovascular ultrasound in endocarditis: Big-
    ger is not better. J Am Coll Cardiol 15:1227, 1990.
26. O'Brien, JT and Geiser, EA: Infective endocarditis and echocardiography. Am Heart J 108:386,
    1984.
27. Buda, AJ, Zotz, RJ, LeMire, MS, et al: Prognostic significance of vegetations detected by two-
    dimensional echocardiography in infective endocarditis. Am Heart J 112:1291, 1986.
28. Stewart, JA, Silimperi, D, Harris, P, et al: Echocardiographic documentation of vegetative lesions
    in infective endocarditis: Clinical implications. Circulation 61:374, 1980.
29. Erbel, R, Rohmann, S, Drexler, M, et al: Improved diagnostic value of echocardiography in
    patients with infective endocarditis by transesophageal approach. A prospective study. Eur
    Heart J 9:45, 1988.
30. Mugge, A, Daniel, WG, Frank, G, et al: Echocardiography in infective endocarditis: Reassessment
    of prognostic implications of vegetation size determined by the transthoracic and the trans-
    esophageal approach. J Am Coll Cardiol 14:631, 1989.
31. Melvin, ET, Berger, M, Lutzker, LG, et al: Non-invasive methods for detection of valve vegetations
    in infective endocarditis. Am J Cardiol 47:271, 1981.
32. Lutas, EM, Roberts, RB, Devereux, RB, et al: Relation between the presence of echocardiographic
    vegetations and the complication rate in infective endocarditis. Am Heart J 112:107, 1986.
33. Ellis, SG, Goldstein, J, and Popp, RL: Detection of endocarditis-associated perivalvular abscesses
    by two-dimensional echocardiography. J Am Coll Cardiol 5:647, 1985.
34. Byrd, BF, III, Shelton, ME, Wilson, BH, III, et al: Infective perivalvular abscess of the aortic ring:
    Echocardiographic features and clinical course. Am J Cardiol 66:102, 1990.
35. Saner, HE, Asinger, RW, Homans, DC, et al: Two-dimensional echocardiographic identification
    of complicated aortic root endocarditis: Implications for surgery. J Am Coll Cardiol 10:859,
    1987.
36. Mulcahy, D, Shapiro, LM, Westgate, C, et al: The diagnosis of aortic root abscess by cross-sectional
    echocardiography. Clin Radiol 37:235, 1986.
37. Daniel, WG, Mugge, A, Martin, RP, et al: Improvement in the diagnosis of abscesses associated
    with endocarditis by transesophageal echocardiography. N Engl J Med 12:795, 1991.
38. Chow, LC, Dittrich, HC, Dembitsky, WP, et al: Accurate localization of ruptured sinus of Valsalva
    aneurysm by real-time two-dimensional Doppler flow imaging. Chest 94:462, 1988.
39. Bansal, RC, Graham, BM, Jutzy, KR, et al: Left ventricular outflow tract to left atrial communi-
    cation secondary to rupture of mitral-aortic intervalvular fibrosa in infective endocarditis:
    Diagnosis by transesophageal echocardiography and color flow imaging. J Am Coll Cardiol
    15:499, 1990.
40. Karalis, DG, Chandrasekaran, K, Wahl, JM, et al: Transesophageal echocardiographic recognition
    of mitral valve abnormalities associated with aortic valve endocarditis. Am Heart J 119:1209,
    1990.
41. Nellessen, U, Schnittger, I, Appleton, CP, et al: Transesophageal two-dimensional echocardiogra-
    phy and color flow velocity mapping in the evaluation of cardiac valve prosthesis. Circulation
    78:848, 1988.
42. Dittrich, HC, McCann, HA, Walsh, TP, et al: Transesophageal echocardiography in the evaluation
    of prosthetic and native aortic valve. Am J Cardiol 66:758, 1990.
43. Pearlman, AS: Transesophageal echocardiography—sound diagnostic technique or two-edged
    sword? N Engl J Med 324:841, 1991.
44. Durack, DT and Beeson, PB: Experimental bacterial endocarditis. II. Survival of bacteria in endo-
    cardial vegetations. Br J Exp Pathol 53:50, 1972.
45. Bisno, AL, Dismukes, WE, Durack, DT, et al: Antimicrobial treatment of infective endocarditis
    due to viridans streptococci, enterococci, and staphylococci. JAMA 261:1471, 1989.
46. Ruoff, KL: Nutritionally variant streptococci. Clin Microbiol Rev 4:184, 1991.
47. Karchmer, AW, Moellering, RC, Jr, Maki, DG, et al: Single antibiotic therapy for streptococcal
    endocarditis. JAMA 241:1801, 1979.
48. Malacoff, RF, Frank, E, and Andriole, VT: Streptococcal endocarditis (nonenterococcal, non-
    group A). Single vs. combination therapy. JAMA 241:1807, 1979.
49. Wilson, WR and Geraci, JE: Treatment of streptococcal infective endocarditis. Am J Med 78:128,
    1985.

50. Wilson, WR: Antimicrobial therapy of streptococcal endocarditis. J Antimicrob Chemother 20 (Suppl A):147, 1987.
51. Hamburger, M and Stein, L: *Streptococcus viridans* subacute bacterial endocarditis: Two week treatment schedule with penicillin. JAMA 149:542, 1952.
52. Sande, MA and Scheld, WM: Combination antibiotic therapy of bacterial endocarditis. Ann Intern Med 92:390, 1980.
53. Enzler, MJ, Rouse, MS, Henry, NK, et al: In vitro and in vivo studies of streptomycin-resistant, penicillin-susceptible streptococci from patients with infective endocarditis. J Infect Dis 155:954, 1987.
54. Wolfe, JC and Johnson, WD, Jr: Penicillin-sensitive streptococcal endocarditis: In vitro and clinical observations on penicillin-streptomycin therapy. Ann Intern Med 81:178, 1974.
55. DiNubile, MJ: Treatment of endocarditis caused by relatively resistant nonenterococcal streptococci: Is penicillin enough? Rev Infect Dis 12:112, 1990.
56. Stein, DS and Nelson, KE: Endocarditis due to nutritionally deficient streptococci: Therapeutic dilemma. Rev Infect Dis 9:908, 1987.
57. Gallagher, PG and Watanakunakorn, C: Group B streptococcal endocarditis: Report of seven cases and review of the literature, 1962–1985. Rev Infect Dis 8:175, 1986.
58. Vatian, C, Lerner, PI, Shlaes, DM, et al: Infections due to Lancefield group G streptococci. Medicine 64:75, 1985.
59. Powderly, WG, Stanley, SI, Jr, and Medoff, G: Pneumococcal endocarditis: Report of a series and review of the literature. Rev Infect Dis 5:786, 1986.
60. Maki, DG and Agger, WA: Enterococcal bacteremia: Clinical features, the risk of endocarditis, and management. Medicine 67:248, 1988.
61. Murray, BE and Mederski-Samoraj, B: Transferable beta-lactamase: A new mechanism for in vitro penicillin resistance in *Streptococcus faecalis.* J Clin Invest 72:1168, 1983.
62. Bush, LM, Calmon, J, Cherney, CL, et al: High-level penicillin resistance among isolates of enterococci. Ann Intern Med 110:515, 1989.
63. Uttley, AH, Collins, CH, Naidoo, J, et al: Vancomycin-resistant enterococci. Lancet 1:57, 1988.
64. Storch, GA, Krogstad, DA, and Parquette, AR: Antibiotic-induced lysis of enterococci. J Clin Invest 68:639, 1981.
65. Krogstad, DJ and Parquette, AR: Defective killing of enterococci: A common property of antimicrobial agents acting on the cell wall. Antimicrob Agents Chemother 17:965, 1980.
66. Mederski-Samoraj, B and Murray, BE: High-level resistance to gentamicin in clinical isolates of enterococci. J Infect Dis 147:751, 1983.
67. Wilson, WR, Wilkowski, CJ, Wright, AJ, et al: Treatment of streptomycin-susceptible and streptomycin-resistant enterococcal endocarditis. Ann Intern Med 100:816, 1984.
68. Chambers, HF, Korzeniowski, OM, Sande, MA, et al: *Staphylococcus aureus* endocarditis: Clinical manifestations in addicts and nonaddicts. Medicine 62:170, 1983.
69. Kaye, D: Infecting microorganisms. In Kaye, D (ed): Infective Endocarditis. University Park Press, Baltimore, 1976, p 43.
70. Caputo, GM, Archer, GL, Calderwood, SB, et al: Native valve endocarditis due to coagulase-negative staphylococci. Clinical and microbiologic features. Am J Med 83:619, 1987.
71. Korzeniowski, OM and Sande, MA: The National Collaborative Endocarditis Study Group. Combination antimicrobial therapy for *Staphylococcus aureus* endocarditis in patients addicted to parenteral drugs and in nonaddicts. A prospective study. Ann Intern Med 97:496, 1982.
72. Schlesinger, LS, Ross, SC, and Schaberg, DR: *Staphylococcus aureus* meningitis: A broad-based epidemiologic study. Medicine 66:148, 1987.
73. Chambers, HF, Miller, RT, and Newman, MD: Right-sided *Staphylococcus aureus* endocarditis in intravenous drug abusers: Two-week combination therapy. Ann Intern Med 109:619, 1988.
74. Small, PM and Chambers, HF: Vancomycin for *Staphylococcus aureus* endocarditis in intravenous drug users. Antimicrob Agents Chemother 34:1227, 1990.
75. Garvey, GJ and New, HC: Infective endocarditis—an evolving disease: A review of endocarditis at the Columbia-Presbyterian Medical Center, 1968–1973. Medicine 57:105, 1978.
76. Pelletier, LL, Jr and Petersdorf, RG: Infective endocarditis: A review of 125 cases from the University of Washington Hospitals, 1963–72. Medicine 56:287, 1977.
77. Threlkeld, MG and Cobbs, CG: Infectious disorders of prosthetic valves and intravascular devices. In Mandell, GL, Douglas, RG, and Bennett, JE (eds): Principles and Practices of Infectious Diseases. Churchill Livingstone, New York, 1990, p 705.

78. Cohen, PS, Maquire, JH, and Weinstein, L: Infective endocarditis caused by gram-negative bacteria: A review of the literature, 1945–1977. Prog Cardiovasc Dis 22:205, 1980.

79. Carruthers, M: Endocarditis due to enteric bacilli other than salmonellae: Case reports and literature review. Am J Med Sci 273:203, 1977.

80. Levine, DP, Crane, LR, and Zervos, MJ: Bacteremia in narcotic addicts at the Detroit Medical Center II. Infectious Endocarditis: A prospective comparative study. Rev Infect Dis 8:374, 1986.

81. Wieland, M, Lederman, MM, Kline-King, C, et al: Left-sided endocarditis due to *Pseudomonas aeruginosa.* A report of 10 cases and review of the literature. Medicine 65:180, 1986.

82. Reyes, MP and Lerner, AM: Current problems in the treatment of infective endocarditis due to *Pseudomonas aeruginosa.* Rev Infect Dis 5:314, 1983.

83. Jemsek, JG, Greenberg, SB, Gentry, LO, et al: *Haemophilus parainfluenzae* endocarditis. Two cases and review of the literature in the past decade. Am J Med 66:51, 1979.

84. Murray, BE, Karchmer, AW, and Moellering, RC, Jr: Diphtheroid prosthetic valve endocarditis: A study of clinical features and infecting organisms. Am J Med 69:838, 1980.

85. Fort, S, Fraser, AG, and Fox, KA: Extensive aortic valve ring abscess formation: A rare complication of Q fever endocarditis. Postgrad Med J 65:384, 1989.

86. Vosti, K: Serum bactericidal test: Past, present, and future use in the management of patients with infections. In Remington, JS and Swartz, MN: Current Clinical Topics in Infectious Diseases 10:43, 1989.

87. Reller, LB: The serum bactericidal test. Rev Infect Dis 8:803, 1986.

88. Reller, LB and Stratton, CW: Serum dilution test for bactericidal activity. II. Standardization and correlation with antimicrobial assays and susceptibility tests. J Infect Dis 136:196, 1977.

89. Stratton, CW: The role of the microbiology laboratory in the treatment of infective endocarditis. J Antimicrob Chemother 20(Suppl A):41, 1987.

90. Weinstein, MP, Stratton, CW, Ackley, A, et al: Multicenter collaborative evaluation of a standardized serum bactericidal test as a prognostic indicator in infective endocarditis. Am J Med 78:262, 1985.

91. Pruit, AA, Rubin, RH, Karchmer, AW, et al: Neurologic complications of bacterial endocarditis. Medicine 57:329, 1978.

92. Wallace, AG, Young, WG, and Osterhout, S: Treatment of acute bacterial endocarditis by valve excision and replacement. Circulation 31:450, 1965.

93. Karchmer, AW: Surgical therapy for infective endocarditis. Medguide Infect Dis 9:1, 1989.

94. Alsip, SG, Blackstone, EH, Kirklin, JW, et al: Indications for cardiac surgery in patients with active infective endocarditis. Am J Med (Suppl 6B):138, 1985.

95. D'Agostino, RS, Miller, DC, Stinson, EB, et al: Valve replacement in patients with native valve endocarditis: What really determines operative outcome? Ann Thorac Surg 40:429, 1985.

96. Mann, T, McLaurin, L, Grossman, W, et al: Assessing the hemodynamic severity of acute aortic regurgitation due to infective endocarditis. N Engl J Med 293:108, 1975.

97. Omari, B, Shapiro, S, Ginzton, L, et al: Predictive risk factors for periannular extension of native valve endocarditis: Clinical and echocardiographic analyses. Chest 96:1273, 1989.

98. Douglas, A, Moore-Gillon, J, and Eykyn, S: Fever during treatment of infective endocarditis. Lancet 1:1341, 1986.

99. DiNubile, MJ, Calderwood, SB, Steinhaus, DM, et al: Cardiac conduction abnormalities complicating native valve endocarditis. Am J Cardiol 58:1213, 1986.

100. Mayrer, AR, Brown, A, Weintraub, RA, et al: Successful medical therapy for endocarditis due to *Candida parapsilosis.* Chest 73:546, 1978.

101. Faix, RG, Feick, HJ, Frommelt, P, et al: Successful medical treatment of Candida parapsilosis endocarditis in a premature infant. Am J Perinatal 7:272, 1990.

102. Jaffe, WM, Morgan, DE, Pearlman, AS, et al: Infective endocarditis: Echocardiographic findings and factors influencing mortality and morbidity. J Am Coll Cardiol 15:1227, 1990.

103. Steckelberg, JM, Murphy, JG, Ballard, D, et al: Emboli in infective endocarditis: The prognostic valve of echocardiography. Ann Intern Med 114:635, 1991.

104. Lewis, HS and Greenberg BH: Does the patient with infective endocarditis and a large vegetation on the mitral or aortic valve need surgery? Cardiovasc Clin 21:215, 1990.

105. DiNubile, M: Surgery for addition-related tricuspid valve endocarditis: Caveat emptor. Am J Med 82:811, 1987.

106. Chamber, HF and Mills, J: Endocarditis associated with intravenous drug abuse. In Sande, MA,

Kaye, D, and Root, RK (eds): Contemporary Issues in Infectious Diseases. Churchill Livingstone, New York, 1984, p 183.

107. Barbour, DJ and Roberts, WC: Valve excision only versus valve excision plus replacement for active infective endocarditis involving the tricuspid valve. Am J Cardiol 57:475, 1986.

108. Arbulu, A and Asfaw, I: Tricuspid valvulectomy without prosthetic replacement. Ten years of clinical experience. J Thorac Cardiovasc Surg 82:684, 1981.

109. Arbulu, A, Asfaw, I, and Homes, RJ: Tricuspid valvulectomy without replacement: 20 years experience. Abstract No. 31. 71st Annual Meeting of the American Association for Thoracic Surgery, Washington, DC, 1991.

110. Evora, PRB, Brasil, JCF, Elias, MLC, et al: Surgical excision of the vegetation as treatment of tricuspid valve endocarditis. Cardiology 75:287, 1988.

111. Huges, CF and Noble, N: Vegetectomy: An alternative surgical treatment for infective endocarditis of the atrioventricular valves in drug addicts. J Thorac Cardiovasc Surg 95:857, 1988.

112. Chandraratna, PAN, Reagan, RB, Imaizumi, T, et al: Infective endocarditis cured by resection of a tricuspid valve vegetation. Ann Intern Med 89:517, 1978.

113. Yee, ES and Khonsari, S: Right-sided infective endocarditis: Valvuloplasty, valvectomy or replacement. J Cardiovasc Surg 30:744, 1989.

114. Tanaka, M, Abe, T, Hosokawa, S, et al: Tricuspid valve candida endocarditis cured by valve-sparing debridement. Ann Thorac Surg 48:857, 1989.

115. Richardson, JV, Karp, RB, Kirklin, JW, et al: Treatment of infective endocarditis: A 10 year comparative analysis. Circulation 78:589, 1978.

116. Mayer, KH and Schoenbaum, SC: Evaluation and management of prosthetic valve endocarditis. Prog Cardiovasc Dis 25:48, 1982.

117. Karchmer, AW, Dismukes, WE, Buckley, MJ, et al: Late prosthetic valve endocarditis: Clinical features influencing therapy. Am J Med 64:199, 1978.

118. Meyer, DJ and Gerding, DN: Favorable prognosis of patients with prosthetic valve endocarditis caused by gram-negative bacilli of the HACEK group. Am J Med 85:104, 1988.

119. Bisno, AL: Antimicrobial prophylaxis for infective endocarditis. Hosp Pract 24(3):209, 1989.

120. Everett, ED and Hirschmann, JV: Transient bacteremia and endocarditis prophylaxis. A review. Medicine 56:61–77, 1977.

121. LeFrock, JL and Molavi, A: Transient bacteremia associated with diagnostic and therapeutic procedures. Comp Surg 8:65, 1982.

122. Durack, DT: Prophylaxis of infective endocarditis. In Mandell, GL, Douglas, RG, Jr, Bennett, JE (eds): Principles and Practice of Infectious Diseases, ed 3. Churchill Livingstone, New York, 1990, pp 716–721.

123. Imperiale, TF and Horwitz, RI: Does prophylaxis prevent postdental infective endocarditis? A controlled evaluation of protective efficacy. Am J Med 88:131, 1990.

124. Horstkotte, D, Friedrichs, W, Pippert, H, et al: Benefit of endocarditis prevention in patients with prosthetic heart valves. Z Kardiol 75:8, 1986.

125. Guntheroth, WG: How important are dental procedures as a cause of infective endocarditis? Am J Cardiol 54:797, 1984.

126. Durack, DT, Bisno, AL, and Kaplan, EL: Apparent failures of endocarditis prophylaxis. Analysis of 52 cases submitted to a national registry. JAMA 250:2318, 1983.

127. Dajani, AS, Bisno, AL, Chung, KJ, et al: Prevention of bacterial endocarditis. Recommendations by the American Heart Association. JAMA 264:2919, 1990.

128. Working Party of the British Society for Antimicrobial Chemotherapy: The antibiotic prophylaxis of infective endocarditis. Lancet 335:88, 1990.

129. Prevention of bacterial endocarditis. Med Lett Drugs Ther 31:112, 1989.

130. Nolan, CM, Kane, JJ, and Grunow, WA: Infective endocarditis and mitral prolapse. A comparison with other types of endocarditis. Arch Intern Med 131:477, 1981.

131. Clemens, JD, Horwitz, RI, Jaffee, CC, et al: A controlled evaluation of the risk of bacterial endocarditis in persons with mitral valve prolapse. N Engl J Med 307:776, 1982.

132. McKinsey, DS, Ratts, TE, and Bisno, AL: Underlying cardiac lesions in adults with infective endocarditis: The changing spectrum. Am J Med 82:681, 1981.

133. Baddour, LM and Bisno, AL: Infective endocarditis complicating mitral valve prolapse. Epidemiologic, clinical, and microbiologic aspects. Rev Infect Dis 8:117, 1986.

134. Danchin, N, Briancon, S, Mathieu, P, et al: Mitral valve prolapse as a risk factor for infective endocarditis. Lancet 1:743, 1989.

135. MacMahon, SW, Hickey, AJ, Wilcken, DEL, et al: Risk of infective endocarditis in mitral valve prolapse with and without precordial systolic murmurs. Am J Cardiol 58:105, 1986.
136. Marks, AR, Choong, CY, Sanfilippo, AJ, et al: Identification of high-risk and low-risk subgroups of patients with mitral-valve prolapse. N Engl J Med 320:1031, 1989.
137. Baltch, AL, Pressman, HL, Hammer, MC, et al: Bacteremia following dental extractions in patients with or without penicillin prophylaxis. Am J Med Sci 283:129, 1982.
138. Kelson, SR and White, PD: Notes on 250 cases of subacute bacterial (streptococcal) endocarditis studied and treated between 1927 and 1939. Ann Intern Med 22:40, 1945.
139. Meyer, GW: Endocarditis prophylaxis and gastrointestinal procedures. Am J Gastroenterol 84:1492, 1989.
140. Fleischer, D: Recommendations for antibiotic prophylaxis before endoscopy. Am J Gastroenterol 12:1489, 1990.
141. Botoman, VA and Surawicz, CM: Bacteremia with gastrointestinal endoscopic procedures. Gastrointest Endosc 32:342, 1986.

CHAPTER 9

Valvular Disease in the Elderly

Kevin P. Marzo, M.D.
Irving M. Herling, M.D.

Medical practice in the United States is gradually becoming dominated by the health-care needs of the elderly. During the past 80 years, the proportion of persons in our society older than 65 years of age has increased from 4% to 12%. The number of elderly persons is expected to be 51 million by 2020, and the number of very aged (80 years and older) will triple. In addition, as the mortality from coronary artery disease continues to decline, many more patients are surviving to develop degenerative valvular heart disease.[1]

As aging occurs, physiologic changes develop that impact upon the ability of the elderly to respond to pathologic processes.[2] Some variables of physiologic function, such as cardiac output, glomerular filtration rate, and carbohydrate tolerance change dramatically with age. The variability in response to aging among different individuals may be substantial as well. The changes associated with aging influence the presentation of illness, ensuing complications, and the response to treatment. The clinical features, natural history, diagnosis, and management of valvular heart disease in the elderly will be reviewed in this chapter.

NORMAL CARDIOVASCULAR EFFECTS OF THE AGING PROCESS

It is important to review the normal cardiovascular changes that occur with aging before discussing disease processes (Table 9–1).[3] Left ventricular hypertrophy and increased cardiac mass develop uniformly as a consequence of the increased arterial pressure that accompanies aging. In the elderly, diastolic dysfunction is common resulting in prolongation of isovolumic relaxation and incomplete diastolic filling, with compensatory increased late filling mediated by atrial contraction. Slowing of the intrinsic heart rate occurs as a result of reduced sinoatrial (SA) nodal fibers as well as diminished responsiveness of the aging myocardium to catecholamines. The reduced elasticity of the larger arteries in the elderly alters the carotid pulse contour causing a more rapid upstroke and a higher peak systolic pressure. During exercise, the elderly's cardiac responses are characterized by

Table 9–1. Cardiovascular
Responses to Aging

- ♠ Vascular stiffness and systolic hypertension
- ♠ Impedance to left ventricular ejection
- ♠ Contraction and relaxation times
- ♠ Late diastolic filling
- ♥ Early diastolic filling
- ♥ Adrenergic responsiveness
- ♥ Myocardial compliance
- ♥ Heart rate

---

decreased adrenergic responsiveness and are similar to those of younger patients treated with beta-blocking drugs.[4] The rate of development of these changes in cardiovascular function, however, varies dramatically and is influenced by life style as well as concomitant medical illnesses. As a consequence of this variability, chronologic age is frequently not concordant with biologic age. The latter, not the former, determines the cardiovascular impact of valvular pathology and provides a framework for the therapeutic plan developed by the physician.

NONCARDIOVASCULAR EFFECTS OF THE AGING PROCESS

In addition to the cardiovascular changes of aging, other physiologic parameters are altered that may substantially impact upon the ability of the elderly to tolerate cardiovascular surgery.

The elderly are more susceptible to infection than younger persons as a result of a decline in host defense mechanisms.[5] Both B- and T-cell–mediated immunity decline with age. Other host factors contribute to immune senescence, including decreased bacterial clearance, less effective intracellular killing of microbes, and impaired leukocyte and febrile responses to infection. Urinary tract, gastrointestinal, and respiratory infections occur more commonly in the elderly and disseminate more quickly than in their younger counterparts. Unfortunately, in the environment of the surgical intensive care unit (ICU), patients having multiple portals of entry for bacteria are at risk for frequent and, at times, overwhelming infection. These infections and their sequelae may be the greatest source of morbidity and mortality in the elderly who have undergone cardiovascular surgery.

The central nervous system is also affected by the aging process, with elderly persons being particularly susceptible to acute confusion and delirium. Almost any significant alteration, such as a new environment, new or worsening illness, or change in medications, can precipitate confusion.[6] The ICU environment alone may be sufficient to precipitate delirium in the elderly, not withstanding the potential contribution of medications known to produce confusion, such as sedatives, antihypertensives, and H_2 blockers that are frequently used in postoperative management. Electrolyte abnormalities commonly encountered after surgery, including hyper- or hyponatremia, azotemia, hypocalcemia, or hypophosphatemia, may cause acute confusion in this group of patients.

Depression, the most frequent psychiatric problem encountered in the elderly, may occur following cardiac surgery and may frequently contribute to delayed convalescence. Geriatric psychiatric consultation is often helpful in diagnosing and managing both delirium and postoperative depression. Postural hypotension attributable to diminished baroreceptor responsiveness is common and may result in cerebral hypoperfusion during convalescence from heart surgery.[7]

Age-related losses of taste and olfaction occur and may, in part, explain the frequent difficulty in providing adequate enteral nutrition to the elderly who are recovering from cardiovascular surgery.

Iatrogenic illness may contribute substantially to morbidity and mortality in the elderly undergoing surgery. Altered drug metabolism, decreased volume of distribution of water-soluble drugs, increased volume of distribution for fat-soluble drugs, and decreased hepatic and renal drug clearance may result in iatrogenic complications of drug therapy.[8] The elderly also appear to be more susceptible to drug side effects than younger patients.

The changes of aging thereby result in multiple abnormalities that increase morbidity and mortality following any surgical procedure, especially cardiovascular surgery. Therefore, the potential benefits of such surgery in these patients must be substantial and greatly exceed nonsurgical options in regard to symptom relief and improved survival in order to outweigh potential risks.

AORTIC STENOSIS

Aortic stenosis remains the most common valvular lesion in the elderly. As large numbers of elderly survive, degenerative aortic stenosis has come to exceed rheumatic valvular disease in frequency (Fig. 9–1).[9] Unfortunately, hemodynamically significant aortic stenosis is frequently underdiagnosed in the elderly for reasons that will be described. Since aortic valve replacement in this population now

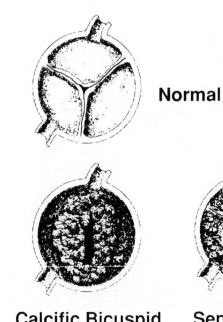

Normal Aortic Valve

Rheumatic   **Calcific Bicuspid**   **Senile/Calcific**

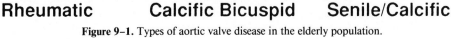

Figure 9–1. Types of aortic valve disease in the elderly population.

entails an acceptable risk and results in significant clinical improvement, the accurate diagnosis of aortic stenosis is mandatory.

ETIOLOGY AND PATHOLOGY

Valvular aortic stenosis may be a congenital or an acquired malformation. In 1904, Mönckeberg described a degenerative process affecting the aortic cusps leading to acquired aortic stenosis.[10] The term *calcific aortic stenosis* has been applied to this process. Stenosis is produced by calcium deposits that prevent the cusps from opening normally during systole. In younger adults in the United States, most cases of aortic stenosis result from the dense calcification of a congenitally bicuspid valve. Patients with "senile" calcification of a previously normal tricuspid valve develop symptoms at a more advanced age (>65 years) than those with calcified bicuspid valves. Among patients older than 65 years of age with calcific aortic stenosis, the aortic valve is tricuspid in more than 90% and congenitally malformed or bicuspid in less than 10%.[11] The consequences of the two conditions are, however, identical.

Calcific aortic stenosis appears to result from years of normal mechanical "wear and tear" upon the valvular apparatus (Fig. 9–2). Solid amorphous masses of calcium deposits usually begin at the bases of the cusps where flexion is greatest.[12] As the process advances, the calcific masses expand along the fibrosa, sometimes breaking through but rarely extending distally beyond the linea alba. In contrast to rheumatic valvular disease, degenerative calcification rarely involves the valvular endocardium and free edges of the valve.[13] The commissures are usually unaffected

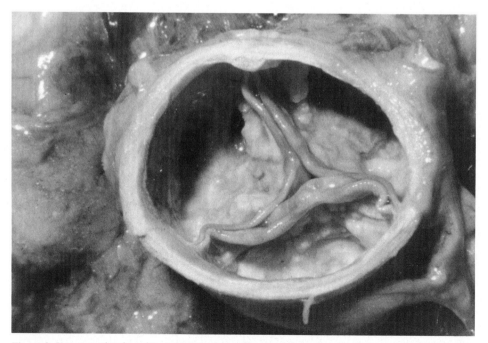

Figure 9–2. A stenotic tricuspid aortic valve in an 87-year-old woman. Aortic stenosis in the elderly is characterized by calcific deposits on the aortic surface of the cusps and absence of commissural fusion.

by calcific aortic stenosis. The valve becomes more stenotic as increasing deposition of calcium reduces the mobility of the valve. Because the commissures are usually not fused in degenerative calcific aortic stenosis, associated significant aortic regurgitation (AR) is infrequent.

Approximately 50% of patients older than age 65 have evidence of a systolic murmur arising from these degenerative changes; however, the occurrence of critical or hemodynamically significant aortic stenosis is much less frequent.[14] The incidence of critical aortic stenosis in the aged remains unknown, although estimates of up to 1% of the elderly population have been made.[15] Although degenerative aortic valve calcification is clearly an age-related condition, it is not known why it develops to a greater degree in some individuals than in others. Conditions associated with increased mechanical stress, such as hypertension or metabolic derangements predisposing to hypercalcemia, have not been associated with an increased incidence of this disorder.

PATHOPHYSIOLOGY

As the aortic valve becomes stenotic, the left ventricle compensates for the pressure load by developing concentric hypertrophy to normalize wall stress and overcome the increased afterload. Left ventricular function remains preserved until late in the natural history of the disease even with the most severely stenotic valves. End-systolic and end-diastolic volumes likewise remain normal until the late stages of the disease. Obstruction to outflow from aortic stenosis usually evolves slowly and progresses gradually. Some patients, however, especially those with degenerative calcification, may demonstrate more rapid progression.[16] The hypertrophied left ventricle can sustain a large pressure gradient across the aortic valve, preserving cardiac output without left ventricular dilation. A peak systolic pressure gradient exceeding 50 mm Hg in the presence of a normal cardiac output or an aortic valve area less than 0.7 to 0.8 cm^2 is generally considered to represent critical obstruction. Left ventricular compliance decreases as a result of increasing hypertrophy. Left atrial hypertrophy occurs as atrial contraction plays a greater role in diastolic filling. Therefore, the loss of the atrial systole consequent to development of atrial fibrillation in aortic stenosis frequently leads to markedly compromised left ventricular filling and the abrupt onset of pulmonary venous congestion.

The symptoms of aortic stenosis initially result from obstruction to left ventricular outflow when left ventricular function is normal.[17] Effort-related angina and syncope are common early symptoms. If the outflow obtruction is not relieved, left ventricle function deteriorates and symptoms of congestive heart failure develop. Angina may occur as a result of subendocardial ischemia even in the absence of coronary artery disease—a consequence of a diminished coronary flow reserve.[18] However, more than half the elderly population with significant calcific aortic stenosis and angina will have coexistent coronary artery disease.

Syncope may result from peripheral vasodilation due to faulty baroreceptor function.[19] An arrhythmia or an abrupt failure of the overloaded left ventricle during stress and exercise are less likely explanations for aortic stenosis-associated syncope.

The cardiac alterations that result from the normal aging process, including increased arterial stiffness, left ventricular hypertrophy, and decreased left ventricular compliance, further exacerbate the pathophysiologic response to aortic stenosis and may explain why symptoms often progress more rapidly in the elderly than in younger individuals. These processes may in part explain why heart failure may occur early in the natural history of aortic stenosis in the elderly.

CLINICAL MANIFESTATIONS

The clinical presentation of elderly patients with symptomatic aortic stenosis often differs from that of younger patients. Typical symptoms of angina, heart failure, and of effort-related syncope may be the result of other processes in the elderly. Because many elderly patients are physically inactive, exertionally provoked symptoms may not be noted. In contrast to younger patients who most commonly present with angina, left ventricular failure is the most common presenting symptom in the elderly.[20] Furthermore, coexistent disease, such as hypertension, lung disease, and coronary artery disease, may obscure the clinical manifestations of aortic stenosis in these patients. Other less common presentations of calcific aortic stenosis include infective endocarditis, cerebral emboli resulting in stroke, or even occasionally amaurosis fugax.[21,22]

The mortality of patients with symptomatic severe aortic stenosis treated medically is high (Fig. 9–3).[23] Symptoms of angina or syncope predict an average survival of 2 to 3 years The prognosis of those with congestive heart failure is even worse, with their survival averaging 1½ years. Sudden death is not uncommon in symptomatic patients with aortic stenosis but is more frequent in those with previous syncopal events. The etiology of sudden death is not well defined; it may reflect irreconcilable syncope or malignant ventricular dysrhythmias, especially in the setting of severe left ventricular dysfunction.

The natural history of critical stenosis in the asymptomatic patient is less well defined.[24] Available data suggest that the asymptomatic adult patient with hemodynamically severe aortic stenosis and normal left ventricular function is not likely

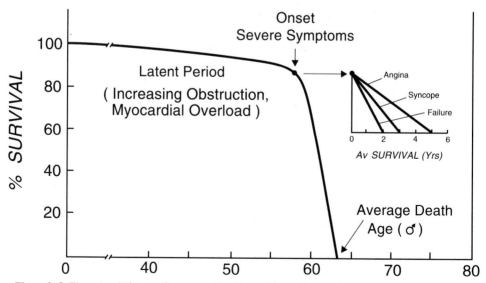

Figure 9–3. The natural history of unoperated patients with aortic stenosis. (From Ross, J Jr and Braunwald, E,[23] with permission of American Heart Association, Inc.)

to die suddenly. Therefore, such asymptomatic patients should not be referred for surgical therapy but require close follow-up for the onset of symptoms. Data, in fact, suggest that "operative treatment is the most frequent cause of sudden death in asymptomatic patients with aortic stenosis."[25]

PHYSICAL EXAMINATION

Aortic ejection murmurs are appreciated in approximately 30% of patients older than 65 years of age and an even higher percentage of elderly hypertensives.[26] The clinician must learn to distinguish these benign murmurs from the less common and often unsuspected critical aortic stenosis murmur. The common basal systolic murmur of aortic sclerosis results from fibrotic thickening of the aortic valve cusps and mild calcification involving the base of the leaflets. Although the cusps may not open fully, they do open sufficiently to prevent a significant gradient across the valve orifice. These aortic ejection murmurs are associated with a brisk carotid upstroke and typically begin with S1, are crescendo-decrescendo and peak in the first one third of systole, end before the A2, and become louder after long diastolic cycles.

The physical findings of significant aortic stenosis, however, may be atypical in the elderly.[27] In these patients, the decreased arterial compliance may cause the carotid upstroke to appear brisk and may cause systolic hypertension despite significant aortic stenosis. The aortic ejection click heard in younger patients is not heard in the elderly because the severely calcified valves are immobile. The characteristic high-frequency basal systolic murmur of degenerative aortic stenosis may be heard along the lower-left sternal border throughout most of systole and is often appreciated best at the left ventricular apex; thus the murmur may be mistaken for that of mitral regurgitation (MR), especially when A2 is inaudible. Post–premature-beat augmentation, which does not occur with the murmur of MR, may be helpful in distinguishing the two murmurs. Because of the increased anterior-posterior chest diameter commonly found in the aged, the sustained ventricular impulse may not be palpable and the murmur of critical aortic stenosis may be nearly inaudible. Additionally, the reduced cardiac output that frequently accompanies critical aortic stenosis in the symptomatic elderly patient, may markedly diminish the intensity of the murmur.

Hypertrophic obstructive cardiomyopathy (HOCM) also may cause the systolic murmurs in the elderly.[28] In HOCM, however, the carotid impulse frequently reveals a characteristic bifid pulse with a primary spike and secondary dome impulse, and the systolic murmur usually does not radiate to the neck. This murmur intensifies with the straining phase of the Valsalva maneuver whereas the murmur of aortic stenosis diminishes.

DIAGNOSIS

Elderly patients with a systolic murmur and symptoms that might be of cardiac origin need a careful evaluation to exclude significant aortic stenosis. Because the history may be unreliable and the physical examination difficult to interpret, non-invasive cardiac studies are often necessary to diagnose the presence of significant valvular obstruction. The electrocardiogram (ECG) in patients with significant aortic stenosis usually reveals evidence of left ventricular hypertrophy, but the frequent occurrence of systolic hypertension in the elderly also may explain this finding. The absence of ECG criteria for left ventricular hypertrophy, though uncommon, does not always exclude aortic stenosis in these patients. The frequent occurrence of coronary disease and conduction disease in the elderly also may make the electrocardiographic findings nonspecific. Conduction disease may result from contiguous calcification of the atrioventricular (AV) node and His bundle from the base of the cusps.[29,30] Left-anterior hemiblock occurs most frequently although first-degree AV block, left bundle branch block, and complete heart block are also encountered. Atrial fibrillation is uncommon early in the course of aortic stenosis. Its occurrence in a well-compensated patient should suggest alternative etiologies, such as coexistent mitral stenosis, hypertensive heart disease, or coronary artery disease.

The chest x-ray in patients with isolated aortic stenosis frequently reveals a normal cardiac silhouette with post-stentotic dilation of the aorta. Valvular calcification is found invariably on fluoroscopic examination in the adult patient with significant aortic stenosis although it may not be apparent on chest x-ray.[31] Its absence virtually excludes significant aortic stenosis. Its presence, however, does not necessarily confirm that significant valvular obstruction exists.

Echocardiography is the most important noninvasive technique in assessing the severity of aortic stenosis in the elderly.[32] M-mode and two-dimensional (2-D) echocardiographic tracings can reveal valvular characteristics, such as thickening of valve leaflets, the number of leaflets and leaflet mobility, evidence of pressure overload (e.g., concentric left ventricular hypertrophy), and other coexistent valvular disease. Both M-mode and 2-D echocardiography, however, are significantly limited in their ability to quantitate the severity of stenosis, particularly in the elderly patient with extensive valvular calcification (Fig. 9–4). Heavily calcified valve leaflets are not likely to be clearly visualized so that their separation during systole may not be accurately assessed. If, however, leaflet excursion is visualized and is normal, severe valvular obstruction can be excluded. Reduced leaflet separation alone, however, does not differentiate among mild, moderate, or severe degrees of stenosis.

Doppler echocardiography allows more accurate assessment of valvular obstruction and is currently the procedure of choice for the routine evaluation of aortic valvular disease.[33] Peak instantaneous and mean transaortic valve gradients can be calculated using the modified Bernoulli equation (Fig. 9–4). The peak pressure gradient (P) is calculated from the peak velocity (V) obtained by continuous-wave Doppler echocardiography ($P = 4 \times V^2$). Studies during the past decade have confirmed an excellent correlation between echo-derived gradients and those obtained during cardiac catheterization.[34] The clinician must be aware, however, that certain technical factors may lead to an underestimation of the severity of aortic stenosis and that catheterization may be necessary in these patients for an accurate assessment of the magnitude of the outflow obstruction.[35] Careful interrogation of the aortic outflow tract with the continuous-wave Doppler transducer from multiple locations must be performed to assure that the highest velocity jet has been identified. Aortic valve replacement has been undertaken using echo-derived data alone in some selected patients.[36] Although this approach may be acceptable in younger patients, the presence of unrecognized coronary disease mandates coronary arteriography be performed in all adults older than 35 to 40 years of age. Furthermore, cardiac catheterization should be performed to assess the transaortic gradient and valve area in any symptomatic patient in whom the severity of aortic stenosis remains uncertain—a not uncommon occurrence in the patient with severe left ventricular dysfunction and low cardiac output.[37]

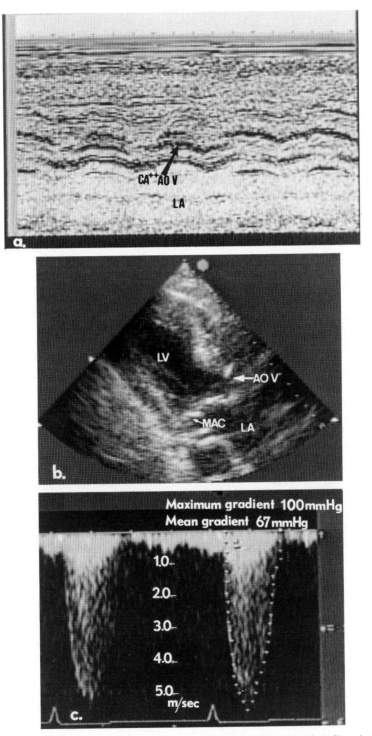

Figure 9–4. Echocardiogram of an 86-year-old man with severe aortic stenosis (AS) and progressive congestive heart failure. M-Mode (*a*) and 2D-echo (*b*) demonstrate marked thickening and calcification of aortic valve (AoV). Leaflet motion is not discernible and there is severe concentric left ventricular hypertrophy. Mitral annular calcification (MAC) is also present. Continuous wave Doppler (*c*) demonstrates a peak AoV gradient of 5.2 m/sec indicating a peak instantaneous gradient of 100 mmHg and a mean AoV gradient of 67 mmHg. LA = left atrium; LV = left ventricle.

MANAGEMENT

Medical therapy for symptomatic aortic stenosis is associated with a poor prognosis. Symptoms of aortic stenosis are usually associated with substantial valvular obstruction. Recently, O'Keefe and associates[38] provided evidence of the high mortality associated with medical management of aortic stenosis. The 1-year mortality of patients who refused aortic valve replacement or who were too ill for such surgery was approximately 45%. Valvular surgery in the elderly is clearly associated with a greater operative mortality than that of younger patients.[39] Despite increased surgical risk, valve replacement often results in prolonged clinical improvement, which may make the risk acceptable in many patients. The marked clinical improvement likely after successful valve replacement, even in patients with severe preoperative heart failure, may be attributable to the reduction in afterload that results from relief of the outflow obstruction.[40] Aortic percutaneous balloon valvuloplasty now appears to provide an alternative intervention for a selected subset of patients who may not be ideal operative candidates. Physiologic age may not be concordant with chronologic age, so the therapeutic approaches must be thoughtfully individualized.

Aortic valve replacement in the elderly before 1970 was associated with a 15% to 20% operative risk.[41,42] The operative mortality currently for aortic valve replacement has fallen to between 5% and 15%.[43-47] The improvement in operative mortality likely results from improved operative techniques and better postoperative care. Selection bias may also, in part, explain improved operative mortality. Therefore, many symptomatic elderly patients apparently can tolerate valvular surgery that will result in marked symptomatic improvement and improved survival. Octogenarians who had undergone aortic valve replacement for aortic stenosis had survival rates of 83% and 67% at 1- and 5-years, respectively, in a series reported by Levinson and coworkers[47] (Fig. 9–5).

Certain subsets of patients undergoing valvular surgery appear, however, to have substantially poorer outcomes (Table 9–2). A series of octogenarians undergoing aortic valve surgery reported by Edmunds and colleagues[48] noted a 48% early and late mortality rate. When high-risk patients were excluded, early mortality fell to 15%. Factors associated with greater operative risk included emergency surgery, left ventricular dysfunction, significant coronary disease, cachexia, or additional valve replacement. Women appear to have higher mortality than men after aortic valve replacement in several series—perhaps a consequence of their greater likelihood of requiring aortaplasty or annuloplasty to enlarge their anatomically smaller aortic roots.[44,49]

Concomitant coronary artery bypass surgery in the elderly increases surgical risk by between 8% and 21%; however, unreconciled coronary lesions increase mortality to an even greater degree.[49-51] The combination of ventricular hypertrophy and coronary artery obstruction may compromise the ability to maintain adequate cardioplegia when coronary revascularization is not undertaken. As a consequence, myocardial protection may be inadequate and left ventricular dysfunction may result. Thus, combined valve replacement and coronary revascularization are required when both conditions coexist.

Another group of patients exists in which the risk of aortic valve replacement may be prohibitive. These patients have extensive calcification of the aortic root, which may be recognized during cardiac catheterization or on routine chest x-ray

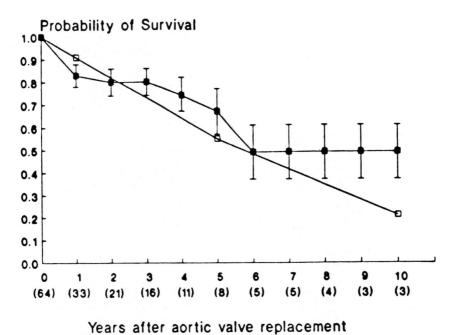

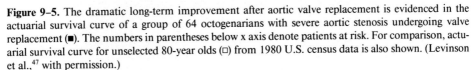

Figure 9–5. The dramatic long-term improvement after aortic valve replacement is evidenced in the actuarial survival curve of a group of 64 octogenarians with severe aortic stenosis undergoing valve replacement (■). The numbers in parentheses below x axis denote patients at risk. For comparison, actuarial survival curve for unselected 80-year olds (□) from 1980 U.S. census data is also shown. (Levinson et al.,[47] with permission.)

examination. This entity, described as "egg-shell calcification" of the aorta, may result in catastrophic disruption of the aorta after aortic cross-clamping that is not amenable to repair and results in death. We believe that "egg-shell calcification" should be considered a strong contraindication to aortic valve replacement and should mandate alternative management (Fig. 9–6).

The choice of which prosthetic valve should be implanted in the elderly patient also must be individualized.[52] With bioprosthetic valves, there is no need for the usual systemic anticoagulation, which appears to have substantial mortality and morbidity in the elderly. However, tissue degeneration necessitating reoperation is a distinct disadvantage of these devices and may approach 30% to 40% at 10 years.

Table 9–2. Risk Factors for
Valvular Surgery in Elderly
Patients

Emergent surgery
Multiple valve surgery
Coronary artery disease, especially if nongrafted
Female gender
Left ventricular dysfunction
Cachexia or malnutrition

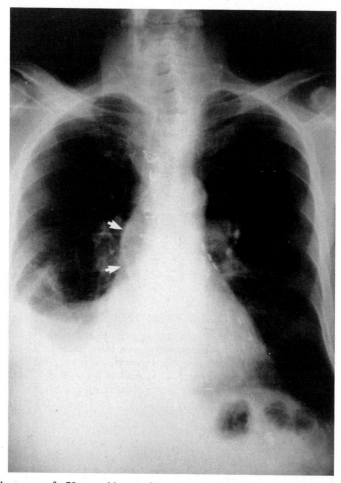

Figure 9–6. Chest x-ray of a 79-year-old man with progressive heart failure due to critical aortic stenosis demonstrating extensive calcification or "egg-shell calcification" of the ascending aorta *(arrows)*. Because of this finding, aortic valve replacement was considered "high risk."

Mechanical valves are extremely durable and are likely to have better hemodynamic profiles than their bioprosthetic counterparts, but all require lifelong anticoagulation, resulting in ongoing hemorrhagic risk. Improved survival in elderly patients receiving a bioprosthesis appears to result from the elimination of anticoagulation-related hemorrhagic events. Recent studies also suggest that bioprosthetic durability may be improved in the elderly compared with that of younger patients.[53] Nonetheless, an active patient less than 70 years of age with an actuarial life survival greater than 10 years and with no contraindication to anticoagulation may be better served with a mechanical prosthesis.

The development of aortic balloon valvuloplasty (ABV) appeared to offer an alternative to valvular replacement in the elderly with aortic stenosis.[54,55] Initial enthusiasm for ABV has been tempered, however, by the recognition of rapid restenosis in patients with degenerative aortic stenosis.[56] Additional deficiencies of this procedure have been defined. The final post-ABV valve area frequently ranges from 0.7 to 1.0 cm², representing substantial residual outflow obstruction. Absolute increases in area are generally 0.2 to 0.4 cm². The strongest predictor of the final aortic valve area appears to be the pre-ABV area. However, because of the curvilinear relationship of gradient to valve area, a small increase in valve area may be sufficient to alter the loading conditions of the heart, improve hemodynamics, and alleviate symptoms. The mechanism of successful valvuloplasty in calcific aortic stenosis appears to result from the following structural changes: increased flexibility of the leaflets owning to fracture of calcific nodules, cusp and aorta stretching, and tearing of the cusps.[57] Complications of ABV have been acceptably low given the generally poor medical condition of these patients, but include death, stroke, access-related complications, and severe AR. Hospital mortality has ranged from 2.8% to 8.9%.[58–60] Unfortunately, restenosis defined as a 50% reduction in valve area from the initial improvement occurs in most patients (approaching 50% to 60%) by 6 months.[61] All patients with recurrent symptoms are likely to have restenosis. Additionally, a significant number of those with persistent clinical improvement also will have restenosis. Mortality in the first 9 months after successful ABV is substantial, with reports ranging from 17% to 28%.[57,62] Despite these somewhat unfavorable results, a substantial number of patients will have significant, although short-lived, symptomatic improvement after ABV.[60,63] Therefore, it may be difficult to decide which patients should be offered palliation by ABV and which should be referred for valvular replacement. Perhaps the most frequent indication for ABV in the elderly is a palliative procedure for the symptomatic patient with significant aortic stenosis who refuses aortic valve replacement because of the inherent operative surgical risks. In contrast, a patient who might be offered ABV initially might be a frail, cachetic elderly patient with symptomatic aortic stenosis and severe left ventricular dysfunction with or without coexisting medical illnesses that limit his or her short-term life span (Table 9–3). For such patients, a palliative procedure may well be preferred to a much higher risk surgical procedure. Such a patient might well be offered ABV repeatedly (Fig. 9–7). Unfortunately, patients undergoing a second procedure have a substantial rate of subsequent failure, which may be even more likely if the interval between procedures is short.[64]

Aortic balloon valvuloplasty also may be considered as a bridge to surgery in a critically ill patient presenting in cardiogenic shock due to aortic stenosis.[65] It can temporarily improve the patients' clinical condition and allow valvular replacement to be undertaken on a nonemergent basis, which would likely reduce the sur-

Table 9–3. Indications for Aortic PBV in Elderly with Symptomatic Aortic Stenosis

Limited life span 2° to noncardiac illness
Cardiac surgery undesirable
    Patient refusal
    Dementia
    Severe cachexia
    Surgical high risk: coexistent nonrevascularizable coronary artery disease, severe pulmonary
      hypertension, "egg-shell aorta"
"Bridge" before future surgery
    Valve replacement (cardiogenic shock or severe congestive heart failure 2° to aortic stenosis)
    Urgent noncardiac surgery
Assessment of aortic stenosis severity in patients with left ventricular dysfunction and low cardiac
  output and gradient

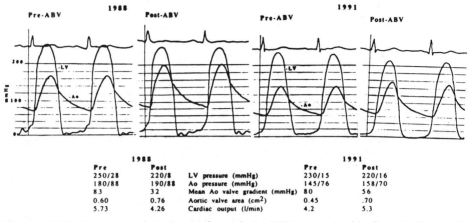

			1988			1991	
	Pre	Post				Pre	Post
	250/28	220/8	LV pressure (mmHg)			230/15	220/16
	180/88	190/88	Ao pressure (mmHg)			145/76	158/70
	83	32	Mean Ao valve gradient (mmHg)			80	56
	0.60	0.76	Aortic valve area (cm^2)			0.45	.70
	5.73	4.26	Cardiac output (l/min)			4.2	5.3

Figure 9–7. Simultaneous aortic (Ao) and left ventricular (LV) pressure tracings from the 86-year-old man whose echocardiographic findings are shown in Figure 9–4. The patient underwent ABV in 1988 for symptomatic AS resulting in an increase in aortic valve area from 0.60 to 0.76 cm^2 with subsequent clinical improvement. In 1991 he developed recurrent heart failure symptoms and had echocardiographic evidence of restenosis. Repeat ABV was performed resulting in an increase in valve area from 0.45 to 0.70 cm^2 (data provided by H. C. Herrmann, M.D.).

gical risk substantially. The use of ABV as a bridge in patients with severe symptomatic aortic stenosis undergoing noncardiac surgery also has been suggested because these patients are at substantial risk with their valvular lesion unaddressed.[66] In the patient with dense aortic root calcification, ABV may be the only procedure that can be undertaken with an acceptable level of risk.

The role of ABV or aortic valve replacement before noncardiac surgery in patients with asymptomatic but hemodynamically significant aortic stenosis is even more uncertain and requires further study. The mortality risk of performing prophylactic aortic valve replacement or ABV on an asymptomatic patient may be greater than the risk associated with undergoing noncardiac surgery without these interventions.

AORTIC REGURGITATION

ETIOLOGY AND PATHOLOGY

In contrast to aortic stenosis, isolated severe aortic regurgitation (AR) is uncommon in the elderly. Of elderly patients undergoing aortic valve replacement, less than 20% have primary AR. The etiology of chronic AR in the elderly is often uncertain. The etiologies may be grouped, however, into two general categories: (1) those associated with intrinsic valvular disease and (2) those related to pathology of the aortic root (Table 9–4).[67]

Although rheumatic heart disease is a common cause of AR, it is usually associated with mitral valve disease and typically becomes clinically manifest before the age of 65. Myxomatous degeneration of the aortic valve is another cause but is usually evident by the third and fourth decades of life.[68] The congenitally bicuspid valve is a rare cause of isolated severe AR unless endocarditis has been contribu-

Table 9–4. Etiology of Aortic
Regurgitation in the Elderly

Valvular	Aortic Root Disease
Rheumatic	Progressive idiopathic dilation
Bicuspid	Hypertension
Senile calcific	Aortic dissection
Infective endocarditis	Syphilitic aortitis
Myxomatous degeneration	Connective tissue disorders
	Anuloaortic ectasia
	Marfan's syndrome

tory. Degenerative calcific aortic stenosis in the elderly is rarely associated with significant AR.

Aortic root abnormalities may be the most common cause for valvular incompetence in the elderly. Degenerative dilation of the aortic root can result in regurgitation as stretching and bowing of the valve cusps and widening of the commissures occurs. Idiopathic dilation may result from cystic medial necrosis and be exacerbated by systemic hypertension.[69] A variety of other diseases, such as Marfan's syndrome, annuloaortic ectasia, syphilitic aortitis, and connective tissue disorders, may produce AR by causing aortic root dilation. Acute severe AR in the elderly also may result from aortic dissection or infective endocarditis.

PATHOPHYSIOLOGY

Chronic severe AR results in left ventricular volume overload. Compensatory left ventricular dilation occurs early and hypertrophy develops over time. Dilation increases preload so that stroke volume is augmented by the Starling principle. Eventually fibrosis and myocardial fiber slippage develop resulting in irreversible left ventricular dysfunction and depressed contractility if AR is not reconciled. The aging ventricle may be less likely to tolerate volume overload as a consequence of impaired diastolic function. Pulmonary venous congestion may develop earlier in the course of the process than in younger patients. Furthermore, the slower heart rate that occurs with aging may increase the duration of diastole and the magnitude of regurgitation.

CLINICAL MANIFESTATIONS

Patients with severe chronic AR, in contrast to those with aortic stenosis, may remain asymptomatic for many years. Initially, common symptoms may be those of a forceful heartbeat or arterial pulsation resulting from the increased stroke volume and widened pulse pressure. Exertional dyspnea is common and may arise from elevated left ventricular end-diastolic pressures resulting in pulmonary venous congestion. Angina may occur early in the disease process and appears to result from diminished diastolic coronary perfusion pressures and impaired coronary flow reserve. Coexistent coronary disease is common in the elderly and may dominate the clinical symptomatology.

The presentation of acute severe regurgitation differs greatly from that of chronic regurgitation inasmuch as left ventricular compensation and stroke volume changes have not yet occurred.[70] Pulmonary venous congestion and tachycardia dominate the clinical syndrome. The pulse pressure may be narrow, and the regurgitant murmur barely audible. Not infrequently, pneumonia is suspected when the elderly febrile patient presents with dyspnea, an abnormal chest x-ray and a normal cardiac silhouette, when, in fact, the fever is due to aortic valve endocarditis and the x-ray findings reflect pulmonary edema. Echocardiography may be required to diagnose the unsuspected valvular lesion.

DIAGNOSIS

The ECG in chronic severe regurgitation is characterized by left ventricular hypertrophy without repolarization abnormalities. The chest x-ray reveals left ventricular enlargement and dilation of the ascending aorta. Echocardiography is the most reliable noninvasive method of detecting the presence of AR.[71] In addition, it provides an objective evaluation of left ventricular size and function and allows the ongoing assessment of the changes occurring with chronic left ventricular overload. Fine diastolic fluttering of the anterior mitral leaflet may alert the physician to the presence of AR on M-mode echocardiogram. Premature closure of the mitral valve may occur in patients with acute severe regurgitation owing to the elevated left ventricular end-diastolic pressure. Two-dimensional echocardiography may assist in determining whether pathology involves the valve or the aortic root. Both can be used to measure chamber dimensions, ventricular function, and wall thickness. A significant and persistent enlargement of end-diastolic and end-systolic dimensions may be an indicator of the onset of irreversible left ventricular dysfunction, identifying the point at which surgery is mandated. An end-systolic dimension of >55 mm and fractional shortening of <25% appeared in one study to identify patients likely to have irreversible left ventricular dysfunction. The authors suggested that these criteria be used to recommend valve replacement even in asymptomatic patients.[72] Other studies subsequently, however, demonstrated that even these findings in asymptomatic patients were not predictors of a poor surgical outcome. Serial measurements may be valuable in identifying impending decompensation but must be assessed in the context of other clinical parameters before considering valve replacement.[73]

Doppler echocardiography is useful for the semiquantitative assessment of the severity of AR as well as in the determination of the regurgitant fraction.[74] The size of the regurgitant jet may be assessed by careful mapping of the left ventricular cavity by pulsed-wave Doppler. This technique is limited because only the length of the regurgitant jet is measured rather than its area. Color-flow imaging is more accurate in assessing AR inasmuch as it permits visualization of both jet area and width. It has been shown to correlate well with the angiographic severity of AR. However, the size of the regurgitant jet by color-flow mapping must be interpreted with caution because it is heavily dependent on technical factors.

Radionuclide angiography also may assist in the assessment of patients with AR.[75] Cardiac catheterization should be performed in elderly patients with symptomatic chronic AR or those with acute severe regurgitation who are considered potential surgical candidates to assess left ventricular performance and to examine the coronary anatomy. Angiographic evaluation allows an assessment of the severity of regurgitation as well as a gross assessment of the aortic valve leaflets, ascending aorta, and any associated abnormalities of the aorta (dissection, root abscess, sinus of Valsalva aneurysm) or intraventricular septum.[76]

MANAGEMENT

The prognosis of patients with chronic AR correlates with the severity of regurgitation and the presence of symptomatology. Those with mild-to-moderate regurgitation have a 10-year mortality rate of approximately 5% to 15% whereas those with severe regurgitation have a mortality of 30%.[77] Symptoms of angina and heart failure identify worsening prognosis, with death occurring 4 years after the development of angina and within 2 years after the onset of heart failure.

The timing of aortic valve replacement for chronic AR remains controversial.[78] Preoperative resting left ventricular dysfunction continues to identify patients with AR at increased risk of death or heart failure after valve replacement.[79] Identification of early left ventricular dysfunction using clinical and noninvasive assessment may optimize the timing of surgery. Asymptomatic patients with severe regurgitation and normal left ventricular function should not receive prophylactic valve replacement but should be closely monitored for the onset of symptoms or left ventricular dysfunction using noninvasive studies.[80]

Valve replacement for aortic insufficiency in the elderly should be considered only for the severely symptomatic patient who does not respond to medical therapy. As with symptomatic calcific aortic stenosis, age alone should not contraindicate valve replacement. The threshold for recommending surgery in the elderly should be tempered by clinical assessment of the patient in regard to comorbid illnesses, operative risk, functional capacity, and anticipated survival. Patients with predominant regurgitation, however, may not tolerate surgery as well as their counterparts with aortic stenosis because irreversible left ventricular dysfunction occurs more commonly in these patients. In the carefully selected elderly patient, surgical mortality for regurgitation is similar to that of valve replacement for aortic stenosis with a mortality of 5% to 15% and a favorable long-term clinical outcome.[44,45] Thus, the active, otherwise healthy elderly patient with chronic regurgitation, increasing symptomatology, and progressively enlarging left ventricular dimensions who does not respond to medical therapy should undergo assessment for potential valve replacement.

The role of medical therapy in altering the natural history of chronic AR is presently under investigation. Mild heart failure may be treated with digitalis and diuretics. Vasodilator therapy appears to be the most useful pharmacologic approach inasmuch as it may favorably influence cardiac performance by altering left ventricular loading conditions. Afterload reducing agents will often improve symptoms. Recent studies have suggested that vasodilators also may alter the natural history of the disease and should be used before surgery in anyone who can tolerate them.[81] At this time, vasodilator therapy should not be considered an alternative to surgery unless operative risk is high, inasmuch as valve replacement generally results in a favorable long-term prognosis. Vasodilators may be most effectively used to relieve early symptoms of heart failure or as an alternative to valve replacement in patients in whom surgical risk is excessive.

MITRAL STENOSIS

ETIOLOGY AND PATHOLOGY

Rheumatic heart disease, the predominant cause of mitral stenosis, is almost always acquired before the age of 20 and becomes clinically apparent in most cases in the third, fourth, and fifth decades of life.[82] Rheumatic fever results in inflammation and fibrosis of the mitral valve apparatus leading to stenosis. When rheumatic fever results predominantly in contraction and fusion of the chordae tendineae and minimal fusion of valvular commissures, MR predominates. An uncommon cause of nonrheumatic mitral stenosis has been described in elderly patients with mitral anular calcification.[83] Despite the presence of structurally normal leaflets, inflow obstruction may result from a "shelf" of calcification beneath the posterior mitral valve leaflet in patients with small, hypertrophied, noncompliant left ventricles.

CLINICAL MANIFESTATIONS

Inasmuch as rheumatic disease frequently permits survival to old age, mitral stenosis is not an uncommon clinical problem in the elderly population.[84] The clinical spectrum of the disease may be one of little disability to one of severe symptomatology.[85] Once a patient with mitral stenosis develops limiting, disabling symptoms, the downhill progression is frequently rapid. From initial diagnosis, patients with symptomatic mitral stenosis have a mortality of 20% at 5 years. New York Heart Association class IV heart failure symptomatology is associated with a 15% 5-year survival.[86]

Approximately one third of patients with rheumatic mitral disease will have predominant stenosis, whereas two thirds will have predominant regurgitation, although a combination of the two lesions is common. Symptoms due to mitral stenosis result from elevated left atrial and pulmonary venous pressures. They include exertional dyspnea, paroxysmal nocturnal dyspnea, and orthopnea. The clinical features of mitral stenosis in the elderly differ little from those of younger patients except for the frequent occurrence of valvular calcification and the higher frequency of atrial fibrillation.[84] Symptoms of dyspnea on exertion and lethargy are common and are generally associated with valve areas of less than 1.5 cm^2.

Mitral stenosis is frequently not diagnosed in the elderly because of the absence of the usual physical findings.[87] Elderly patients may initially present with evidence of a systemic embolus, such as a stroke. Because of the coexistence of such conditions as hypertension and chronic atrial fibrillation, the diagnosis of mitral stenosis is often not entertained. Additionally, severe pulmonary hypertension and right heart failure in some elderly patients may be incorrectly ascribed to chronic obstructive lung disease. Careful examination and review of the ECG and chest x-ray may provide clues to the existence of mitral stenosis.

Auscultatory findings of mitral stenosis in the elderly population include the characteristic apical diastolic rumbling murmur.[88] In contrast to younger patients, an opening snap is rare because of the stiffness and calcification of the valve. A presystolic murmur and accentuation of S1 are also less commonly found in older patients due to absence of a pliable valve. In all age groups, especially the elderly, there are patients in whom the diastolic murmur is difficult to auscultate or may actually be absent ("silent" mitral stenosis). The severely depressed cardiac output that has been found in these patients results in a very soft murmur as a consequence of the minimal gradient despite the presence of a severely stenotic valve. In others, obesity, obstructive pulmonary disease, or senile kyphosis may limit access to effective auscultation of the left ventricular apex.

DIAGNOSIS

The ECG often provides the first clue to the presence of mitral stenosis by revealing left atrial enlargement, right ventricular hypertrophy, or atrial fibrillation. On chest x-ray, left atrial enlargement is suggested by posterior bulging of the left atrium, straightening of the left-upper heart border, a double contour of the right heart border, and elevation of the left mainstem bronchus.

The presence and severity of mitral stenosis can almost invariably be diagnosed by echocardiography.[89] Mitral leaflet M-mode findings include thickening, reduced motion, and parallel movement of anterior and posterior leaflets in diastole. The severity of mitral stenosis can be assessed by 2-D and Doppler echocardiography. Two-dimensional imaging of the mitral valve often will reveal the characteristic "doming" appearance of the mitral valve and restricted leaflet opening in diastole (Fig. 9–8). Evaluation of valvular morphology and the presence or absence of subvalvular involvement is crucial in determining what therapeutic options may be available. The mitral orifice can be visualized in diastole and the area directly planimetered. In approximately 20% of patients, particularly those with heavily calcified valves and densely fibrotic commissures, these planimetered valve areas may be inaccurate. Doppler interrogation provides effective supplemental data to further assess the severity of mitral stenosis. The peak velocity of transmitral flow is increased when the valve is stenotic and the rate of decline of the flow during diastole is reduced. The time course for peak velocity to reach half its initial value correlates with the size of the mitral orifice (pressure half-time technique). In the elderly, an overestimation of valve area may occur as the mitral pressure half-time is significantly affected by the changes in atrial and ventricular compliance that occur with the aging process.[90] Coexisting conditions, such as MR, aortic valve disease, left atrial thrombus, and pulmonary hypertension also can be assessed echocardiographically. Transesophageal echocardiography is uniquely suited to assess these parameters and provides an important adjunct to transthoracic assessment in patients with a technically limited standard echocardiographic assessment.[91]

Cardiac catheterization should be performed in any elderly patient with symptomatic mitral stenosis considered for valvuloplasty or surgery or those patients in whom the severity of mitral stenosis remains uncertain after noninvasive studies. Coronary arteriography also should be performed in adult patients referred for therapeutic interventions. Right and left heart catheterization are necessary to confirm the severity of mitral stenosis, assess the degree of pulmonary hypertension, and aid in the exclusion of other coexistent valvular lesions.

MANAGEMENT

The therapeutic options for elderly patients with symptomatic mitral stenosis include medical therapy, commissurotomy (percutaneous balloon or surgical), and mitral valve replacement. Antibiotic prophylaxis against bacterial endocarditis is indicated regardless of age, especially if MR coexists. Mild heart failure symptom-

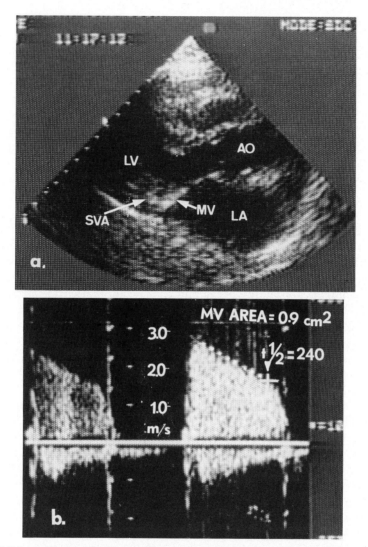

Figure 9–8. Echocardiogram of a 73-year-old woman with class III heart failure secondary to rheumatic mitral stenosis. (*a*) There is substantial thickening and "doming" of the mitral valve leaflets (MV). The subvalvular apparatus (SVA) is also markedly thickened. (*b*) Doppler revealed a mitral valve area of 0.9 cm^2 by the pressure 1/2 time method. The echo score was calculated to be 9.

atology is managed in the standard manner with diuretics and salt restriction. Atrial fibrillation eventually occurs in most patients with moderate or severe mitral stenosis. Electrical or chemical cardioversion should be attempted at least once although long-term maintenance of sinus rhythm is infrequent.[92] Before cardioversion, patients should be anticoagulated for several weeks if the duration of atrial fibrillation exceeds several days or if there is a history of embolism.[93]

Digoxin remains the drug of choice for the control of the ventricular rate in patients with atrial fibrillation, although beta-blockers and calcium channel blockers may be more effective in controlling the ventricular rate during exercise or stress.[94] However, the use of these agents may be associated with untoward side effects in the elderly and should be used cautiously.

Systemic embolism may be a devastating consequence of rheumatic valve disease. Systemic anticoagulation should be considered in all patients with a history of embolism unless contraindicated. Patients with atrial fibrillation (chronic or paroxysmal) are also at increased risk for systemic embolization.[93,95] Unfortunately, anticoagulation-related mortality and morbidity increase with age so that the physician must carefully weigh the relative risk versus benefit. Factors contributing to the decision to anticoagulate include the individual's physiologic age, coexisting disease processes, social environment, life style, and actuarial survival. Generally, less aggressive anticoagulation (prothrombin 1.2 to 1.4 times control) should be employed in the elderly compared with younger, lower risk patients.

Elderly patients with severely symptomatic pure mitral stenosis should be considered for valve replacement or commissurotomy (surgical or balloon). The operative mortality of selected patients older than 70 years of age undergoing mitral valve replacement is approximately 10% to 15%.[96-98] Mortality in elderly patients with other coexistent medical illness is generally significantly higher. Mortality also relates to functional class, concomitant coronary artery disease, and need for additional valvular surgery. Surgical commissurotomy is now less frequently performed on elderly patients because of the emergence of percutaneous balloon mitral valvuloplasty (PMV).

In the past 6 years, PMV has become established as a nonsurgical alternative for the treatment of mitral stenosis.[99] Successful PMV most likely results from the separation of adherent commissures and fracture of nodular calcium.[100] The advantages of PMV compared with valve replacement include shorter hospitalizations, initial lower mortality and morbidity, and the avoidance of complications associated with the implantation of a prosthetic mitral valve, such as endocarditis and valve-associated thromboembolism. Most patients experience immediate clinical improvement, although there is considerable interpatient variability. Concomitant mitral stenosis and severe MR preclude the use of this procedure. In patients with echocardiographically identified left atrial thrombus, PMV is contraindicated although the procedure may be undertaken at a later date if the thrombus resolves subsequent to a course of systemic anticoagulation.

Echocardiography is valuable in identifying patients who are most likely to benefit from PMV.[101] The morphologic characteristics of the mitral valve and subvalvular apparatus appear to influence the immediate results of PMV. Patients with pliable valves and minimal calcification have better initial and long-term clinical benefit. The extent and severity of involvement of the mitral apparatus has been quantitated using an echocardiographic scoring system assessing four morphologic variables (see Fig. 9–8). These include valvular thickening, valvular mobility, valvular calcification, and subvalvular thickening. Each variable is analyzed and assigned a score. The total score is then calculated. A high total score, indicating markedly limited leaflet motion, extensive valvular thickening, and subvalvular disease, is associated with less favorable immediate and long-term outcome after PMV.[102] Complications of PMV, including mortality, the need for emergent surgery, post-PMV severe MR, and the development of a significant left-to-right shunt, occur more frequently in patients with higher scores. Although elderly patients are more likely to have higher scores, these findings do not always preclude a good response to PMV (Fig. 9–9). Favorable immediate outcome is supported by the results of the eight valvuloplasties on elderly patients with mitral stenosis performed at our institution (mean age 77 ± 2). In this group, the mean transmitral gradient decreased from 15 ± 2 to 5 ± 1 mm Hg, and the calculated mitral valve

196 CLINICAL CONSIDERATIONS

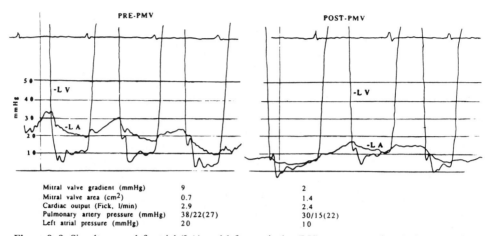

	PRE-PMV	POST-PMV
Mitral valve gradient (mmHg)	9	2
Mitral valve area (cm²)	0.7	1.4
Cardiac output (Fick, l/min)	2.9	2.4
Pulmonary artery pressure (mmHg)	38/22(27)	30/15(22)
Left atrial pressure (mmHg)	20	10

Figure 9–9. Simultaneous left atrial (LA) and left ventricular (LV) pressure tracings before and after percutaneous balloon mitral valvuloplasty (PMV) of the elderly female whose echocardiogram is shown in Figure 9–8. The PMV resulted in an increase in mitral valve area from 0.7 to 1.4 cm² (provided by H. C. Herrmann, M.D.).

area increased from 0.7 ± 0.1 to 1.6 ± 0.1 cm² (personal communication H. C. Herrmann). Future studies in larger numbers of elderly patients are necessary to better define the role of this procedure in this population. Furthermore, improved equipment and techniques including the self-positioning Inoue balloon have reduced the influence of age and echocardiographic morphology on the immediate results of PMV.[103]

Successful PMV typically results in an increase of the mitral valve orifice by approximately 1.0 cm² and is associated with a substantial improvement in functional class that is often maintained at least through the first year of followup. There does appear to be an inverse relationship between age and enlargement in mitral area after PMV. Inhospital mortality after PMV is reported as being less than 1% to 3% with few complications.[104] These studies, however, included only small numbers of elderly patients. In contrast, a procedural mortality of 9% was recently reported by Lefevre and associates[105] in a series of 34 surgical high-risk patients with severe mitral stenosis. *High risk* was defined as patients older than 70 years, ejection fraction <35%, New York Heart Association class IV, severe pulmonary hypertension, or those requiring coronary revascularization or additional valvular surgery. Despite the increased mortality, the clinical status in the majority of patients was significantly improved 6 months after valvuloplasty. Specific conclusions regarding the elderly in this series were limited because these patients comprised less than one third of the total study population, and subgroup analysis was not performed. Nonetheless, the data demonstrate that PMV may be a viable alternative to surgery in elderly high-risk patients.

The management of patients with severe symptomatic mitral stenosis must be individualized. Although there are many elderly patients whose stenotic mitral valves can be successfully dilated with PMV, there are others who are likely better served with mitral valve replacement. If the valvular and subvalvular assessment is favorable, then PMV should be considered as the procedure of choice. Patients with very high echocardiographic scores indicating severe disease of the mitral valve apparatus and who are otherwise well should be considered for surgery.

The type of valve offered should depend upon the patient's anticipated longevity as well as the need and safety of anticoagulation. Inasmuch as many patients will likely require long-term anticoagulation for chronic atrial fibrillation, a mechanical prosthesis is most often employed. In those in whom anticoagulation must be avoided, a bioprosthesis may be advised although the diminutive left ventricular dimensions associated with mitral inflow obstruction may well preclude the insertion of these high-profile valves. Surgical valvuloplasty or open commissurotomy, specifically directed at the relief of commissural fusion and debridement of calcium deposits, may also be viable options.[106] Assessment of the final result of such procedures may be made intraoperatively with transesophageal echocardiography. If the result is inadequate, then valve replacement can be undertaken.

MITRAL REGURGITATION

Mitral valve disease in the elderly more commonly presents with mitral regurgitation than with mitral stenosis. Mitral regurgitation may result from dysfunction of one or more components of the mitral valve apparatus (Table 9–5). Causes include mitral annular calcification, rheumatic heart disease, papillary muscle dysfunction from coronary artery disease, infectious endocarditis, and myxomatous degeneration of the mitral valve.[107]

The normal physiologic changes of the mitral valve apparatus result from chronic "wear and tear" related degeneration.[12] These degenerative changes occur on both atrial and mural aspects of the leaflets. The atrial surfaces of the valve become thickened and opaque. Elastic fiber and collagen proliferation with progressive fragmentation and disorganization are apparent on microscopic examination. The leaflet edges develop degenerative nodules. In contrast to rheumatic valvular involvement, commissural fusion does not occur. Yellow plaques are frequently visualized on the mural aspect of the leaflets. Microscopically, these changes are the consequence of foamy vacuolation of the fibrous elements of the cusp by lipid droplets. These deposits resemble atheroma although there is no associated presence of hemorrhage or thrombosis. Minimal leaflet calcification is commonly seen. As aging progresses, pathologic changes may occur which impact upon the functional integrity of the valve apparatus.

MITRAL ANNULAR CALCIFICATION

Mitral annular calcification (MAC) is a degenerative disease that is, with rare exceptions, unique to the elderly. Most affected patients are older than 60 years of age.[108] The prevalence of this condition increases with increasing age. For unclear

Table 9–5. Etiology of Mitral Regurgitation in the Elderly

Myxomatous degeneration of the mitral valve
Mitral annular calcification
Rheumatic heart disease
Papillary muscle dysfunction 2° to coronary artery disease
Infectious endocarditis
Chordae tendineae rupture

reasons, woman are affected two to three times more frequently than men.[109] MAC is reported in 8% to 13% of autopsy series in the elderly. The gross appearance of MAC may vary from small localized spicules of calcium to a rigid C- or J-shaped bar up to 2 cm in thickness (Fig. 9–10). Initially, calcification begins at the mid-portion of the posterior leaflet attachment of the mitral annulus (Fig. 9–11). As calcification progresses, the leaflets become deformed upward, stretching the chordae tendineae and causing the leaflets to protrude into the left ventricular inflow tract. MAC also can erode into the myocardium and impinge on the closely related conduction system. When examined microscopically, calcification appears first in the fibrosa of the annulus, and then may extend to expand into the myocardium. The etiology of this process is not clearly understood, but hemodynamic stress upon the anulus appears contributory to its presence and magnitude. The association of MAC with hypertension, hypertrophic cardiomyopathy, aortic stenosis, and mitral valve replacement supports this relationship. Additional predisposing conditions for the development of MAC include chronic renal failure and diabetes mellitus.

Clinical Manifestations

MAC causes MR by two mechanisms. It may displace the mitral leaflets from their normal anatomic position and may impair systolic mitral anular contraction. As MAC worsens and MR intensifies, left ventricular volume overload progresses resulting in heart failure. Atrial fibrillation may develop as a consequence of left

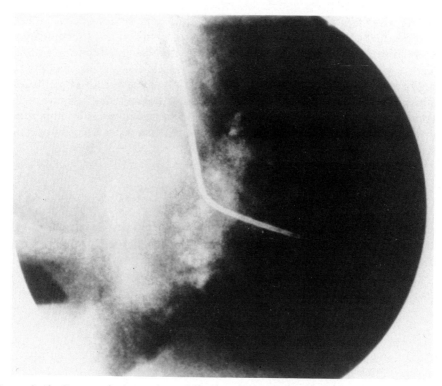

Figure 9–10. Severe mitral annular calcification in an elderly patient noted during cardiac catheterization.

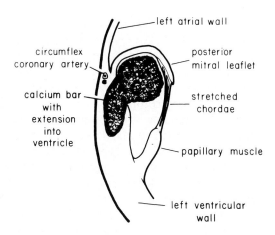

Figure 9–11. Schema of pathologic features of mitral annular calcification (MAC). Extension of calcium into the subvalve angle is common and may form a prominent ridge over which the posterior mitral cusp becomes stretched and to which the chordae tendineae may become adherent.

atrial enlargement. Heart block also may occur as the conduction system is invaded by the calcific process.[110] Second-degree and complete heart block, which may require pacemaker implantation, have been reported in as many as 50% of patients with severe MAC in some series.[111] Coexistent diffuse sclerodegenerative disease of the conduction system also may contribute to these conduction disturbances.

Systemic embolization of calcific debris has been reported with extensive MAC resulting in retinal and cerebral emboli.[112] Bacterial endocarditis has been described in patients with severe MAC, but because MR coexists, it is unclear whether MAC itself is the cause.[113]

MYXOMATOUS DEGENERATION OF THE MITRAL VALVE

Myxomatous degeneration of the mitral valve is a common etiology of symptomatic MR in the elderly population.[114] Although a variety of terms have been used to describe this entity, mitral valve prolapse (MVP) is the most common. It has become recognized as one of the most prevalent of cardiac abnormalities. The manifestations of MVP are frequently more serious in the elderly than in younger patients. The pathologic findings of myxomatous degeneration are well described and will not be reviewed here.

Clinical Manifestations

It is difficult to define the natural history of such a common disorder as MVP.[115] The majority of patients are asymptomatic. Most long-term studies demonstrate that the vast majority of patients remain stable without progression of the severity of MR. Nonetheless, studies from countries in which the prevalence of rheumatic heart disease has markedly decreased have reported that MVP is the most common etiology of MR for which valvular surgery is necessary.[116]

In the elderly, MVP is often overlooked or misdiagnosed because of the frequent occurrence of systolic ejection murmurs, although the diagnosis of MVP can be made by a careful physical examination and can be confirmed by echocardiography. Auscultation reveals the characteristic midsystolic click and mid-to-late systolic murmur, although these findings may be intermittently present. If MVP is substantial, a classic MR murmur is appreciated.

Progressive mitral regurgitation occurs in approximately 5% to 10% of patients with MVP. The risk of progressive MR increases with age and is greater in men than in women. Hypertension, especially in men, is associated with a greater likelihood of progressive regurgitation. In one study, 4% of men and 1.5% of women with MVP required mitral valve surgery before the age of 70.[117] Heart failure may be the presenting complaint in 25% to 40% of symptomatic elderly patients with MVP.[118] Severe chronic MR may result from enlargement of the mitral anulus or from the redundant prolapsing leaflets. Congestive heart failure appears to occur earlier in elderly patients with MVP, but this observation may, in part, be due to attributing the insidious symptoms of MR to advancing age or depression. Additionally, diminished left ventricular compliance may result in higher diastolic left ventricular pressures and earlier occurrence of pulmonary venous congestion than in younger individuals. Acute or subacute decompensation in a patient with MVP may result from rupture of the chordae tendineae.[119] This rupture may be spontaneous or be associated with bacterial endocarditis. Flail chordae may be identified by echocardiographic studies. Blood cultures should be obtained in such patients to exclude endocarditis.

Chest pain (atypical or typical), palpitations, and dizziness are common symptoms in all patients with MVP, including the elderly. Because coronary artery disease is so common in the elderly, angina and MVP may coexist. The physician must not attribute symptoms consistent with angina pectoris as being due to MVP alone and should perform additional studies to assess the presence of coronary artery disease.

Endocarditis prophylaxis is mandated in all patients with MR. Although the need for prophylaxis in the absence of regurgitation is controversial, we believe that the elderly should receive such prophylaxis if the leaflets are substantially abnormal inasmuch as these patients may have impaired host defenses.

PAPILLARY MUSCLE DYSFUNCTION

Clinical Manifestations

Coronary artery disease is the predominant cause of papillary muscle dysfunction that results in symptomatic MR.[120] The severity of MR relates to the magnitude of papillary muscle compromise. Rupture of the whole muscle or one head is usually associated with acute inferior infarction and results in catastrophic hemodynamic deterioration that may be irreconcilable. More frequently, however, the base of the muscle becomes compromised, and valve coaption is impaired.[121] The posteromedial muscle is more commonly affected because its blood supply originates from the posterior descending branch of the right coronary artery only. In contrast, the anterolateral papillary muscle receives a dual blood supply from both the left anterior descending and circumflex arteries. Transient papillary muscle dysfunction, which may occur during episodes of reversible ischemia, often results in intermittent MR and, at times, acute pulmonary venous congestion. Left ventricular dilation and papillary muscle fibrosis from chronic ischemic heart disease can cause papillary muscle malalignment leading to moderate MR. The diagnosis of papillary muscle involvement as the etiology of MR is made by echocardiography.

MANAGEMENT OF MITRAL REGURGITATION

The symptoms of chronic MR are subtle and often insidious, frequently resulting in unrecognized left ventricular dysfunction before the development of clinical heart failure. Medical management with digoxin, diuretics, and vasodilator therapy is useful to ameliorate symptoms and reduce the regurgitant volume.[122] Mitral valve surgery should, however, be considered in symptomatic elderly patients with chronic progressive MR before development of severe irreversible left ventricular dysfunction. The appropriate timing of surgery, as in younger patients, is a matter of considerable controversy.[78] The risk of mitral valvular surgery in the elderly is greater than that of aortic valvular surgery but should not be considered prohibitive in those carefully selected patients in whom a favorable clinical outcome is anticipated. The increased surgical mortality of mitral compared with aortic valvular surgery is likely multifactorial, including the higher incidence of irreconcilable but unrecognized left ventricular dysfunction, adverse alterations in left ventricular afterload resulting from restored mitral valve competence, and the adverse impact of mitral valve replacement on contractile function of the base of the left ventricle. Mortality in most recent studies for valve replacement approximates 10% to 15%[45,96] but has been reported to be as high as 50% in higher risk patients.[123] Such high-risk patients include those with severe left ventricular dysfunction, concomitant coronary artery disease requiring revascularization, multivalvular surgery, emergent surgery, and advanced age. Mitral valve reconstruction or repair may offer advantages over valve replacement and has been performed with reduced operative mortality compared with replacement. Scott and associates[124] have reported an operative mortality of 13% in patients undergoing valvular repair and bypass surgery in contrast to a 22% mortality when valve replacement and bypass were required.[124] The apparent benefit may result from better left ventricular performance in those with a preserved mitral valve apparatus. Late surgical outcome likewise may be improved by repair because prosthetic valve complications may be obviated. Mitral valvular repair data in the elderly, however, are not uniform. Fremes and associates[46] reported no difference in operative mortality in the elderly undergoing repair compared with those undergoing mitral valve replacement. In addition, mitral valvular repair in the elderly is often technically more demanding or not possible as a consequence of the friability and calcification of the leaflets in these patients. Future studies using transesophageal echocardiography may assist in defining the role of mitral valve repair in the elderly.

In itself, MAC is an infrequent cause of isolated, severe MR. The presence of severe MAC, however, imposes substantial technical difficulties for the surgeon attempting mitral valve repair, as demonstrated by the operative mortality of 27% reported in the recent series by Cammack and colleagues.[125] Medical management may be more prudent than surgery in the minimally symptomatic elderly patient with severe MAC and MR. In a few small series, newer surgical techniques, including ultrasonic debridement of the calcification and reconstruction of the AV groove, have been reported to improve outcome in these patients.[126]

Patients with acute MR resulting from papillary muscle rupture or chordal rupture are frequently in cardiogenic shock. Attempts should be made to stabilize these patients with medical therapy and intraaortic balloon counterpulsation. Cardiac catheterization and coronary angiography should be performed emergently to identify the coronary anatomy and exclude concomitant septal rupture. Although operative mortality is high, the prognosis is bleak with medical therapy alone.

Table 9–6. Endocarditis Prophylaxis
Recommendations in Elderly*

Acquired valvular dysfunction, even after surgery
All prosthetic cardiac valves
MVP with valvular regurgitation
MVP associated with thickening or redundancy of leaflets†
History of bacterial endocarditis
Most congenital malformations
Hypertrophic cardiomyopathy

*This table is not meant to be all inclusive (see American Heart Association recommendation, reference 127).
†Controversial.

INFECTIVE ENDOCARDITIS

The elderly constitute an increasing percentage of patients with infective endocarditis, thus emphasizing the importance of appropriate endocarditis prophylaxis in this age group (Table 9–6).[127] Presently, patients older than the age of 60 years comprise approximately 40% to 60% of all patients with endocarditis.[128] The reasons for this increase are multifactorial and include the significant increase in number of elderly patients who also have a high prevalence of acquired valvular disease, an increase in intravascular procedures and urologic procedures performed upon these patients, and an increase in the number of elderly patients who have prosthetic valves. In the elderly, as in younger patients, the percentage of cases of endocarditis caused by staphylococci and streptococci are similar. Certain organisms, including enterococci, *Streptococcus bovi,* and coagulase-negative staphylococci, appear more likely to cause endocarditis in the elderly than in younger patients. Invasive vascular procedures, in particular intravenous catheters, are the most common source of bacteremia. Unfortunately, errors and delay in diagnosis are frequent in the elderly. Although most patients have a murmur, they are often overlooked and considered benign. The elderly often are poor historians, have fewer symptoms, and commonly demonstrate a diminished febrile response. Initial presentations of endocarditis in the elderly may include confusion, renal failure, acute neurologic events, pneumonia, or pulmonary edema secondary to acute valvular incompetence. The diagnosis, once suspected, should be made with documentation of bacteremia by blood cultures. Echocardiography may be helpful in visualizing vegetations and the extent of valvular involvement.

SUMMARY

As patients survive to advanced age, they commonly develop degenerative valvular heart disease as well as degenerative diseases of other organ systems. In addition, a reservoir of patients with other forms of valvular heart disease develop progressive symptomatology with advancing age. These patients often present a challenge to the cardiologist in both diagnosis and management. Inasmuch as these patients tolerate cardiovascular surgery less well than their younger counterparts, criteria for surgical intervention may often need modification. Chronologic age must be recognized as but one of many factors affecting physiologic function. Knowledge of aging-related alterations in function must be employed in both diagnostic and therapeutic algorithms. At times, input from other health-care providers who specialize in the care of the elderly may assist in the assessment of these patients.

Surgery should be reserved for higher-risk patients who are severely symptomatic or for those in whom severe symptoms are likely to soon develop based on the natural history of the disease process involved. Those less symptomatic elderly patients with otherwise preserved physiologic functions also may be offered valvular surgery. The availability of nonsurgical, albeit at times palliative, techniques to relieve aortic or mitral stenosis provides an alternative therapeutic option to cardiothoracic surgery. Advances in understanding the pathophysiology and medical therapy of heart failure will continue to contribute to an improved quality of life for those for whom only medical options exist.

REFERENCES

1. Rowe, JW: Health care of the elderly. N Engl J Med 312:827, 1985.
2. Wenger, NK, O'Rourke, RA, and Marcus, FI: The care of elderly patients with cardiovascular disease. Ann Intern Med 109:425, 1988.
3. Lakatta, EG, Mitchell, JH, Promerance, A, et al: Human aging: Changes in structure and function. J Am Coll Cardiol 10(Suppl A):42, 1987.
4. Rodeheffer, RJ, Gerstenblith, G, Becker, LC, et al: Exercise cardiac output is maintained with advancing age in healthy human subjects: Cardiac dilation and increased stroke volume compensate for a diminished heart rate. Circulation 69:203, 1984.
5. Garibaldi, RA and Nurse, BA: Infections in the elderly. Am J Med 81(Suppl 1A):53, 1986.
6. Gillick, MR, Serrell, N, and Gillick, LS: Adverse consequences of hospitalization in the elderly. Soc Sci Med 16:1033, 1982.
7. Robbins, AS and Rubenstein, LZ: Postural hypotension in the elderly. J Am Geriatr Soc 32:769, 1984.
8. Vestel, RE: Drug use in the elderly: A review of problems and special considerations. Drugs 16:358, 1978.
9. Selzer, A: Changing aspects of the natural history of valvular aortic stenosis. N Engl J Med 317:91, 1987.
10. Mönckenberg, JG: Der normale histologische Bau und die Sklerose der Aortenklappen. Virchows Arch [Pathol Anat] 176:472, 1904.
11. Roberts, WC: The structure of the aortic valve in clinically isolated aortic stenosis. Circulation 42:91, 1970.
12. Pomerance, A: Ageing changes in human heart valves. Br Heart J 29:222, 1967.
13. Edwards, JE: Calcific aortic stenosis: Pathologic features. Mayo Clin Proc 36:444, 1961.
14. Wong, M, Tel, C, and Shah, PM: Degenerative calcific valvular disease and the systolic murmurs in the elderly. J Am Geriatr Soc 31:156, 1983.
15. Wenger, NK: Selected cardiac problems in the elderly patient. J Med Assoc Ga 68:1033, 1979.
16. Wagner, S and Selzer, A: Patterns of progression of aortic stenosis: A longitudinal hemodynamic study. Circulation 65:709, 1982.
17. Lombard, JT and Selzer, A: Valvular aortic stenosis: Clinical and hemodynamic profile of patients. Ann Intern Med 106:292, 1987.
18. Marcus, ML, Doty, DB, Hiratzka, LF, et al: Decreased coronary reserve: A mechanism for angina pectoris in patients with aortic stenosis and normal coronary arteries. N Engl J Med 307:1362, 1982.
19. Johnson, AM: Aortic stenosis, sudden death, and the left ventricular baroceptors. Br Heart J 33:1, 1971.
20. Roberts, WC, Perloff, JK, and Costantino, T: Severe valvular aortic stenosis in patients over 65 years of age: Clinicopathologic study. Am J Cardiol 27:497, 1971.
21. Holley, KE, Bahn, RC, McGoon, DC, et al: Spontaneous calcific embolization associated with calcific aortic stenosis. Circulation 27:197, 1963.
22. Brockmeier, LB, Adolph, RJ, Gustin, BW, et al: Calcium emboli to the retinal artery in calcific aortic stenosis. Am Heart J 101:32, 1981.

23. Ross, J and Braunwald, E: Aortic stenosis. Circulation 38(suppl V):V-61, 1968.
24. Pellikka, PA, Nishimura, RA, Bailey, KR, et al: The natural history of adults with asymptomatic, hemodynamically significant aortic stenosis. J Am Coll Cardiol 15:1012, 1990.
25. Braunwald, E: On the natural history of severe aortic stenosis. J Am Coll Cardiol 15:1018, 1990.
26. Perloff, JK: Clinical recognition of aortic stenosis. Prog Cardiovasc Dis 10:323, 1968.
27. Kotler, MN, Mintz, GS, Parry, WR, et al: Bedside diagnosis of organic murmurs in the elderly. Geriatrics 36:107, 1981.
28. Albin, EL, Chandraratna, PA, Littman, BB, et al: Idiopathic hypertrophic subaortic stenosis in the elderly. Am J Med Sci 274:163, 1977.
29. Nair, CK, Aronow, WS, Stokke, K, et al: Cardiac conduction defects in patients older than 60 years with aortic stenosis and without mitral annular calcium. Am J Cardiol 53:169, 1984.
30. Thompson, R, Mitchell, A, Ahmed, M, et al: Conduction defects in aortic valve disease. Am Heart J 98:3, 1979.
31. Szamosi, A and Wassberg, B: Radiologic detection of aortic stenosis. Acta Radiol [Diagn] (Stock) 24:201, 1983.
32. Seigel, RJ, Maurer, G, Navatpumin, T, et al: Accurate noninvasive assessment of critical aortic valve stenosis in the elderly. J Am Coll Cardiol 1:639, 1983.
33. Currie, PJ, Seward, JB, Reeder, GS, et al: Continuous-wave Doppler echocardiographic assessment of severity of calcific aortic stenosis: A simultaneous Doppler-catheter correlative study in 100 adult patients. Circulation 71:1162, 1985.
34. Yeager, M, Yock, PG, and Popp, RL: Comparison of Doppler-derived pressure gradient to that determined at cardiac catheterization in adults with aortic stenosis: Implications for management. Am J Cardiol 57:644, 1986.
35. Rijsterborgh, H and Roelandt, J: Doppler assessment of aortic stenosis: Bernoulli revisited. Ultrasound Med Biol 13:241, 1987.
36. St. John Sutton, MG, St. John Sutton, M, Oldershaw, P, et al: Valve replacement without preoperative cardiac catheterization. N Engl J Med 305:1233, 1981.
37. Ramsdale, DR, Faragher, EB, Bennet, DH, et al: Preoperative prediction of significant coronary artery disease in patients with valvular heart disease. Br Med J 284:223, 1982.
38. O'Keefe, JH, Vlietstra, RE, Bailey, KR, et al: Natural history of candidates for balloon aortic valvuloplasty. Mayo Clin Proc 62:986, 1987.
39. Christakis, GT, Weisel, RD, David, TE, et al: Predictors of operative survival after valve replacement. Circulation 78(suppl I):I-25, 1988.
40. Smith, N, McAnulty, JH, and Rahimtoola, SH: Severe aortic stenosis with impaired left ventricular function and clinical heart failure: Results of valve replacement. Circulation 58:255, 1978.
41. Austen, WG, DeSanctis, RW, Buckley, MJ, et al: Surgical management of aortic valve disease in the elderly. JAMA 211:624, 1970.
42. Ahmad, A and Starr, A: Valve replacement in geriatric patients. Br Heart J 31:322, 1969.
43. Jamieson, WR, Dooner, J, Munro, A, et al: Cardiac valve replacement in the elderly: A review of 320 consecutive cases. Circulation 64(suppl II)II-177, 1981.
44. Bessone, LN, Pupello, DF, Blank, RH, et al: Valve replacement in patients over 70 years of age. Ann Thorac Surg 24:417, 1977.
45. Blakeman, BM, Pifarre, R, Sullivan, HJ, et al: Aortic valve replacement in patients 75 years and older. Ann Thorac Surg 44:637, 1987.
46. Fremes, SE, Goldman, BS, Ivanov, J, et al: Valvular surgery in the elderly. Circulation 80(suppl I): I-77, 1989.
47. Levinson, JR, Akins, CW, Buckley, MJ, et al: Octogenarians with aortic stenosis: Outcome after aortic valve replacement. Circulation 80(suppl I):I-49, 1989.
48. Edmunds, LH, Stephenson, LW, Edie, RN, et al: Open heart surgery in octogenarians. N Engl J Med 319:131, 1988.
49. Lytle, BW, Cosgrove, DM, Loop, FD, et al: Replacement of aortic valve combined with myocardial revascularization. Determinants of early and late risk for 500 patients, 1967–1981. Circulation 68:1149, 1983.
50. Tsai, TP, Matloff, JM, Chaux, A, et al: Combined valve and coronary artery bypass procedures in septuagenarians and octogenarians: Results in 120 patients. Ann Thorac Surg 42:681, 1986.
51. MacGovern, JA, Pennock, JL, Campbell, DB, et al: Aortic valve replacement and combined aortic valve replacement and coronary artery bypass grafting: Predicting high risk groups. J Am Coll Cardiol 9:38, 1987.

52. Borkon, AM, Soule, LM, Baughman, KL, et al: Aortic valve selection in the elderly patient. Ann Thorac Surg 46:270, 1988.

53. Jamieson, WR, Rosado, LJ, Muriro, AI, et al: Carpentier-Edwards standard porcine bioprosthesis: Primary tissue failure (structural valve deterioration) by age groups. Ann Thorac Surg 46:155, 1988.

54. Cribier, A, Savin, T, Rocha, P, et al: Percutaneous transluminal valvuloplasty of acquired aortic stenosis in elderly patients: An alternative to valve replacement? Lancet 1:68, 1986.

55. Schneider, JF, Wilson, M, and Gallant, TE: Percutaneous balloon valvuloplasty for aortic stenosis in elderly patients at high risk for surgery. Ann Intern Med 106:696, 1987.

56. Safian, RD, Berman, AD, Diver, DJ, et al: Balloon aortic valvuloplasty in 170 consecutive patients. N Engl J Med 319:125, 1988.

57. Safian, RD, Mandell, VS, Thurer, RE, et al: Postmortem and intraoperative balloon valvuloplasty of calcific aortic stenosis in elderly patients: Mechanism of successful dilation. J Am Coll Cardiol 9:655, 1987.

58. Block, PC and Palacios, IF: Restenosis after percutaneous aortic valvuloplasty in elderly patients: Clinical and catheterization follow-up. Am J Cardiol 62:760, 1988.

59. Sherman, W, Hershman, R, Lazzam, C, et al: Balloon valvuloplasty in aortic stenosis: Determinants of clinical outcome. Ann Intern Med 110:421 1989.

60. Brady, ST, Davis, CA, Kussmaul, WG, et al: Percutaneous aortic balloon valvuloplasty in octogenarians: Morbidity and mortality. Ann Intern Med 110:761, 1989.

61. Nishishmura, RA, Holmes, DR, Reeder, GS, et al: Doppler evaluation of results of percutaneous aortic balloon valvuloplasty in calcific aortic stenosis. Circulation 78:791, 1988.

62. Letac, B, Bribier, A, Koning, R, et al: Results of percutaneous transluminal valvuloplasty in 218 patients with valvular aortic stenosis. Am J Cardiol 62:598, 1988.

63. Safian, RD, Warren, SE, Berman, AD, et al: Improvement in symptoms and left ventricular performance after balloon aortic valvuloplasty in patients with aortic stenosis and depressed left ventricular ejection fraction. Circulation 78:1181, 1988.

64. Ferguson, JJ and Garza, RA: Efficacy of multiple balloon aortic valvuloplasty procedures. J Am Coll Cardiol 17:1430, 1991.

65. Desnoyers, MR, Salem, DN, Rosenfield, K, et al: Treatment of cardiogenic shock by emergency aortic balloon valvuloplasty. Ann Intern Med 108:833, 1988.

66. Roth, RB, Palacios, F, and Block, PC: Percutaneous aortic valvuloplasty: Its role in the management of patients with aortic stenosis requiring major noncardiac surgery. J Am Coll Cardiol 13:1039, 1989.

67. Olson, LJ, Subramanian, R, and Edwards, WD: Surgical pathology of pure aortic regurgitation: A study of 255 cases. Mayo Clin Proc 59:835, 1984.

68. Allen, WM, Matloff, JM, and Fishbein, MC: Myxoid degeneration of the aortic valve and isolated severe aortic regurgitation. Am J Cardiol 55:429, 1985.

69. Waller, BF, Kishel, JC, and Roberts, WC: Severe aortic regurgitation from systemic hypertension. Chest 82:365, 1982.

70. Morganroth, J, Perloff, JK, Zeldis, SM, et al: Acute severe aortic regurgitation: Pathophysiology, clinical recognition, and management. Ann Intern Med 87:223, 1977.

71. Grayburn, PA, Smith, MD, Handshoe, R, et al: Detection of aortic insufficiency by standard echocardiography, pulsed Doppler echocardiography, and auscultation. Ann Intern Med 104:599, 1986.

72. Henry, WL, Bonow, RO, Borer, JS, et al: Observations on the optimum time for operative intervention for aortic regurgitation. Serial echocardiographic evaluation of asymptomatic patients. Circulation 61:471, 1980.

73. Fioretta, P, Roelandt, J, Bos, RJ, et al: Echocardiography in chronic aortic insufficiency: Is valve replacement too late when left ventricular end-systolic dimension reaches 55 mm? Circulation 67:216, 1983.

74. Perry, GJ, Helmcke, F, Nanda, NC, et al: Evaluation of aortic insufficiency by Doppler color flow mapping. J Am Coll Cardiol 9:952, 1987.

75. Manyari, DE, Nolewajka, AJ, and Kostuk, WJ: Quantitative assessment of aortic valvular insufficiency by radionuclide angiography. Chest 81:170, 1982.

76. DePace, NL, Nestico, PF, and Kotler, MN: Comparison of echocardiography and angiography in determining the cause of severe aortic regurgitation. Br Heart J 51:36, 1984.

77. Turina, J, Hess, O, Sepulcri, F, et al: Spontaneous course of aortic valve disease. Eur Heart J 8:471, 1987.

78. Grossman, W: Aortic and mitral regurgitation: How to evaluate the condition and when to consider surgical intervention. JAMA 252:2447, 1984.

79. Greves, J, Rahimtoola, SH, McAnulty, JH, et al: Preoperative criteria predictive of late survival following valve replacement for severe aortic regurgitation. Am Heart J 101:300, 1981.

80. Bonow, RO, Rosing, DR, McIntosh, CL, et al: The natural history of asymptomatic patients with aortic regurgitation and normal left ventricular function. Circulation 68:509, 1983.

81. Greenberg, BH, Massie, B, Bristow, JD, et al: Long-term vasodilator therapy of chronic aortic insufficiency: A randomized double-blinded, placebo-controlled clinical trial. Circulation 78:92, 1988.

82. Wood, P: An appreciation of mitral stenosis. Br Med J 1:1113, 1954.

83. Hammer, WJ, Roberts, WC, DeLeon, AL: "Mitral stenosis" secondary to combined "massive" mitral annular calcific deposits and small, hypertrophied left ventricles. Am J Med 64:371, 1978.

84. Hargreaves, T: Rheumatic mitral valve disease in the elderly: Incidence found at necropsy. Br Med J 2:342, 1961.

85. Selzer, A and Cohn, KE: Natural history of mitral stenosis. Circulation 45:878, 1972.

86. Rowe, JC, Bland, EF, Sprague, HB, et al: The course of mitral stenosis without surgery: Ten and twenty year perspectives. Ann Intern Med 52:741, 1960.

87. Limas, CT: Mitral stenosis in the elderly. Geriatrics 26:75, 1971.

88. Reichek, N, Shelburne, JD, and Perloff, JR: Clinical aspects of rheumatic valve disease. Prog Cardiovasc Disc 15:491, 1973.

89. Nichol, PM, Gilbert, BW, and Kisslo, JA: Two-dimensional echocardiographic assessment of mitral stenosis. Circulation 55:120, 1977.

90. Thomas, JD and Weyman, AE: Mitral pressure half-time: In search of theoretical justification. J Am Coll Cardiol 10:932, 1987.

91. Seward, JB, Khandheria, BK, Oh, JK, et al: Transesophageal echocardiography: Technique, anatomic considerations, implementation and clinical applications. Mayo Clin Proc 63:649, 1988.

92. Brye-Quinn, E and Wing, AJ: Maintenance of sinus rhythm after DC revision of atrial fibrillation: A double blind controlled trial of long-acting quinidine bisulphate. Br Heart J 32:370, 1970.

93. Casella, L, Abelmann, WH, and Ellis, LB: Patients with mitral stenosis and systemic emboli. Arch Intern Med 114:773, 1964.

94. Klein, HO, Sareli P, Schamroth, CL, et al: Effects of atenolol on exercise capacity in patients with mitral stenosis and sinus rhythm. Am J Cardiol 56:598, 1985.

95. Levine, HJ: Which atrial fibrillation patients should be on chronic anticoagulation? J Cardiovasc Med 6:483, 1981.

96. Scott, WC, Miller, DC, Haverich, A, et al: Operative risk of mitral valve replacement: Discriminant analysis of 1,329 procedures. Circulation 72(Suppl II)II-108, 1985.

97. Christakis, GT, Kormos, RL, Weisel, R, et al: Morbidity and mortality in mitral valve surgery. Circulation 72(suppl II):II-120, 1985.

98. Hochberg, MS, Derkac, WM, Conkle, DM, et al: Mitral valve replacement in elderly patients: Encouraging postoperative clinical and hemodynamic results. J Thorac Cardiovasc Surg 77:422, 1979.

99. Palacios, I, Block, PC, Brandi, S, et al: Percutaneous balloon valvotomy for patients with severe mitral stenosis. Circulation 75:778, 1987.

100. Block, PC, Palacios, IF, Jacobs, M, et al: The mechanism of successfull percutaneous mitral valvotomy in humans. Circulation 80:282, 1989.

101. Herrmann, HC, Wilkins, GT, Block, PC, et al: Percutaneous balloon mitral valvotomy for patients with mitral stenosis: Analysis of factors influencing early results. J Thorac Cardiovasc Surg 96:33, 1988.

102. Abscal, VM, Wilkins, GT, O'Shea, JP, et al: Prediction of successful outcome in 130 patients undergoing percutaneous balloon mitral valvotomy. Circulation 82:448, 1990.

103. Feldman, T, Carroll, JD, Isner, JM, et al: Effect of valve deformity on results and mitral regurgitation after Inoue balloon commissurotomy. Circulation 85:180, 1992.

104. Herrmann, HC, Kleaveland, JP, Hill, JA, et al: The M-heart percutaneous balloon mitral valvuloplasty registry: Initial results and early follow-up. J Am Coll Cardiol 15:1221, 1990.

105. Lefevre, T, Bonan, R, Serra, A, et al: Percutaneous mitral valvuloplasty in surgical high risk patients. J Am Coll Cardiol 17:348, 1991.

106. Cohn, LH, Allred, EN, Cohn, LA, et al: Long term results of open mitral valve reconstruction for mitral stenosis. Am J Cardiol 55:731, 1985.

107. Roberts, WC and Perloff, JF: Mitral valvular disease. A clinical pathologic survey of the conditions causing the mitral valve to function abnormally. Ann Intern Med 77:939, 1972.
108. Korn, D, DeSanctis, RW, and Sell, S: Massive calcification of the mitral annulus: A clinicopathological study of 14 cases. N Engl J Med 367:900, 1962.
109. Nestico, PF, Depace, NL, Morganroth, J, et al: Mitral annular calcification: Clinical, pathophysiology, and echocardiographic review. Am Heart J 107:989, 1984.
110. Fulkerson, PK, Beaver, BM, Auseon, JC, et al: Calcification of the mitral annulus—etiology, clinical associations, and therapy. Am J Med 66:967, 1979.
111. Zoneraich, S, Zoneraich, O, and Patel, M: Conduction disturbances in patients with calcified mitral annulus diagnosed by echocardiography. J Electrocardiol 12:137, 1979.
112. DeBono, DP and Warlow, CP: Mitral annulus calcification and cerebral or retinal ischemia. Lancet 25:383, 1979.
113. Burnside, JW and DeSanctis, RW: Bacterial endocarditis on calcification of the mitral annulus fibrosus. Ann Intern Med 76:615, 1972.
114. Tresch, DD, Siegel, R, Keelan, MH, et al: Mitral valve proplapse in the elderly. J Am Geriatr Soc 28:421, 1979.
115. Devereux, RB, Kramer-Fox, R, and Kligfield, P: Mitral valve prolapse: Causes, clinical manifestations, and management. Ann Intern Med 111:305, 1989.
116. Waller, BF, Morrow, AG, Maron, BJ, et al: Etiology of clinically isolated, severe, chronic, pure mitral regurgitation: Analysis of 97 patients over age 30 having mitral valve replacement. Am Heart J 104:279, 1982.
117. Wilcken, DE and Hickey, AJ: Lifetime risk for patients with mitral prolapse of developing severe valve regurgitation requiring surgery. Circulation 78:10, 1988.
118. Nagger, CZ, Pearson, WN, Seljan, MP, et al: Frequency of complications of mitral valve prolapse in subjects aged 60 years or older. Am J Cardiol 1209, 1986.
119. Hickey, AJ, Wilcken, DE, Wright, JS, et al: Primary (spontaneous) chordal rupture: Relation to myxomatous valve disease and mitral valve prolapse. J Am Coll Cardiol 5:1341, 1985.
120. Morrow, AG, Cohen, LS, Roberts, WL, et al: Severe mitral regurgitation following acute myocardial infarction and ruptured papillary muscle. Circulation 37(Suppl II):II-124, 1968.
121. Godley, RW, Wann, LS, Rogers, EW, et al: Incomplete mitral leaflet closure in patients with papillary muscle dysfunction. Circulation 63:565, 1981.
122. Yoran, C, Yellin, EL, Becker, RM, et al: Mechanism of reduction of mitral regurgitation with vasodilator therapy. Am J Cardiol 43:773, 1979.
123. Sethi, GK, Miller, DC, Souchek, J, et al: Clinical, hemodynamic, and angiographic predictors of operative mortality in patients undergoing single valve replacement. J Thorac Cardiovasc Surg 93:884, 1987.
124. Scott, ML, Stowe, CL, Nunnally, LC, et al: Mitral valve reconstruction in the elderly population. Ann Thorac Surg 48:213, 1989.
125. Cammack, PL, Edie, RN, and Edmunds, LH: Bar calcification of the mitral anulus: A risk factor in mitral valve operations. J Thorac Cardiovasc Surg 94:399, 1987.
126. Vander Salm, TJ: Mitral annular calcification: A new technique for valve replacement. Ann Thorac Surg 48:437, 1989.
127. Dajani, AS, Bisno, AL, Chung, KJ, et al: Prevention of bacterial endocarditis: Recommendations by the American Heart Association. JAMA 264:2919, 1990.
128. Terpenning, MS, Buggy, BP, and Kauffman, CA: Infective endocarditis: Clinical features in young and elderly patients. Am J Med 83:626, 1987.

CHAPTER 10

Timing of Surgery for Valvular Heart Disease

Richard J. Gray, M.D.
Richard H. Helfant, M.D.

The era of surgical treatment of valvular heart disease began in 1960 with the first reports of successful complete replacement of the aortic valve[1] and mitral valve.[2] Previous work had included largely unsuccessful attempts at repair or partial valve replacement and did not lead to patient survival. Despite these successes, mortality for valve replacement remained high, and because of that, clinicians of the time exercised conservative judgment, preferring to wait as long as possible before referring their patients for surgery. This resulted in advanced cardiac disease, contributing to high surgical risk and influencing results throughout the 1960s and early 1970s. Since then, the results of surgery have been a function of continually evolving technical factors and patient- or host-related factors. Initially, dramatic changes in surgical management occurred. These included a whole new array of prostheses types and designs, revamped surgical techniques and procedures for postoperative care, and, most importantly, an understanding of the need for chronic anticoagulation therapy.

As with most surgical procedures, the results do affect the indications, and as results have improved, patients are referred to surgery earlier and for different reasons than during the 1960s and early 1970s. The nature of the cardiac valve population has changed dramatically in the past 2 decades as well. In the United States, rheumatic and infection-related heart diseases have given way to the valve pathology of degenerative and aging-associated conditions—myxomatous degeneration and ischemic heart disease in the mitral valve and calcific stenosis of the elderly in the aortic valve. These factors, along with changing life-style expectations of the elderly, have altered surgical thinking in this rapidly growing population. Thus, although patients may be referred to surgery earlier in the course of their chronic valvular heart disease, it is usually later in life, and is more often associated with other serious cardiac conditions.

Because technical improvements have continued—for example, better anesthetic agents, membrane oxygenators, bileaflet and homograft valves, repair procedures—recommendations about the timing of surgery as a function of results is at best a changing proposition. For these reasons, and because of improvements in the medical treatment of valvular heart disease, one must be cautious in relying too heavily upon early natural history studies or early reports of surgical results. Furthermore, it appears very unlikely that the natural history of today's valve patients in the United States will be charted for future use.

Nowadays, patients are treated surgically to alleviate symptoms or to avoid irreversible cardiac dysfunction. In the absence of symptoms, controversy arises over how best to assess cardiac function, especially in the regurgitant lesions, and what level or duration of cardiac dysfunction will still allow a meaningful recovery after surgery. Although there are tremendous similarities between the management of patients with regurgitant valvular lesions and those with stenotic ones, tradition dictates that mitral and aortic valve disease be treated as separate entities. Further, it must be recognized that both types of lesions coexist in a sizable proportion of patients. The somewhat arbitrary separation into regurgitation and stenosis categories allows for meaningful discussion of the specific effects these lesions have upon cardiac function and surgical timing. Obviously, the clinician is required to exercise great judgment in individual patients who present with varying admixtures of valve abnormalities or multiple valve involvement.

MITRAL VALVE DISEASE

MITRAL REGURGITATION

Natural History

Nowhere have more changes in patient population and surgical techniques occurred than in patients with chronic mitral regurgitation (MR). The ultimate effectiveness and timing of mitral valve replacement (MVR) surgery must be judged in light of the natural history of the disease, which is dramatically variable from one patient to another. The specific type of symptoms and rate of progression will be influenced by the underlying pathology and by regurgitant volume and left ventricular functional reserve.

The ultimate results of severe MR are progressive signs and symptoms of congestive heart failure with debilitation and cardiac death. Rapaport[3] reported that of 70 patients with chronic MR, as many as 80% survived 5 years and almost 60% survived 10 years from the time of diagnosis. The reported operative mortality for MVR has varied from 2% to as high as 30% for certain patient subgroups.[4-6] Postoperative survival rates at 5 years have ranged from 82% for patients without coronary artery disease (CAD),[7] to 50% for patients with predominantly ischemic-based regurgitation.[6] Although an individual can remain asymptomatic with reasonably well-compensated cardiac function for many years, this is somewhat uncommon. More often, signs of left ventricular dysfunction begin to appear shortly after diagnosis, if they are not already present. Even then, many patients remain minimally symptomatic and, when symptoms do develop, a gratifying response is usually observed with diuretic and vasodilator therapy. Unfortunately, an otherwise stable, slowly progressing course can be punctuated by a sudden onset of pulmonary edema, sometimes traceable to atrial fibrillation or a coronary event, or rupture of chordae tendineae leading to massive regurgitation.

There are no conclusive data that MVR actually prolongs life in patients with

MR. A controlled clinical trial of early MVR has been proposed,[4] but it is unlikely that such a study can be conducted in the United States. One uncontrolled study found that in patients with MR who had MVR or valvuloplasty, survival at 10 years was better than that in medically treated patients; however, the difference was of borderline significance.[8]

Predictors of Clinical Outcome

Predictors of mortality and functional status following MVR for MR have been analyzed retrospectively by several groups of investigators (Table 10–1). Patient age at the time of MVR significantly correlated with poorest survival, with patients older than 60 years of age at higher risk for operative death and complications.[7–10] While age is also associated with other indicators of advanced disease, age by itself represents a risk, especially over age 70.[11,12] Patients with advanced New York Heart Association (NYHA) functional class (III, IV) have higher postoperative mortality and poorer long-term survival. Associated CAD reduces perioperative and late postoperative survival as well; it appears that simultaneous coronary revascularization, when indicated, improves this otherwise adverse outcome (Fig. 10–1).[6]

Several preoperative hemodynamic variables also have been correlated with poorer survival following MVR. Cardiac index <2.0 L/min/m^2 and left ventricular end-diastolic pressure >12 mmHg have been related to both early and late postoperative deaths.[9,10] Elevated pulmonary vascular resistance and mean pulmonary artery pressure have been associated with perioperative mortality.[9,10] Interestingly, elevated right ventricular end-diastolic pressure in chronic MR was an important hemodynamic predictor of operative mortality and poor symptomatic response

Table 10–1. Indications for Surgery: Predictors of Survival and Symptoms after Mitral Valve Replacement for Mitral Regurgitation

	Predictors of:	
	Poor Survival	**Poor Symptomatic Outcome**
Clinical	Age	Symptom duration
	NYHA class	
	Associated CAD	
Hemodynamic	Cardiac index ≤ 24 mm/m^2	
	LVEDP ≥ 12 mm Hg	
	PA pressure elevated	
	RVEDP elevated	RVEDP
Cath	ESVI >60 ml/m^2	ESVI >100 ml/m^2
	Ejection fraction $<40\%$	EDVI
	ESWS/ESVI ratio	ESWS/ESVI ratio
Echo		ESD >2.6 cm/m^2
		Fractional shortening $<31\%$
		ESWS index >195 mm Hg

Key: NYHA = New York Heart Association; CAD = coronary artery disease; LVEDP = left ventricular end-diastolic pressure; PA = pulmonary artery; RVEDP = right ventricular end-diastolic pressure; ESVI = end-systolic volume index; ESWS = end-systolic wall stress; EDVI = end-diastolic volume index; ESD = end-systolic dimension.

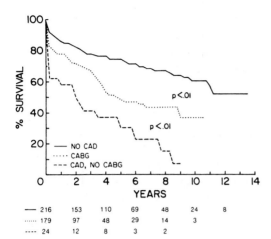

Figure 10–1. Survival after valve replacement in three cohorts of patients, stratified by presence or absence of CAD and coronary artery bypass grafting (CABG). The 5- and 8-year survival rates and standard errors were: $75 \pm 3\%$ and $68 \pm 4\%$ in patients with no CAD, $49 \pm 5\%$ and $44 \pm 5\%$ in patients with bypassed CAD, and $31 \pm 10\%$ and $15 \pm 9\%$ in patients with unbypassed CAD. The numbers below the figure indicated the patients at risk during follow-up. (From Czer et al.[6] with permission.)

to MVR, possibly as a result of right ventricular failure and pulmonary hypertension.[13]

Echocardiographic and angiographic descriptors of preoperative left ventricular function also have been linked to postoperative survival and functional status. In one study, end-systolic volume index >60 ml/m² predicted all perioperative cardiac deaths as well as persistent heart failure symptoms (Fig. 10–2).[14] End-diastolic volume index >100 ml/m² also has predicted a poorer postoperative outcome.[15] Depressed resting ejection fraction ($<40\%$) has been associated with higher early and late mortality.[6,7] Other investigators have found that the preoperative ratio of end-systolic wall stress to end-systolic volume index—a systolic functional parameter relatively independent of loading conditions—was superior to the variables of age, ejection fraction, and end-diastolic volume index in predicting perioperative death and symptomatic improvement after surgery.[16] Zile and associates[17] described a triad of echocardiographic indices of left ventricular function that predicted continued symptoms of congestive heart failure following MVR for chronic MR in 20 patients. These were end-systolic dimension >2.6 cm/m², fractional shortening $<31\%$, or end-systolic wall stress index >195 mmHg.[17] One or more of these echocardiographic parameters correctly characterized four patients who remained symptomatic after MVR. There were no false–positive results in 16 patients who became asymptomatic.

Ventricular Function

Assessment of left ventricular myocardial function is a highly complex task in the setting of MR. In MR, the presence of a low-resistance outflow path to the left atrium in parallel with systemic outflow to the aorta reduces impedance to left ventricular emptying.[18,19] At any given level of left ventricular end-diastolic volume or preload, MR reduces afterload, and thus, myocardial wall tension. This permits contractile energy to be used more in fiber shortening and ventricular emptying and less in tension development. As a result, in an acute experimental model of MR with myocardial contractility held fixed, left ventricular ejection fraction increases.[18,19]

Chronic MR is accompanied by left ventricular dilation and hypertrophy. Cardiac catheterization studies reveal increased end-diastolic volume with normal ejection fraction and normal extent of fiber shortening.[20,21] However, velocity of shortening may be abnormal, indicating a depressed contractile state that may be masked by early systolic unloading of the ventricle.[20] In addition, a normal ejection fraction also may mask significant left ventricular dysfunction.[22] Because of the low impedance leak during systole, systolic phase parameters for cardiac function will appear normal even though myocardial function may be severely depressed. For this reason, the end-systolic wall stress/end-systolic volume index (ESWS/ESVI) ratio is useful in volume overload states. Extensive experimental data indicate that this parameter is independent of alterations in preload. Applying this measurement, Carabello and coworkers[16] found that the ESWS/ESVI ratio in normal persons was 5.6 ± 0.9, and a smaller ratio indicated progressively worse left ventricular function. Four of five patients with ESWS/ESVI values ≤2.2 died after MVR for MR, and a fifth patient did not improve his functional status.

Following successful MVR for MR, left ventricular end-diastolic volume has

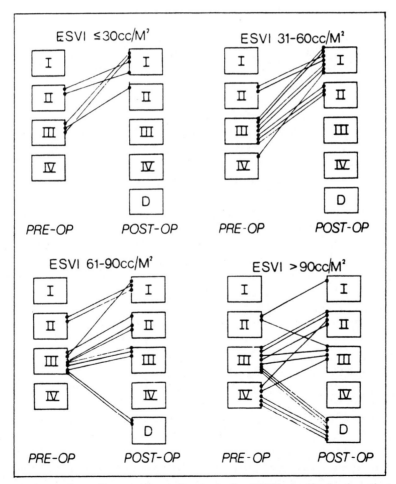

Figure 10–2. Comparison of preoperative and postoperative NYHA classification in patients divided according to their preoperative end-systolic volume index (ESVI). D designates perioperative cardiac death. (From Borow et al.[14] with permission.)

been reported to decrease,[23,24] or not to change significantly.[25,26] Left ventricular mass has been estimated to decrease variably following MVR.[17,23,27] Ejection fraction generally decreases.[7,23,24,28] Dubroff and associates[29] demonstrated intraoperatively that correction of MR resulted in an immediate decrease in ejection fraction, estimated echocardiographically, with no change in end-diastolic cavity size. Significant postoperative depression of resting ejection fraction, lack of postoperative ejection fraction response to exercise, or lack of resolution of cardiac hypertrophy after surgery are of concern. These factors have been interpreted as indicating that ventricular function, at least during exercise, remained abnormal after apparently successful MVR, despite obvious hemodynamic and symptomatic improvement.[30] This may represent afterload mismatch as a result of surgery.[22]

Another factor initially reported by Lillehei and colleagues[31] in 1964, and currently receiving much more attention, is the importance of the subvalvular mitral apparatus and its contribution to cardiac function. Much credit for the superior surgical survival and cardiac functional benefits of mitral valve repair is given to this technical feature, in contrast to the typical approach used in MVR, wherein all of the valve and subvalvular apparatus is removed.[26] Some of the left ventricular functional differences between mitral valvuloplasty and typical MVR can be explained by the loss of continuity between the mitral anulus and left ventricular wall. Thus, post-MVR left ventricular function nearly equivalent to that after valve anuloplasty has been demonstrated when much or all of the chordal attachments are left intact, a novel approach to MVR used by some surgeons.[32]

There are considerable data allowing for prediction of poor symptomatic outcome or continued left ventricular dysfunction after surgery. Short duration congestive heart failure symptoms are associated with significant functional improvement postoperatively.[15] A poor symptomatic response to medical therapy preoperatively, in patients with congestive heart failure for 3 years or more, implies a $<25\%$ likelihood of complete reversal of symptoms following MVR.[5] Echocardiographic measurements indicating a large left ventricular end-diastolic dimension (>7.0 cm or >4.0 cm/m^2) or end-systolic dimension (>5.0 cm or >2.6 cm/m^2), reduced fractional shortening ($<30\%$) or increased end-systolic wall stress index (>195 mmHg) have been associated with substantial postoperative functional deterioration in small groups.[17,27] Similarly, preoperative angiographic findings of end-diastolic volume index (>100 ml/m^2, end-systolic volume index >60 ml/m^2, or reduced resting ejection fraction ($<55\%$) have been associated with poor left ventricular function following MVR.[14,15,22]

Unfortunately, waiting until some or many of the aforementioned indices are present also would spell a poor prognosis for the patient. In the absence of symptoms that compellingly indicate surgery, the physician is obliged to consider surgery before the onset of the aforementioned endpoints.

Mitral Valve Repair

The emergence of repair procedures for both MR and stenosis casts an entirely different light on the timing of surgery for mitral valve disease. Using a variety of surgical techniques, extremely attractive surgical mortality and long-term survival results have been reported. The best of these have reported a stunning 10-year actuarial survival of 90%, with a 15-year probability survival of 72.5%.[33] Valvuloplasty also is associated with marked improvement of ventricular function over conventional valve repair, as demonstrated both in the experimental animal and in patients.[26,34-36] Of nearly equal importance is the striking lack of valve-associated complications during the expected long survival. Freedom from reoperation and probabilities of freedom from thromboembolism, anticoagulation-related hemorrhage, and endocarditis is in excess of 90% at 15-year follow-up.[33] Surgeons with the skill and experience to perform intricate mitral valve repair procedures are found increasingly in larger medical centers throughout the United States. Reports have begun to appear that substantiate Carpentier's superb results.[37,38]

Coupled with the use of anuloplasty rings, valve repair can be accomplished in more than one-half of patients referred for mitral valve surgery. It is still too early, however, to compare the feasibility and outcome of repair versus replacement because past series of reported cases may have selected better candidates for repair than for replacement. Case-matched series such as those of Craver and colleagues,[38] or an intervention trial, may be required to confirm this approach. Nevertheless, the potential for valve repair should always be in the clinician's mind and could have a major impact on the timing of surgery.

With an extremely low surgical mortality, a high likelihood of freedom from prosthesis-related complications, such as thromboembolism, a low likelihood of need for reoperation; and no need for anticoagulation, the rationale for delaying surgery until a significant left ventricular dysfunction occurs must be reconsidered. In fact, the prospect of repair may be lost if left ventricular geometry becomes too deranged due to excessive ventricular remodeling. The prospects for mitral valve repair should allow for earlier consideration of surgery in the mildly symptomatic individual, perhaps one who is intolerant or poorly tolerant of medication required to maintain New York Heart Association class II status. It should lead to surgical consideration in the presence of relatively less severe degrees of left ventricular dysfunction. Lower operative mortality and better postoperative ventricular function should extend the limits of operability to those patients with more severe degrees of left ventricular dysfunction, to the elderly, and to those with comorbidity that renders traditional MVR undesirable.

Table 10–2 provides practical suggestions about surgical decision making in the presence or absence of symptoms or left ventricular dysfunction. It must be emphasized that this refers to chronic MR. Four possible combinations of symptomatic status and ventricular function status are proposed. For the purposes of this table, which may be somewhat oversimplified, symptoms are defined as those of early NYHA class III, despite medical therapy consisting of diuretics and vasodilators. Left ventricular dysfunction consists of the presence of one or more of the measures of left ventricular function mentioned earlier, detected on a singular invasive study or on two successive noninvasive studies.

In category A, surgery is clearly indicated. Category B represents a consideration for surgery. If left ventricular dysfunction is quite severe, the operability of the patient may be questionable. In category C, surgery must be considered. In pure MR, absence of significant symptoms in the presence of severe dysfunction should prompt the investigation for additional factors such as CAD, cardiomyopathy, or the like. In category D, the patient should be followed with noninvasive testing at 6-month to 1-year intervals.

MITRAL STENOSIS

In contrast to MR, in which the etiologies are varied, the cause of mitral stenosis in the adult is almost without exception rheumatic heart disease.

Table 10–2. Indications for
Surgery: Chronic Mitral
Regurgitation

Symptoms	+	+	−	−
LV dysfunction	−	+	+	−
	A	B	C	D

SYMPTOMS
Early NYHA class III, despite medical therapy
LV DYSFUNCTION
Criteria in text, seen invasively or on two
   successive noninvasive studies
     A: Refer for surgery.
     B: Consider surgery. Is the patient
       operable?
     C: Consider surgery. Is mitral
       regurgitation the only problem?
     D: Follow-up with noninvasive studies at
       6-month to 1-year intervals.

Key: LV = left ventricular; NYHA = New York
Heart Association.

Natural History

The natural history of rheumatic mitral stenosis includes a significant latent period, lasting up to 8 years or so, during which there are no signs or symptoms, despite the gradual development of stenosis. The next phase is the asymptomatic or subclinical phase, lasting up to 10 years, in which physical signs of stenosis have begun to appear. After that, symptoms manifest and progressively worsen, ending with NYHA class IV status and cardiac death in an additional 10 years or so.

Olesen[39] studied 271 patients with mitral stenosis treated between 1933 and 1949. He found that survival was related to functional status at the time of entrance into the study. His classification is somewhat different from that of the current NYHA system, but symptoms most consistent with class III were associated with 5-year survival of 62% and 10-year survival of 38%; patients similar to class IV at entry had a 15% 5-year survival, and all were dead by 8 years. Rapaport[3] has reported a series of 133 patients with mitral stenosis, treated medically, who exhibited a 5-year survival of 80% and 10-year survival of 60%.

The symptomatic phase of disease results from pulmonary venous congestion and low cardiac output and typically results in indolent, very slowly progressive symptoms, consisting of fatigue and breathlessness. Classically, symptoms are so insidious in their progression that the patient may not be aware of their presence. Associated with this disease are several potential events of a more dramatic nature. Atrial fibrillation may be present in one-third to one-half of patients with either pure mitral valve stenosis, mixed mitral stenosis, or MR.[40] Neilson and colleagues[40] also reported a 17% incidence of thromboembolism in pure mitral stenosis and 19% in patients with mixed mitral stenosis/MR. In more advanced stages of disease, hemoptysis occurs, and recurrent pleural effusions also may be noted.

Ventricular Function

Issues of preoperative and postoperative ventricular function are generally not as critical in mitral stenosis as they are in MR. Unlike other valve lesions, the left ventricle is neither pressure nor volume overloaded. Some patients do develop left ventricular dysfunction, however, due to recurrent myocarditis or other factors resulting in fibrosis and producing a restrictive cardiac filling pattern. The ventricle takes on a foreshortened, more globular shape in chronic severe mitral stenosis. These changes rarely dictate the timing of surgery nor dominate surgical outcome.

Pulmonary hypertension, however, has important adverse prognostic indications and can be important clinically as it may result in life-threatening hemoptysis. Often the result of excess interstitial pulmonary water, pulmonary hypertension is often reversible with well-timed surgical repair.[41]

Results of Surgery

Commissurotomy is the traditional procedure designed for this lesion and is appropriate in patients with relatively little calcification and no significant MR. In such patients, either open or closed valvuloplasty can have an operative mortality of between 1% and 3%.[42] In a series of 3,724 patients reported from India, John and colleagues[43] noted a 1.5% mortality and actuarial survival of 89.5% in 15 years, with excellent functional improvement in 85% of long-term survivors at 15 years. Importantly, this group reported that commissurotomy reduced the incidence of systemic embolization by approximately 50%.

The only shortcoming with this otherwise remarkably effective procedure is the occurrence of restenosis and need for repeat surgery in approximately 10% of patients at 5 years.[44] Indicators that commissurotomy is feasible include evidence of mobility on echocardiography without significant calcification or physical evidence of regurgitation either by examination or by echocardiographic Doppler.

Recommendations for Surgery

When valve replacement is needed, indications ought to be somewhat stringent and include (1) symptomatic classification of early NYHA class III, (2) severe mitral stenosis in the absence of symptoms when atrial fibrillation is present for 1 year or less (when atrial fibrillation is present for 1 year or more resumption of sinus rhythm after surgery is unlikely), and (3) recurrent systemic embolization despite anticoagulation.

If commissurotomy is feasible, indications are much more liberal and include (1) NYHA symptomatic class II or poor tolerance of imposed life-style restrictions, (2) the onset of atrial fibrillation, and (3) the presence of any episode of systemic embolus with or without anticoagulation.

When valve replacement is needed, mortality will be in the range of 5% to 10%. Scott and associates[45] reported an 8% mortality rate in their series from Stanford. Whether commissurotomy or replacement is performed, symptoms are overwhelmingly relieved with 85% to 90% of patients achieving a NYHA class I or II status.

AORTIC VALVE DISEASE

AORTIC REGURGITATION

Natural History

Goldschlager and colleagues[46] have characterized the time course of chronic aortic regurgitation (AR) in 126 patients. Patients are generally asymptomatic for decades, develop dyspnea and fatigue in the fourth or fifth decade, and then become progressively disabled during 5 to 10 years. Very often the appearance of congestive heart failure will be signaled by pulmonary congestion or pulmonary edema, which responds rapidly to medical therapy. Additional symptoms include exertional angina as well as non–Q-wave infarction and exertional syncope. Ventricular arrhythmias often correlate with advancing cardiac dysfunction and may lead to sudden death. The survival rate without surgery has been found to be 75% at 5 years, 50% at 10 years from the time of diagnosis,[3] or 50% at 7 years from the onset of "diminished working capacity."[47] Even lower survival rates have been documented in patients who have abnormal systemic blood pressure, cardiac enlargement by x-ray, and left ventricular hypertrophy by electrocardiogram (ECG).[48]

Results of Surgery

Aortic valve replacement (AVR) for chronic AR has been associated with an operative mortality of 4.4%,[49] and 6%[50] in two studies. Reported late survival results vary widely and probably reflect differences in patient selection, surgical expertise, presence or absence of coronary disease, and the surgical era. Two-year survival has ranged from 60% to 90%.[50,51] Five-year survival after AVR has been reported between 50% and 86%.[52–57] Unfortunately, there is no prospective or well-controlled comparison of medical and surgical therapy for chronic aortic insufficiency. A retrospective study found that 127 patients who had AVR for chronic AR had a 5-year survival of 86%, and 28 patients had apparently similar clinical characteristics, but when unoperated had an 87% survival. A trend toward improved survival following AVR was seen for those who were in NYHA class IV, or who had abnormal left ventricular function at rest.[57] A retrospective study, especially involving nonconcurrent series of patients, is not likely to adequately address this issue. Nevertheless, the lack of evidence for dramatic survival benefits with surgery (compared with medical therapy) has shifted the emphasis for surgical timing toward the onset of symptoms that typically respond dramatically to surgery. More than 70% to 80% of patients experience symptomatic improvement, and 40% achieve complete relief of symptoms.[50,58,59]

Predictors of Clinical Outcome

A variety of clinical variables and physiologic parameters have been correlated with postoperative survival and symptomatic improvement in chronic AR (Table 10–3). Age older than 65 years and male gender have been associated with reduced 5-year survival.[52,53] The presence of congestive heart failure preoperatively confers an increased long-term mortality risk following AVR.[53,55,60] NYHA functional class IV also portends a high (29%) short-term mortality, and both functional class III and class IV are associated with higher long-term mortality risk.[53–55] Bonow and coworkers[61] found that poor exercise capacity in patients who had reduced echocardiographic fractional shortening identified all nine patients who died following

Table 10–3. Indications for Surgery: Predictors of Survival
and Symptoms after Aortic Valve Replacement

	Predictors of:	
	Poor Survival	Poor Symptomatic Outcome
Clinical	Age $\geq$65	
	Sex, male	
	Heart failure	
	NYHA class III, IV	
	Exercise capacity $\leq$22.5 min	
	Cardiothoracic ratio $\geq$0.60	Cardiothoracic ratio $\geq$0.60
Hemodynamic:	Cardiac index <2.5 L/min/m^2	
	LVEDP	
	PCW	
	PA pressure	
Cath	ESVI >60 ml/m^2	ESVI >60 ml/m^2
	Ejection fraction <50%	LV eccentricity
	Vcf	
Echo	EDDI $\geq$38 mm/m^2	EDDI $\geq$38 mm/m^2
	ESD >55 mm	ESD >55 mm
	Fractional shortening <25%	Fractional shortening <25%
	Ejection fraction <60%	Ejection fraction <60%

Key: NYHA = New York Heart Association; LVH = left ventricular hypertrophy; LVEDP = left ventricular end-diastolic pressure; PCW = pulmonary capillary wedge; PA = pulmonary artery; ESVI = end-systolic volume index; Vcf = velocity of circumferential fiber shortening; EDDI = end-diastolic dimension index; ESD = end-systolic dimension.

AVR for AR. In that study, no patient who completed the 22.5 minute first stage of the National Institutes of Health (NIH) exercise protocol died postoperatively (Fig. 10–3).

The presence of significant cardiomegaly on chest x-ray has been associated with higher mortality and with poor symptomatic response after AVR.[60,62] Severe left ventricular hypertrophy by ECG also correlates with increased risk.[52] Conversely, cardiac index >2.5 L/min/m^2 predicts a high long-term survival rate.[49,60,63] Left ventricular end-diastolic pressure correlates inversely with postoperative survival.[49,52,63] Patients who die following AVR for AR have a higher preoperative pulmonary capillary wedge pressure and pulmonary artery pressure than those who survive.[52,53,60]

Angiographically, Borow and associates[14] found that in AR, as in MR, end-systolic volume index >60 ml/m^2 predicted all perioperative cardiac deaths. In addition, all patients with an index <60 ml/m^2 achieved NYHA class I or class II following AVR (see Fig. 10–2). Long-term survival following AVR also has been substantially better in patients who had preoperative ejection fraction >45%[49] or >50%,[63] than in patients with lower ejection fraction. Mean velocity of circumferential fiber shortening measured angiographically was of borderline significance as a predictor of postoperative survival.[49]

Several echocardiographic studies have been published relating to operative and postoperative risk. One such study found that left ventricular end-systolic dimension >55 mm and fractional shortening of <25% characterized two of three perioperative deaths and seven of eight late deaths from heart failure, among 49

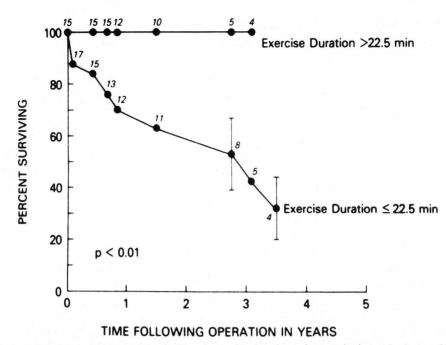

TIME FOLLOWING OPERATION IN YEARS

Figure 10–3. Survival after operation in 32 patients with chronic aortic regurgitation and subnormal left ventricular fractional shortening (<29%) by echocardiography. The 15 patients who completed stage I of the National Institutes of Health protocol (exercise duration >22.5 min) had better postoperative survival than the 17 patients who failed to complete stage I (exercise duration ≤22.5 min), with a 3-year survival of 100% vs. 53%. Numbers of patients at risk are indicated. (Bonow et al.[61] with permission.)

symptomatic patients operated for aortic regurgitation.[64] Another study showed that echocardiographic fractional shortening of <31% or ejection fraction (from calculated echocardiographic volumes) of <60% identified all patients who were dead 5 years after AVR.[65] Gaasch and coworkers[66] found, using serial echocardiography, that persistent ventricular dilation and a 29% mortality rate at 4 years after AVR, were predicted by an end-diastolic dimension of >3.8 cm/m² or an index of end-diastolic wall stress. Others have shown that postoperative symptoms of congestive heart failure correlated with preoperative left ventricular end-diastolic dimension, end-systolic dimension, fractional shortening, and left ventricular mass.[62,65]

Ventricular Function

In chronic AR, the left ventricle adapts to the volume load by dilation, thus increasing compliance so that end-diastolic pressure is not elevated. Compensatory hypertrophy provides for maintenance or increase in wall thickness, thus preventing any marked increase in wall stress. The moderate tachycardia associated with exercise is especially well tolerated for most because of the shortened diastolic filling time and lessened regurgitant fraction. As AR becomes severe and prolonged, an increase in dilation is no longer compensatory; the limits of preload reserve are reached, leading to a decrease in ejection fraction at rest. Eventually, further hypertrophy no longer occurs and systolic wall stress increases a condition termed *afterload mismatch* by Ross.[22]

Following AVR for chronic AR, left ventricular end-diastolic pressure uniformly falls,[67,68] cardiac index increases after surgery,[24,63,66-75] and left ventricular ejection fraction either increases[71,68,76] or does not change significantly.[70,72-74] Early postoperative ejection fraction, at least intraoperatively, appears to fall after surgery.[29] Progression of hypertrophy and other morphologic improvements, such as reduction of muscle fiber diameter, percent interstitial fibrosis, and volume fraction of myofibrils also have been reported.[77,78]

The extent to which these morphologic and functional improvements are linked to preoperative and postoperative cardiac function—all of which appear related to clinically important outcomes such as survival and quality of life—has led to the recommendation by many that surgery should be planned before development of irreversible left ventricular dysfunction in spite of absence of symptoms. This particular aspect of timing of surgery for AR has been singularly controversial in the past and led to extensive experimental work and editorial review. Adding to the confusion is the disagreement over which of several cardiac functional indices most accurately predicts postoperative status. Unfortunately, among all of the available data relatively little prospective comparison of surgical timing strategies for the asymptomatic patient exist.

Henry and colleagues[64] from the National Institutes of health were among the first to propose surgery in the minimally symptomatic or asymptomatic patient based upon specific echocardiographic criteria. In many ways, their recommendations sparked much of this controversy. They reported that echocardiographic measurement of left ventricular end-systolic dimension of >55 mm and fractional shortening of <25% partitioned patients into those who experienced the predominance of postoperative early and late deaths, those who remained symptomatic, and those who did well. However, in an accompanying editorial, a warning against accepting these recommendations as the sole criteria for surgery was issued.[79] Subsequently, others disagreed with this finding as a definite indication for surgery.[59,80] Fioretti and associates,[80] for instance, reported 47 consecutive symptomatic patients undergoing AVR for isolated AR, 20 of whom had preoperative end-systolic diameters of ≥55 mm, and 27 with end-systolic diameters of <55 mm. Half of the group with large end-systolic diameters had left ventricular fractional shortening of <25%, a finding noted in only one group with the smaller end-systolic diameter. No early or late deaths were found during follow-up averaging 41 months. Reduction of left ventricular dimension and mass was similar in both groups. Unfortunately, this is a relatively small series of patients, and the high-risk group did not have both of the indications as suggested by Henry and colleagues.[64]

An important cautionary note for the clinician is the variability of echcoardiographic measurements of left ventricular dimension. The coefficient of variation for end-diastolic and end-systolic dimension has been reported at 6.1% and 10.1%, respectively, and 17.1% for fractional shortening.[81]

Angiographically measured end-systolic volume index correlated directly with postoperative echocardiographic fractional shortening.[14] Preoperative end-systolic volume estimated by radionuclide angiography correlated with postoperative end-diastolic volume and ejection fraction, and a postoperative decrease in end-diastolic volume correlated modestly with both the ejection fraction and regurgitatant fraction in AR.[74] Echocardiographic end-diastolic dimension and systolic wall stress have been shown in retrospective studies to correlate with left ventricular size and function following AVR.[62,66,75]

Ejection fraction has been the subject of much investigation in chronic AR and has now become, along with echocardiographic measurement of left ventricular dimension, one of the most commonly used modalities for assessing and following patients with chronic AR. Although it is afterload dependent and to some extent preload dependent, the value in any given patient is very much a function of cardiac reserve. It is readily available by both invasive and noninvasive means and is quite well understood by most clinicians.

Thompson[82] reported that left ventricular ejection fraction of <55% had predictive accuracy of 95% in identification of a high-risk subgroup of asymptomatic patients with severe AR.[82] Left ventricular end-systolic volume index >70 ml/m^2 added 90% accuracy in this same study. In their experience, left ventricular end-systolic dimension of >55 had 79% accuracy.

Bonow[83] reported that in addition to his left ventricular end-systolic and fractional shortening criteria, resting ejection fraction of >50% was associated with a significantly higher 3-year postoperative survival. Importantly, in two-thirds or more of asymptomatic patients with left ventricular dysfunction, symptoms were incurred within 2 to 3 years.

In minimally symptomatic patients with left ventricular dysfunction, preserved exercise capacity before surgery confers a greater reduction in echocardiographic left ventricular end-diastolic dimension than in those with poor exercise capacity. An additional determinant of reversal of left ventricular dysfunction is the duration of time during which this dysfunction is present before surgery is performed.

For any given degree of dilation of the left ventricle and decrease in fractional shortening or resting ejection fraction, patients with a brief duration of preoperative left ventricular dysfunction (<14 months) have demonstrated a significant decrease in left ventricular diastolic size after surgery, as compared with patients in whom the duration of preoperative dysfunction was more prolonged (>18 months), and despite similar preoperative hemodynamic, echocardiographic, or radionuclide indexes, including resting ejection fraction.[84] This gives hope for improvement in left ventricular function in those patients in whom it has been depressed for a relatively brief period of time.

Other less commonly obtained indices have been found to have excellent independent predictive value for postoperative left ventricular improvement. A regurgitant stroke volume to end-diastolic volume ratio of <0.28 was as good as, or better than, other catheterization or echocardiographic variables in predicting regression of left ventricular dimensions after AVR.[85] Japanese investigators have found that the ratio of ESWS/ESVI is an excellent index of myocardial contractility, and its preoperative measurement correctly predicts postoperative contractile improvement in those patients with a preoperative ESS/ESVI of ≥2.9.[86]

A few prospective studies have begun to confirm the body of largely retrospective descriptive data indicating the benefits of intervention based upon left ventricular dysfunction. Roman and associates[87] did serial preoperative and postoperative echocardiography and radionuclide angiography on 38 patients having AVR for severe AR. Left ventricular end-diastolic dimension normalized in 58% of patients by 9 months postoperatively at which time one-half had normalized mass. Overall normalization of these two parameters was observed in two-thirds of patients upon further follow-up. All patients with normalized end-diastolic dimension also had normal postoperative ejection fractions. Conversely, 42% of patients with a persistently dilated left ventricle had an abnormal postoperative left ventricular ejection fraction. Preoperative left ventricular end-systolic dimension of <55 mm identified 86% of patients in whom end-diastolic dimension was normalized; preoperative end-systolic dimension was >55 mm in 81% of those with persistent dilation. Numerous other preoperative indicators of outcome identified lower proportions of patients whose left ventricular dimensions did or did not normalize.

Tornos and colleagues[88] found that in 53 patients with severe chronic AR, those with significant symptoms and left ventricular dysfunction continued to have dilated hearts, as did both an asymptomatic group and a group with moderate symptoms whose preoperative end-systolic diameter was >55 mm. Radionuclide ejection fraction increased in most patients with preoperative values <50%, except in those with preoperative values <30%.

A fascinating study of decision analysis, based upon extensive review of the existing literature and expert opinion, used a hypothetical case scenario of a 40-year-old man with chronic aortic insufficiency to compare early surgery (timed at the onset of left ventricular dysfunction) with delayed surgery (timed at the onset of symptoms). The early surgery approach was preferred based upon superiority of quality-adjusted life years. Interestingly, to change the preference to the delayed surgery approach, the delayed surgery operative mortality rate had to be almost as low as the early surgery rate. It could also change if survival were much more important to the patient in the first 5 years than after 5 years or if the patient strongly disliked living on anticoagulants enough to value a year on anticoagulants as worth only 80% of a year not on anticoagulants.[89]

In summary, it is clear from available literature that in symptomatic patients, postoperative outcome is adversely affected by duration and severity of symptoms as well as duration and severity of left ventricular dysfunction. In asymptomatic patients, postoperative outcome is adversely affected by left ventricular dysfunction,[49,65] as well as duration of left ventricular dysfunction and maintenance of exercise capacity. Commonly used measures of left ventricular dysfunction, favored by many, include a resting ejection fraction of <50% and a left ventricular end-systolic dimension of >55 mm on a repeated noninvasive measurement. Based on the ability of recovery of left ventricular function, in those in whom it is abnormal for 14 months or less, it seems unnecessary to seek measures of diminished left ventricular functional reserve such as exercise ejection fraction and handgrip response in those who are normal at rest.

Recommendation for Surgery

As indicated in Table 10–4, similar to the algorithm for chronic MR, patients with early NYHA class III symptoms should be referred for surgery, even without left ventricular dysfunction, although it is unlikely that many will have normal left ventricular function at this stage (category A). Those with symptoms and left ventricular dysfunction should be referred for surgery. While recognizing that the outcome will be limited if left ventricular dysfunction is severe (ejection fraction <30%), benefit is still achieved in substantial numbers of such patients (category B). Patients with no significant symptoms, but who evidence left ventricular ejection fraction <50% to 55% or left ventricular end-systolic dimension >50 to 55 mmHg on repeated assessment should be referred for surgery within 12 months of the onset of these findings (category C). Patients with no symptoms or left ventricular dysfunction should have serial clinical follow-up including chest x-ray, physi-

Table 10–4. Indications for
Surgery: Chronic Aortic
Insufficiency

Symptoms	+	+	−	−
LV dysfunction	−	+	+	−
	A	B	C	D

SYMPTOMS
Early NYHA class III
LV DYSFUNCTION
Criteria in text, seen invasively or on two
   successive noninvasive studies
   A. Refer for surgery.
   B. Consider surgery. Is the patient
      operable?
   C. Refer for surgery.
   D. Follow-up with noninvasive studies at
      6-month to 1-year intervals.

Key: LV = left ventricular; NYHA = New York
Heart Association.

cal examination, and periodic echocardiography at 6-month to 1-year intervals,
depending on the status of left ventricular function (category D).

AORTIC STENOSIS

Natural History

As with the other valvular lesions, patients with predominant aortic stenosis
remain asymptomatic for many years, while the degree of obstruction progressively
worsens, along with associated physical findings of left ventricular outflow obstruction. In sharp contrast to AR, cardiac function remains well compensated, owing
to hypertrophy, well into the time when symptoms become apparent. Eventually,
afterload continues to increase to a point at which stroke volume diminishes, at
which time the left ventricle begins to dilate in an attempt to restore stroke volume.
This is when cardiac enlargement begins to appear on chest x-ray, with associated
diminished ejection fraction, as the stroke volume continues to decline with ever
increasing left ventricular diastolic volume. Typically, at the time of these changes,
symptoms will have long since developed, correctly identifying the advanced stage
of disease.

As left ventricular hypertrophy worsens, and if myocardial energetics require
ever-increasing coronary blood flow, angina pectoris is one of the most common
symptoms and often the first to develop. In an early natural history study, compiled
from several previous studies on valvular heart disease, Ross and Braunwald[90]
reported average survival from the time of angina pectoris in aortic stenosis to be
5 years. Syncope and congestive heart failure symptoms are the next most frequent
symptoms and are associated with average survival of 3 and 2 years, respectively
(Fig. 10–4).

In an early report, Harken and associates[91] noted that 90% of 54 patients were

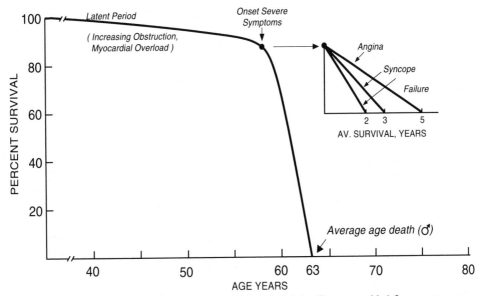

Figure 10–4. Average course of valvular aortic stenosis in adults. Data assembled from postmortem studies. (From Ross et al.[90] with permission.)

dead at 6 months after diagnosis. Schwartz and coworkers[57] reported on 19 patients with hemodynamically severe aortic stenosis who refused surgery and who experienced a 36% mortality in 1 year and a 79% mortality by 2 years. A much more recent study, that of Rapaport, showed that from the time of detection of an aortic stenosis murmur, 40% of patients were dead at 5 years and 80% at 10 years compared with survival in all other valve lesions, in which only 20% were dead at 5 years and 60% at 10 years. Survival, once symptoms do develop, is relatively limited.

Syncope, particularly exertional syncope, is one of the most classic and feared symptoms in aortic stenosis. However, it rarely appears as an initial symptom or causes sudden cardiac death without other preceding symptoms. Therefore, it is seldom a justification for surgery in the asymptomatic adult. This is not the case for children, however.

Results of Surgery

Although operative mortality can exceed 5% or approach 20% with left ventricular dysfunction,[92] improvements in surgical technique and possibly patient selection have led to a dramatic decrease in surgical mortality for AVR from 10.6% during 1970 to 1976, to 2% for surgery performed from 1980 to 1985 at one university hospital.[93] These excellent surgical results are in spite of the unique challenges posed by the typical patient with predominantly aortic stenosis when referred for surgery.

In contrast to those requiring AVR for predominantly aortic insufficiency, patients with aortic stenosis tend to be older, have more significant coronary atherosclerosis, and require a smaller prosthesis, placing a greater emphasis on efficiency of valve prosthesis design. In an earlier study, Miller and colleagues[94] reported a higher operative mortality and perioperative myocardial infarction rate in AVR associated with coronary artery bypass grafting than in AVR alone. However, late follow-up showed no difference between the two groups. More recently, Czer and associates[95] have reported that operative mortality is actually lower in patients undergoing concomitant coronary revascularization when indicated than when AVR alone is performed in patients with significant coronary atherosclerosis.[95] For these reasons, it is currently routine practice to perform coronary angiography in most patients contemplating AVR for predominantly aortic stenosis and to bypass any significant obstructions at the time of surgery.

Predictors of Clinical Outcome

As with most procedures, advanced age confers higher mortality. In a study by Deleuze and coworkers,[96] patients older than 80 years of age undergoing AVR for aortic stenosis experienced a 1-month mortality rate of 28%. In these patients, early mortality was correlated with left ventricular ejection fraction of <40%.

In a comprehensive evaluation of factors associated with late survival after AVR for aortic stenosis, Lund[97] developed a highly successful prognostic index, stratifying patients into eight risk groups and comparing their observed and expected 10-year survival rates to that of the background population in their native Denmark. He found that excess mortality, relative to the background population, was mainly caused by congestive heart failure. He theorized that improved long-term survival during the 22-year study evaluation was related to improved preoperative patient status, and that earlier operation (resulting in a lower prognostic index) inferred a survival rate comparable with that of a matched background population. He found that the peak systolic pressure gradient was the strongest independent risk factor and was inversely related to death rate, possibly because well-maintained ventricular function is required for the blood flow necessary to produce a high gradient. Other at-risk prognostic factors were cardiothoracic index, left ventricular failure, diminished left ventricular ejection fraction, prosthetic orifice diameter of ≤15 mm, advanced patient age, and male gender.

Predictors of Left Ventricular Recovery

Because it is only in comparatively late stages of aortic stenosis that left ventricular dilation occurs, and because much of the afterload excess leading to depressed ejection fraction is corrected at the time of AVR, it is perhaps more appropriate to speak in terms of levels of depressed ejection fraction that may still recover, or how much left ventricular dysfunction is a result of more than simple excessive afterload due to the outflow obstruction. In a series of 103 patients with aortic stenosis undergoing AVR, 58 had an ejection fraction of >46%, and 45 had an ejection fraction <45%. In the group with the good ejection fraction, early mortality was 5.2% and late mortality 5.2%, compared with no early deaths and a 13.3% late death rate in the group with poor ejection fraction. Follow-up was for 12 to 102 months (average 43 months). Both groups showed excellent symptomatic improvement, and ejection fraction improvement was found in 20 of 29 patients with low preoperative ejection fraction.[98] In another smaller study of 19 patients with clinical congestive heart failure and low ejection fraction (mean 37% ± 2%), the surgical mortality was 21% and the 3-year actuarial survival rate was 74%. Repeat catheterization in ten patients revealed a return to normal of left ventricular end-diastolic pressure and an increase in ejection fraction from 34% to 63%.[99] With longstanding hypertrophy, moderate depression of left ventricular myocardial contractility may develop, shifting the end-systolic wall stress volume relationship somewhat to the right.

By the use of the Frank-Starling mechanism, with increased end-diastolic volume, ejection fraction may still be maintained within normal limits at slightly higher wall stress. Eventually, the left ventricle may reach the limit of its preload reserve because of increased diastolic stiffness preventing complete filling. Under these conditions of limited preload reserve, the left ventricle response to further progression of stenosis with marked elevation of systolic wall stress results in further decrease in left ventricular ejection fraction without further depression of myocardial contractility.[22] It is difficult to ascertain how much of the evidence for left ventricular dysfunction is truly the result of diminished contractility or simply due to the adaptive changes to excessive afterload, which can be removed with successful AVR.

An early, modest decrease in myocardial cell hypertrophy is observed postoperatively in patients with aortic stenosis, but left ventricular fibrous content reduction is observed only in later follow-up (5 to 6 years after surgery).[78] Regression of left ventricular hypertrophy after AVR has been tracked and compared with postoperative changes in cardiac function. At least 1½ to 2 years is required for significant regression of hypertrophy to occur.[77]

Recommendations for Surgery

Patients with significant aortic stenosis and symptoms producing limitation of normal activities (NYHA class III) should have surgery. Considering rapid fall-off of survival when symptoms do develop, relatively low surgical mortality and excellent long-term results, surgery also should be considered in patients with lesser symptoms such as NYHA class II, or those who are relatively intolerant of life-style restrictions. Surgery also is recommended with left ventricular dilation or with diminution in resting ejection fraction below normal, in patients in whom, for some reason, symptoms have not yet occurred.

Special Surgical Considerations

Many patients with aortic stenosis will be candidates for a bioprosthesis, and more recently, aortic root homograft, because of their advanced age at the time of surgery. Both of these surgical techniques allow acceptable safety from thromboembolism without the risks of chronic anticoagulation. With a bioprosthesis, the downside is some limitation in durability. With homograft use, this outlook hoped to be improved. In one study, there was a 55%, 15-year actuarial patient survival, and 16% actuarial homograft survival.[100] In another study, 20-year patient survival was 51.6%, freedom from valve-related death was 67%, and freedom from primary tissue failure was 12.4%.[101] Since the initiation of these early studies, marked improvements in tissue preservation have led to heightened enthusiasm for this promising new approach.

Although commissurotomy is a highly successful and low mortality procedure for children, it is not successful for management of aortic stensois in adults. Recent attempts at decalcification of stenotic aortic valves have led to premature valve failure due to aortic insufficiency. Hopefully, future technical advances will allow for the same benefits of valve repair in aortic valve disease as are currently being enjoyed in many patients with mitral valve disease.

REFERENCES

1. Harken, DE, Soroff, HS, Taylor, WJ, et al: Partial and complete prostheses in aortic insufficiency. J Thorac Cardiovasc Surg 40:744, 1960.
2. Braunwald, NS, Cooper, T, and Morrow, AG: Complete replacement of the mitral valve: Successful clinical application of a flexible polyurethane prosthesis. J Thorac Cardiovasc Surg 40:1, 1960.
3. Rapaport, E: Natural history of aortic and mitral valve disease. Am J Cardiol 35:221, 1975.
4. Fowler, NO and Van Der Bel-Kahn, JM: Operations on the mitral valve: A time for weighing the issues. Am J Cardiol 46:159, 1980.
5. Bonchek, LI, Anderson, RP, and Starr A: Mitral valve replacement with cloth-covered composite-seat prostheses. J Thorac Cardiovasc Surg 67:93, 1974.
6. Czer, LSC, Gray, RJ, DeRobertis, MA, et al: Mitral valve replacement: Impact of coronary artery disease and determinants of prognosis after revascularization. Circulation 70(Suppl I):I-198, 1984.
7. Phillips, HR, Levine, FH, Carter, JE, et al: Mitral valve replacement for isolated mitral regurgitation: Analysis of clinical course and late postoperative left ventricular ejection fraction. Am J Cardiol 48:647, 1981.
8. Hammermeister, KE, Fischer, L, Kennedy, JW, et al: Predictors of late survival in patients with mitral valve disease from clinical, hemodynamic, and quantitative angiographic variables. Circulation 57:341, 1978.
9. Salomon, NW, Stinson, EB, Griepp, RB, et al. Patient-related risk factors as predictors of results following isolated mitral valve replacement. Ann Thorac Surg 24:519, 1977.
10. Chaffin, JS and Daggett, WM: Mitral valve replacement: A nine-year follow-up of risks and survivals. Ann Thorac Surg 27:312, 1979.
11. Tsai, TP, Matloff, JM, Chaux, A, et al: Combined valve and coronary artery bypass procedures in septuagenarians and octogenarians. Results in 120 patients. Ann Thorac Surg 42:681, 1986.
12. Tsai, TP, Matloff, JM, Gray, RJ, et al: Cardiac surgery in the octogenarian. J Thorac Cardiovasc Surg 91:924, 1986.
13. Takahashi, S, Kawana, M, and Hirosawa, K: Surgery in severe rheumatic mitral valve disease—Recognition of severity and risk factors. Jpn Circ J 47:1112, 1983.
14. Borow, KM, Green, HL, Mann, T, et al: End-systolic volume as a predictor of postoperative left ventricular performance in volume overload from valvular regurgitation. Am J Med 68:655, 1980.
15. Saltissi, S, Crowther, A, Byrne, C, et al: Assessment of prognostic factors in patients undergoing surgery for non-rheumatic mitral regurgitation. Br Heart J 44:369, 1980.
16. Carabello, BA, Stanton, SP, and McGuire, LB: Assessment of preoperative left ventricular function in patients with mitral regurgitation: Value of the end-systolic wall stress—end-systolic volume ratio. Circulation 64:1212, 1981.
17. Zile, MR, Gaasch, WH, Carroll, JD, et al: Chronic mitral regurgitation: Predictive value of preoperative echocardiographic indexes of left ventricular function and wall stress. J Am Coll Cardiol 3:235, 1984.
18. Urschel, CW, Covell, JW, Sonnenblick, EH, et al: Myocardial mechanics in aortic and mitral valvular regurgitation. The concept of instantaneous impedance and determinants of the performance of the intact heart. J Clin Invest 47:867, 1968.
19. Braunwald, E: Mitral regurgitation: Physiological, clinical and surgical considerations. N Engl J Med 281:425, 1969.
20. Eckberg, DL, Gault, JH, Bouchard, RL, et al: Mechanics of left ventricular contraction in chronic severe mitral regurgitation. Circulation 47:1252, 1973.
21. Vokonas, PS, Gorlin, R, Cohn, PF, et al: Dynamic geometry of the left ventricle in mitral regurgitation. Circulation 48:786, 1973.
22. Ross, J: Afterload mismatch in aortic and mitral valve disease: Implications for surgical therapy. J Am Coll Cardiol 5:811, 1985.
23. Kennedy, JW, Doces, JG, and Stewart, DK: Left ventricular function before and following surgical treatment of mitral valve disease. Am Heart J 97:592, 1979.
24. Boucher, CA, Bingham, JB, Osbakken, MD, et al: Early changes in left ventricular size and function after correction of left ventricular volume overload. Am J Cardiol 47:991, 1981.
25. Morton, MJ, Bohnsted, SW, Pantely, GA, et al: Effect of successful mitral valve replacement on left ventricular function. Circulation 62(Suppl III):III-208, 1980.

26. David, TE, Uden, DE, and Strauss, HD: The importance of the mitral apparatus in left ventricular function after correction of mitral regurgitation. Circulation 68:1176, 1983.

27. Schuler, G, Peterson, KL, Johnson, A, et al: Temporal response of left ventricular performance to mitral valve surgery. Circulation 59:1218, 1979.

28. Huikuri, HV, Ikaheimo, MJ, Linnaluoto, MMK, et al: Left ventricular response to isometric stress and its value in predicting the change in ventricular function after mitral valve replacement for mitral regurgitation. Am J Cardiol 51:1110, 1983.

29. Dubroff, JM, Clark, MB, Wong, CY, et al: Left ventricular ejection fraction during cardiac surgery: A two dimensional echocardiographic study. Circulation 68:95, 1983.

30. Peter, CA, Austin, EH, and Jones, RH: Effect of valve replacement for chronic mitral insufficiency on left ventricular function during rest and exercise. J Thorac Cardiovasc Surg 82:127, 1981.

31. Lillehei, CW, Levy, MJ, and Bonnabeau, RC: Mitral valve replacement with preservation of papillary muscles and chordae tendineae. J Thorac Cardiovasc Surg 47:532, 1964.

32. Shigehito, M and Yutaka, O: Analysis of left-ventricular motion after mitral valve replacement with preservation of all chorda tendineae. Abstract presented at Asia Pacific Symposium, "Current Perspectives in Cardiac Valve Surgery," February 13–17, Napa Valley, California, 1991.

33. Deloche, A, Jebara, VA, Relland, JYM, et al: Valve repair with Carpentier techniques; a second decade. J Thorac Cardiovasc Surg 99:990, 1990.

34. Spence, PA, Peniston, CM, David, TE, et al: Toward a better understanding of the etiology of left ventricular dysfunction after mitral valve replacement: An experimental study with possible clinical implications. Ann Thorac Surg 41:363, 1986.

35. Hansen, DE, Cahill, PD, DeCampli, WM, et al: Valvular-ventricular interaction: Importance of the mitral apparatus in canine left ventricular systolic performance. Circulation 73:1310, 1986.

36. Hansen, DE, Sarris, GE, Niczyporous, MA, et al: Physiologic role of the mitral apparatus in left ventricular regional mechanics, contraction synergy, and global systolic performance. J Thorac Cardiovasc Surg 97:521, 1989.

37. Cosgrove, DM: Surgery for degenerative mitral valve disease. Semin Thorac Cardiovasc Surg 1:183, 1989.

38. Craver, J, Cohen, C, and Weintraub, WS: Case-matched comparison of mitral valve replacement and repair. Ann Thorac Surg 49:964, 1990.

39. Olesen, KH: The natural history of 271 patients with mitral stenosis under medical treatment. Br Heart J 24:349, 1962.

40. Neilson, JH, Galeaeg, EG, and Hossack, KF: Thromboembolic complications of mitral valve disease. Aust NZ J Med 8:372, 1978.

41. Braunwald, E, Braunwald, NS, Ross, J, et al: Effective mitral valve replacement with pulmonary vascular dynamics for patients with pulmonary hypertension. N Engl J Med 273:509, 1965.

42. Boncheck, LI: Current status of mitral commissurotomy: Indications, techniques, and results. Am J Cardiol 52:411, 1983.

43. John, S, Bashi, VV, Jairaj, PS, et al: Closed mitral valvotomy: Early results and long-term follow-up of 3724 consecutive patients. Circulation 68:891, 1983.

44. Smith, WM, Neutze, JM, Barratt-Boyes, BG, et al: Open mitral valvotomy: Effect of preoperative factors on results. J Thorac Cardiovasc Surg 82:738, 1981.

45. Scott, WC, Miller, DC, Haverich, A, et al: Operative risk of mitral valve replacement: Discriminant analysis of 1329 procedures. Circulation 72(Suppl II):II-108, 1985.

46. Goldschlager, N, Pfeifer, J, Cohn, K, et al: The natural history of aortic regurgitation: A clinical and hemodynamic study. Am J Med 54:577, 1973.

47. Dexter, L: Evaluation of the results of cardiac surgery. In Jones, AM (ed): Modern Trends in Cardiology, vol 2. Appleton-Century-Crofts, New York, 1969, pp 311–333.

48. Spagnuolo, M, Kloth, H, Taranta, A, et al: Natural history of rheumatic aortic regurgitation: Criteria predictive of death, congestive heart failure, and angina in young patients. Circulation 44:368, 1971.

49. Greves, J, Rahimtoola, SH, McAnulty, JH, et al: Preoperative criteria predictive of late survival following valve replacement for severe aortic regurgitation. Am Heart J 101:300, 1981.

50. Henry, WL, Bonow, RO, Rosing, DR, et al: Observations on the optimum time for operative intervention for aortic regurgitation: I. Evaluation of the results of aortic valve replacement in symptomatic patients. Circulation 61:471, 1980.

51. Lytle, BW, Cosgrove, DM, Loop, FD, et al: Replacement of aortic valve combined with myocar-

dial revascularization: Determinants of early and late risk for 500 patients, 1967–1981. Circulation 68:1149, 1983.

52. Hirshfeld, JW, Epstein, SE, Roberts, AJ, et al: Indices predicting long-term survival after valve replacement in patients with aortic regurgitation and patients with aortic stenosis. Circulation 50:1190, 1974.

53. Copeland, JG, Griepp, RB, Stinson, EB, et al: Long-term follow-up after isolated aortic valve replacement. J Thorac Cardiovasc Surg 74:875, 1977.

54. Roberts, DL, DeWeese, JA, Mahoney, EB, et al: Long-term survival following aortic valve replacement. Am Heart J 91:311, 1976.

55. Rubin, JW, Moore, HV, Hillson, RF, et al: Thirteen year experience with aortic valve replacement. Am J Cardiol 40:345, 1977.

56. Cohn, LH, Koster, JK, Mee, RBB, et al: Long-term follow-up of the Hancock bioprosthetic heart valve: A 6-year review. Circulation 60(Suppl I):I-17, 1979.

57. Schwartz, F, Baumann, P, Manthey, J, et al: The effect of aortic valve replacement on survival. Circulation 66:1105, 1982.

58. McGoon, MD, Fuster, V, McGoon, DC, et al: Aortic and mitral valve incompetence: Long-term follow-up (10 to 19 years) of patients treated with the Starr-Edwards prosthesis. J Am Coll Cardiol 3:930, 1984.

59. Stone, PH, Clark, RD, Goldschlager, N, et al: Determinants of prognosis of patients with aortic regurgitation who undergo aortic valve replacement. J Am Coll Cardiol 3:1118, 1984.

60. Samuels, DA, Curfman, GD, Friedlich, AL, et al: Valve replacement for aortic regurgitation: Long-term follow-up with factors influencing the results. Circulation 60:647, 1979.

61. Bonow, RO, Borer, JS, Rosing, DR, et al: Preoperative exercise capacity in symptomatic patients with aortic regurgitation as a predictor of postoperative left ventricular function and long-term prognosis. Circulation 62:1280, 1980.

62. Stone, PH, Goldschlager, N, Selzer, A, et al: Determinants of prognosis of patients with aortic insufficiency undergoing aortic valve replacement. Circulation 60(Suppl II):II-38, 1979.

63. Forman, R, Firth, BG, and Barnard, MS: Prognostic significance of preoperative left ventricular ejection fraction and valve lesion in patients with aortic valve replacement. Am J Cardiol 45:1120, 1980.

64. Henry, WL, Bonow, RO, Rosing, DR, et al: Observations on the optimum time for operative intervention for aortic regurgitation. II. Serial echocardiographic evaluation of asymptomatic patients. Circulation 61:484, 1980.

65. Cunha, CLP, Giuliani, ER, Fuster, V, et al: Preoperative M-mode echocardiography as a predictor of surgical results in chronic aortic insufficiency. J Thorac Cardiovasc Surg 79:256, 1980.

66. Gaasch, WH, Carroll, JD, Levine, HJ, et al: Chronic aortic regurgitation: Prognostic value of left ventricular end-systolic dimension and end-diastolic radius/thickness ratio. J Am Coll Cardiol 1:775, 1983.

67. Gault, JH, Covell, JW, Braunwald, E, et al: Left ventricular performance following correction of free aortic regurgitation. Circulation 42:773, 1970.

68. Clark, DG, McAnulty, JH, and Rahimtoola, SH: Valve replacement in aortic insufficiency with left ventricular dysfunction. Circulation 61:411, 1980.

69. Fischl, SJ, Gorlin, R, and Herman, MV: Cardiac shape and function in aortic valve disease: Physiologic and clinical implication. Am J Cardiol 39:170, 1977.

70. Kennedy, JW, Doces, J, and Stewart, DK: Left ventricular function before and following aortic valve replacement. Circulation 56:944, 1977.

71. Schwartz, F, Flameng, W, Thormann, J, et al: Recovery from myocardial failure after aortic valve replacement. J Thorac Cardiovasc Surg 75:854, 1978.

72. Pantely, G, Morton, M, and Rahimtoola, SH: Effects of successful, uncomplicated valve replacement on ventricular hypertrophy, volume, and performance in aortic stenosis and in aortic incompetence. J Thorac Cardiovasc Surg 75:383, 1978.

73. Herreman, F, Ameur, A, DeVernejoul, F, et al: Pre- and postoperative hemodynamic and cineangiographic assessment of left ventricular function in patients with aortic regurgitation. Am Heart J 98:63, 1979.

74. Toussaint, C, Cribier, A, Cazor, JL, et al: Hemodynamic and angiographic evaluation of aortic regurgitation 8 and 27 months after valve replacement. Circulation 64:456, 1981.

75. Gaasch, WH, Andrias, CW, and Levine, HJ: Chronic aortic regurgitation: The effect of aortic valve replacement on left ventricular volume, mass, and function. Circulation 58:825, 1978.

76. Schuler, G, Peterson, KL, Johnson, AD, et al: Serial noninvasive assessment of left ventricular

hypertrophy and function after surgical correction of aortic regurgitation. Am J Cardiol 44:585, 1979.

77. Monrad, ES, Hess, OM, Murakami, T, et al: Time course of regression of left ventricular hypertrophy after aortic valve replacement. Circulation 77:1345, 1988.

78. Krayenbuehl, HP, Hess, OM, Monrad, ES, et al: Left ventricular myocardial structure in aortic valve disease before, intermediate, and late after aortic valve replacement. Circulation 79:744, 1989.

79. O'Rourke, RA and Crawford, MH: Timing of valve replacement in patients with chronic aortic regurgitation (editorial). Circulation 61:493, 1980.

80. Fioretti, P, Roelandt, J, Bos, RJ, et al: Echocardiography in chronic aortic insufficiency: Is valve replacement too late when left ventricular end-systolic dimension reaches 55 mm? Circulation 67:216, 1983.

81. Selachcic, J, Massie, BM, Greenberg, B, et al: Intertest variability of echocardiographic and chest x-ray measurements: Implications for decision making in patients with aortic regurgitation. J Am Coll Cardiol 7:1310, 1986.

82. Thompson, R: Aortic regurgitation—How do we judge optimal timing for surgery? Aust NZ J Med 14:514, 1984.

83. Bonow, RO: Timing of operation for chronic aortic regurgitation: Influence of left ventricular function on clinical management. Herz 9:319, 1984.

84. Bonow, RO, Rosing, DR, Maron, BJ, et al: Reversal of left ventricular dysfunction after valve replacement for chronic aortic regurgitation: Influence of duration of preoperative left ventricular dysfunction. Circulation 10:510, 1984.

85. Fioretti, P, Roelandt, J, Tirtaman, C, et al: Value of the regurgitant volume to end-diastolic volume ratio to predict the regression of left ventricular dimensions after valve replacement in aortic insufficiency. Eur Heart J 8(Suppl C):15, 1987.

86. Taniguchi, K, Nakano, S, Matsuda, H, et al: Timing of operation for aortic regurgitation: Relation to postoperative contractile state. Ann Thorac Surg 50:779, 1990.

87. Roman, MJ, Klein, L, Devereux, RB, et al: Reversal of left ventricular dilatation, hypertrophy, and dysfunction by valve replacement in aortic regurgitation. Am Heart J 118:553, 1989.

88. Tornos, MP, Permanyer-Miralda, G, Evangelista, A, et al: Clinical evaluation of a prospective protocol for the timing of surgery in chronic aortic regurgitation. Am Heart J 120:649, 1990.

89. Biem, HJ, Detsky, AS, and Armstrong, PW: Management of asymptomatic chronic aortic regurgitation with left ventricular dysfunction. A decision analysis. J Gen Intern Med 5:394, 1990.

90. Ross, J and Braunwald, E: The influence of corrective operations on the natural history of aortic stenosis. Circulation 37(Suppl V):V-61, 1968.

91. Harken, DE, Block, H, Taylor, WJ, et al: Surgical correction of calcific aortic stenosis in adults. J Thorac Cardiovasc Surg 36:759, 1958.

92. McAnulty, JH: Timing of surgical therapy for aortic valve stenosis. Herz 9:341, 1984.

93. Di Lello, F, Flemma, RJ, Anderson, AJ, et al: Improved early results after aortic valve replacement: Analysis by surgical time frame. Ann Thorac Surg 47:51, 1989.

94. Miller, DC, Stinson, EB, Oyer, PE et al: Surgical implications and results of combined aortic valve replacement and myocardial revascularization. Am J Cardiol 43:494, 1979.

95. Czer, LSC, Gray, RJ, Stewart, ME, et al: Reduction in sudden late death by concomitant revascularization with aortic valve replacement. J Thorac Cardiovasc Surg 95:390, 1988.

96. Deleuze, P, Loisance, DY, Besnainou, F, et al: Severe aortic stenosis in octogenarians: Is operation an acceptable alternative? Ann Thorac Surg 50:226, 1990.

97. Lund, O: Preoperative risk evaluation and stratification of long-term survival after valve replacement for aortic stenosis: Reasons for earlier operative intervention. Circulation 82:124, 1990.

98. Thompson, R, Yacoub, M, Ahmed, M, et al: Influence of preoperative left ventricular function on results of homograft replacement of the aortic valve for stenosis. Am J Cardiol 43:979, 1979.

99. Smith, N, McAnulty, JH, and Rahimtoola, SH: Severe aortic stenosis with unimpaired left ventricular function and clinical heart failure: Results of valve replacement. Circulation 58:255, 1978.

100. Cohen, DJ, Myerowitz, PD, Young, WP, et al: The fate of aortic valve homografts 12 to 17 years after implantation. Chest 93:482, 1988.

101. Matsuki, O, Robles, A, Gibbs, S, et al: Long-term performance of 555 aortic homografts in the aortic position. Ann Thorac Surg 46:187, 1988.

PART 5

Management

CHAPTER 11

Mechanical Prostheses: Old and New

Robert B. Karp, M.D.
Mark E. Sand, M.D.

In the early 1950s, closed-heart methods to palliate the disability of valvular lesions were limited by several factors, not the least of which was advanced valve pathology. The poor results following open attempts at repair or partial replacement and the greater availability of clinical cardiopulmonary bypass combined to inspire the development of cardiac valve prostheses. A detailed review of the many interesting historical and scientific advancements in cardiac valve development is beyond the scope of this chapter. Several excellent compiled works are available for the interested reader.[1-6]

The factors considered in recommending a valve prosthesis are many and complex. Comparative clinical data on different mechanical valves are not always available and are frequently confounded by patient-specific or institutional factors that importantly affect events after valve replacement and prevent precise conclusions as to the role that a specific device plays in outcome. When one reflects on Harken's[7] "Ten Commandments" for heart valves outlined in the 1950s, it becomes clear that the perfect device has not yet been marketed. However, much progress has been made in a remarkably short time. Valve replacement now is a reproducible operation in most settings. Patients may look forward to many years of functional improvement with currently available devices. The need for anticoagulation, the attendant risk for thromboembolic events, and bleeding complications remain the price to be paid for the durability offered by mechanical prostheses compared with the bioprosthetic options.

The four general categories of mechanical prosthetic designs are reviewed with attention to principles of design and materials selection that have been learned. These are reviewed with particularly attention to suboptimal clinical performance or device failures that might be anticipated in patients still being followed with earlier generation valves. A discussion of considerations in device selection and implantation for currently available devices is presented next. Finally, some thoughts on anticoagulation and valve surveillance are offered.

CAGED BALL VALVES

The caged ball proved to be the first durable mechanical valve replacement. Several investigators modified the design to improve hemodynamic performance, decrease thrombogenicity, and improve durability (Table 11-1). Only the *Starr-Edwards* design (models 1200 and 1260 for aortic and 6120 for mitral) remains available for implantation.

First credit for the concept of a caged ball valve mechanism is given to Williams[8] for his patented bottle stopper in 1858. Drs. J. Moore Campbell and Charles Hufnagel pioneered the concept in the descending aorta as a treatment for aortic incompetence in the early 1950s.[9,10] Harken[11] reported successful human subcoronary aortic valve replacement in 1960. Extensive laboratory collaboration between Starr and Edwards[12] preceded the first successful ball valve replacement of the mitral valve in 1960. Their continued collaboration refined many design features. A few examples include materials selection, ball and cage dimensions to improve hemodynamics without compromising reliability, inclusion of a silicone sponge in the sewing ring to enhance fixation, and extended cloth coverage of the inflow ring to reduce thromboembolism.[13] Improvements of surgical technique and myocardial protection rapidly resulted in better outcomes of valve replacement procedures. Additionally, Starr and his colleagues pioneered the statistical methods that became the foundation for clinical evaluation and reporting of valve-related complications.[14]

Table 11-1. Caged Ball Mechanical Valve Prostheses

Edwards
Stuckey
Ellis
Hufnagel
Harken
Starr-Edwards
    Lucite cage—Silastic poppet
    Stainless Steel—Silastic poppet
    Stellite 21—Silastic poppet
        Aortic models
        Pre 1000, 1000, 1200, 1260
        Mitral models
        Pre 6000, 6000, 6120
    Stellite, Cloth Covered (Dacron, Teflon)—
      Stellite poppet
        Aortic models
        2300, 2310, 2320, 2400
        Mitral models
        6300, 6310, 6320, 6400
    Beaded Metal
Smeloff-Cutter
Braunwald-Cutter
Magovern-Cromie, Sutureless, models A1–A4
DeBakey-Surgitool, models 1–3
Cooley-Liotta-Cromie
Serville-Arbonville

BALL VARIANCE. Lefrak and Starr[15] have nicely outlined the details of this troublesome problem in early generation ball valves as summarized below. Silicone poppet degeneration (ball variance) common to many of the early models, independent of manufacturer, was determined to be the result of abrasion injury to the ball and absorption of water and blood lipids, which altered the weight and physical properties of the ball. The distorted ball was subject to further damage that was manifest by valvular stenosis or incompetence, hemolysis, emboli, or catastrophic failure with poppet sticking or escape. Ball variance was more likely to occur in conditions of high velocity and turbulence that promoted separation of the blood lipids from carrier proteins. Thus, aortic models were more frequently affected than mitral models. Lipid absorption was greatly reduced by changes in the silicone rubber specifications and curing process. Designs combining cloth-covered cages with Silastic balls demonstrated more abrasion injury. Ball variance has been a rare problem since 1966 for valves with bare metal cages and Silastic poppets. However, clinicians should consider the possibility of ball variance in a patient with a caged ball valve and new onset of murmur, hemolysis, emboli, or other clinical change in a previously well-functioning prosthesis. A diminished or absent opening sound is an early clinical sign of ball variance. Radiolucent cracks may be evident on high-resolution x-rays.

Other noncloth caged ball valves implanted include, but are not limited to Magovern-Cromie, DeBakey-Surgitool, and Smeloff-Cutter.

The *Magovern-Cromie* valve is an ingenious sutureless design developed to minimize ischemic time during the era of limited methods of myocardial protection. This stainless steel, closed-cage valve with silicone ball was equipped with two rows of interlocking pins that were extended into the anulus by rotation of an appropriately sized Surgitool insertion instrument. Although earlier models were used in both mitral and aortic positions, the majority of application has been in the aortic position.[16] The incidence of periprosthetic leakage was 13% to 15%, and some cases of prosthesis dehiscence were reported. A recent review of Magovern's institutional experience of 728 patients reported noninfectious paraprosthetic leak in (2.6%) of 588 patients followed. Pacemakers were required in 88 patients perioperatively and 31 in follow-up.[17] Explantation of Magovern-Cromie valve without the appropriately sized Surgitool instrument is extremely difficult.

The *DeBakey-Surgitool* valve marketed in 1969 pioneered the use of a Pyrolyte carbon poppet and in the last of three modifications also had a Pyrolyte inflow orifice with the titanium cage. The Pyrolyte ball was intended to limit the possibility of ball variance. The relatively hard ball and soft titanium cage led to strut wear and instances of strut fracture. Patients with this prosthesis should have periodic radiographic evaluation to detect strut damage before poppet escape.[18]

The *Smeloff-Cutter* (S-C) valve employed a double-cage design with three titanium struts on each of the inflow and outflow regions to contain the Silastic ball. The cages were open at the apex. The full-orifice design was developed to improve hemodynamic performance and to reduce thromboembolic complications. Valve failure was dramatically reduced with the solution of problems related to ball variance. Mechanical failure, late ball variance, and valve thrombosis have been uncommon.[19,20] Rare cases of the open struts engagement by left ventricular muscle and restricted ball motion have been reported.[21,22] The clinical hemodynamic performance, rates of thromboembolism, and bleeding complications have been comparable to the Starr-Edwards noncloth-covered models.[20,23]

The success of caged ball valves was tempered by problems of thromboembolism. On the other hand, early experience with fabric-based flexible leaflet valves showed, after a few months, failure due to leaflet immobility and perforation. The adherent fibrous connective tissue coating the Teflon aortic leaflets was thought to be the basis for the limited thromboembolism observed. These observations and the knowledge that extending fabric covering to the inflow margin of ball valves had substantially decreased thromboembolism stimulated Braunwald and Starr's group to independently develop cloth-covered ball valves during the late 1960s. Braunwald, in collaboration with Cutter Laboratories *(Braunwald-Cutter),* selected a Silastic poppet whereas Starr chose a Stellite ball to limit poppet wear. Results in animal models were encouraging.[24–26] However, the human clinical results without anticoagulation were disappointing, with unacceptable rates of thromboembolism.[27] This was thought to be due to slower and thinner formation of neointima in humans that failed to prevent abrasion injury.[28] Hemolysis, strut cloth wear and fragmentation, impaired hemodynamics, and stuck poppets were observed in both experiences although less in the revised models of later years. Abrasion injury to the Silastic ball created problems leading to poppet escape in the aortic position. This ultimately led to withdrawal of this model of the Braunwald-Cutter valve from the market in 1974 and the recommendation of prophylactic replacement. Performance in the mitral position was not prone to sudden catastrophic poppet escape, and long-term performance of the Braunwald-Cutter mitral prosthesis is comparable to other caged ball valves.[29,30] Other cloth-covered prostheses marketed included the *Cooley-Liotta-Cromie,* which employed a titanium ball and Dacron-covered cage. Hemolysis and cloth fragmentation led to its discontinuation.[31]

CAGED DISC VALVES

Caged ball valves in the mitral position were thought to produce left ventricular outflow tract obstruction and ventricular septal irritation. Caged disc valves were developed as low-profile prostheses to deal with these problems.[32] A number of prostheses in this category were implanted in the 1960s and 1970s (Table 11-2). The majority of models employed lenticular discs that were oriented with the flat surface perpendicular to the axis of flow. The resultant small secondary flow orifice produced relatively high transvalvular gradients at rest and during exercise. The small clearance of the disc made poppet motion susceptible to interference by thrombus or ventricular endocardium leading to marked dysfunction or catastrophic failure. Material incompatibilities between the disc and cage resulted in disc edge wear in some models and strut fracture in others.[33]

The *Kay-Shiley* valve is illustrative of some of the problems with caged disc valves. The original valve design, first implanted in 1965, incorporated a Stellite ring and cage and silicone rubber disc.[34,35] As in the ball valve experience, high thromboembolic rates prompted extension of the knitted Teflon cloth sewing ring to cover the metal of the inflow orifice.[36] Disc entrapment by fibrous ingrowth or thrombus extension over the disc restricted the valve orifice and contributed to accelerated disc wear by the metal struts setting the stage for catastrophic valve failure.[37,38] Subsequent modifications included muscle guards adjacent to the cage to prevent left ventricular muscle impingement on the disc and substitution of a Delrin disc to reduce disc edge wear. Despite these modifications, performance of

Table 11–2. Central Disc
and Central Occluder
Mechanical Prostheses

Kay-Shiley
Beall-Surgitool, models 102–106
Starr-Edwards disc
   Mitral models
     6500 Stellite cage, Stellite disc
     6520 Stellite cage, Polyethylene disc
Cooley-Cutter
   Disc
   Biconal occluder
Cross-Jones
Kay-Suzuki
Barnard-Goosen
Harken-Cromie
Hufnagel-Conrad
Cooley-Bloodwell-Cutter
Lillehei-Nakib (toroidal disc)
Hammersmith
Woodward
Davila
UCT-Barnard
Serville-Arbonville (plate-central axis)
Teardrop Discoid
Pin Teardrop

---

the Kay-Shiley valve has not achieved the design goals. Long-term survival has been reported with this prosthesis.[39,40] Late follow-up suggests survival was less good and thromboembolic complications higher than alternatives available during that era.[41–44] Some authors have recommended elective replacement of the Kay-Shiley valve in the mitral position because of poor performance.[45]

Beall and colleagues[49] working with Surgitool produced five modifications of the *Beall-Surgitool* caged disc valve. Model 102, introduced in 1967, had a Teflon disc and cage. Dacron velour covered the inflow portion to enhance tissue ingrowth and reduce embolism. This valve was plagued by disc edge wear. Model 103 employed a thicker Teflon disc and model 104 also increased the primary and secondary orifice areas to improve hemodynamics. Despite these design changes, disc edge wear led to worsening hemolysis and deteriorating hemodynamic performance sufficiently often to recommend early re-replacement.[46] A Pyrolyte carbon-silicone alloy replaced Teflon for both the disc and cage covering in model 105 (introduced in 1971). Disc wear was improved, but six reported cases of strut fracture in 1974 led to the development of model 106, which has a larger strut wire diameter.[47–49] Late reports concerning early model Beall valves continue to be published.[50–52] Evidence of worsening hemolysis, symptoms of cardiac deterioration, or abnormal disc size or motion by cinefluoroscopy should prompt consideration of prosthesis replacement before further deterioration occurs.[53]

The *Starr-Edwards model 6500* caged disc mitral valve was introduced in 1968 with a hollow stellite-21 poppet and cage struts. This material combination prevented the disc wear problem; however, hemodynamic performance, thromboembolism, and thrombotic poppet entrapment were greater issues than with comparable ball valves.[54]

Model 6520 substituted an ultrahigh molecular weight polyethylene disc that was thinner and lighter and allowed a larger primary and secondary orifice. This valve was implanted beginning in 1970. Hemodynamics were improved but were still not as good as with the model 6120 ball valve.[55] Interference with poppet motion by ventricular endocardium or thrombus was not neutralized by the design changes.

Cooley's contributions to prosthetic valve design with caged ball valves were extended into the caged disc line with the *Cooley-Bloodwell-Cutter* valve in 1966. The first valve employed an open titanium cage concept and a silicone rubber disc. High rates of thromboembolism and disc edge wear of the soft poppet forced discontinued use in 1968. The revised *Cooley-Cutter* valve was introduced in 1971 and was released for general use in 1977. This valve used two sets of open struts similar to the S-C ball valve. The poppet was a biconical shape made of Pyrolyte carbon. The mitral sewing ring was made eccentric to move the valve more anteriorly to reduce mural myocardial entrapment and to increase valve cleansing during systole.[56] *In vitro* studies demonstrated improved flow characteristics for the Cooley-Cutter valve compared with other caged disc models.[57] Clinical results suggest a higher incidence of thromboembolism when compared with the *Björk-Shiley* valve.[58] Strut fracture with poppet escape has been reported and is thought to be due to the combination of a hard poppet material and relatively soft strut material.[59] Insufficient data exist on strut fracture to advise prophylactic removal.

The *Lillehei-Nakib Toroidal* disc valve, which was developed in 1966, incorporated central flow in a caged disc design.[60] Approximately 500 toroidal valves were implanted between 1967 and 1970 primarily in the mitral position. Structural failures have not been reported. Thrombosis or pannus formation and thromboembolism were problems. In Lillehei's personal series of 66 patients, actuarial survival was 50%, 34%, and 22%, and freedom from thrombosis or thromboembolism was 77%, 76%, and 46% at 5, 10, and 15 years, respectively.[60]

TILTING DISC VALVES

Pierce and colleagues[61] demonstrated good *in vitro* hydrodynamics with a tilting disc design and reported his animal experience with the first tilting disc valve in 1968. The insight that thrombus formation at the disc hinge could compromise occluder mobility was gained from this early design.

Wada began clinical implantation of the *Wada-Cutter* valve in 1966. This valve used a hard Teflon disc with a 70° opening angle and titanium ring. Two notches in the disc engaged the claw-like extensions of the metal ring to affix the occluder. Thromboembolism and thrombosis were recognized despite anticoagulation. Valve use was discontinued in 1974 because of disc wear at the hinges, which resulted in valve dysfunction with insufficiency or acute disc embolization.[62]

The improved hemodynamic performance shown possible by these early tilting disc valves met a need for prostheses with improved performance, particularly for small aortic roots and in small subjects. This stimulated development of two additional tilting disc valves that have each evolved through subsequent generations of change, the *Björk-Shiley* and *Lillehei-Kaster (L-K)* valves. A number of other

Table 11–3. Tilting Disc
Mechanical Prostheses

Pierce
Alvarez
Wada-Cutter
Björk-Shiley
    Standard flat disc
    60° Convexo-Concave
    70° Convexo-Concave
    Monostrut
Cruz-Kaster
Lillehei-Kaster
Lillehei-Medical
Omniscience I and II
OmniCarbon
Medtronic-Hall
Sorin Biomedica
Bicer-Valve

tilting disc valves have been implanted (Table 11–3). The evolution of tilting disc valves used extensively in the United States or with pending premarket approval (PMA) are described below. Two other Pyrolite tilting disc valves not discussed in detail include the *Sorin Biomedica* manufactured in Italy and the *Bicer Prosthetic* marketed in Argentina.

Lillehei, a pioneer in many cardiac surgery endeavors, has nurtured the development of a number of cardiac prostheses. The L-K valve is a refinement of the Cruz-Kaster valve constructed at the University of Minnesota by Cruz and Kaster, an innovative engineer. Experimental testing demonstrated downstream stasis in the Cruz-Kaster design.[63] Design changes and further evaluation of disc materials and disc support culminated in a free-floating, tilting Pyrolite carbon disc held within a titanium housing. The sewing ring was knitted Teflon and the maximum disc opening was 80°. Clinical use began in 1970 and general release followed in 1971. An estimated 55,000 L-K valves have been implanted worldwide.[64] In the United States L-K distribution ended on December 9, 1987. This was the Food and Drug Administration (FDA) deadline for valves marketed before 1976 to obtain PMA.

The L-K valve has been a durable prosthesis with only one mechanical failure reported in the literature. This was a mitral disc fracture with embolization, which was managed with successful reoperation.[65] Hemodynamic performance of the L-K valve is comparable to other prostheses of that era. Transvalvular gradients in small aortic sizes and the mitral position are higher than more recently marketed valves.[66,67] This was in part attributed to a less favorable ratio of effective orifice area to tissue anulus diameter.[68]

Extensive research to improve the L-K valve culminated in the *Omniscience I* (OS-I) valve, which increased the disc diameter to tissue anulus diameter ratio, reduced disc mass, and optimized disc curvature and pivot axis eccentricity.[69] The opening angle of 80° was retained. The PMA implantations of the OS-I began in 1978. Whereas clinical results were good in the North American PMA centers, a few European centers experienced high rates of thromboembolism and valve thrombosis in the mitral position.[70,71] Review of data from 19 centers traced the disparity in results to a combination of the following three coexisting factors.[72,69]

1. A thin Dacron sewing ring allowing smaller clearance between the valve disc and ventricular wall
2. Posterior orientation of the large orifice, allowing disc motion against the posterior ventricular wall
3. Oversizing of the prosthesis

In response to these insights, the *Omniscience-II* (OS-II) was introduced in November of 1981. The housing diameter of the larger-size valves (29 and 31 mm) was reduced by 2 mm. A thicker Teflon sewing ring was used to compensate for the reduced housing size. In addition, orientation of the larger orifice toward the aorta (anterior orientation) was recommended to avoid disc interference with posterior structures, particularly when the posterior mitral leaflet is preserved. The OS-II valve was granted PMA in May of 1985.

The *Omnicarbon* (OC) valve is the latest in the evolution of the Medical Incorporated valve line. The major difference between the OS-II and the OC valve is a change in the housing material from titanium to Pyrolite carbon.[69] This design change was predicated on the observation that the earliest bileaflet valves (Kalke-Lillehei) were not clinically successful until a similar conversion in materials was accomplished. The valve was first produced as the *Lillehei-Medical,* but refinements in mass production of an all carbon valves delayed marketing.[73] Medical Incorporated is testing the hypothesis that a hingeless, strutless all-carbon valve design will offer further improvement in thromboresistance. This valve has been in clinical trials outside the United States for 7 years with approximately 12,000 implants.[64] The limited published data available do not yet confirm the hypothesis of superior performance of the OC valve compared with the OS-II valve, but initial results are encouraging.[74–76]

Björk was motivated to try to develop a valve prosthesis in 1968 because of the problem of elevated transvalvular gradients with the Starr-Edwards ball valve and the Kay-Shiley disc valve in patients with small aortic roots.[77] Björk employed the Wada-Cutter valve. He noted the improved systolic valve performance, but confirmed the problem of hinge wear and catastrophic valve dysfunction, particularly in larger valve sizes. In collaboration with Mr. Donald Shiley, the *Björk-Shiley* (B-S) valve was developed. The first valve employed a cast Stellite cage welded to the valve ring suspending a free-floating, nonoverlapping disc made of Delrin. The opening angle was 60°. Implantation began in January of 1969. Delrin was then found to absorb moisture during autoclaving, producing disc swelling and the potential for valve dysfunction.[78] A flat Pyrolite carbon disc was substituted in 1971 *(Standard B-S)* and modified with a radiopaque tantalum marker in 1975. Despite the change to Pyrolite disc material, the rate of thromboembolism remained unchanged. Valve thrombosis was particularly common in the first year in the mitral position (3.25% of 339 valves) in the Karolinska series.[77] Thrombosis was probably due to the fact that the flat disc came in contact with the valve ring in the fully open position producing an area of stasis behind the valve. This prompted development of the *60° Convexo-Concave B-S* valve. The convexo-concave disc permitted the disc to slide out 2.5 mm from the ring in the open position. *In vitro* studies showed a 50% reduction in the low flow areas. There was a 15% reduction in transvalvular gradients in clinical experience in 849 cases. Mitral valve thrombosis in the first year occurred in 0.28% in Björk's series of 380 cases with the 60° Convexo-Concave B-S valve (p <0.01 compared with Standard B-S). This valve was distributed between 1976 and 1986. The 60° Convexo-Concave B-S valve has served many patients well for many years but has been withdrawn from the market because of outlet strut fractures.

STRUT FRACTURE. Recommendations for managing patients with the 60° Convexo-Concave B-S valve have been published by Hiratzka and coworkers[79] and are summarized below. The incidence of strut fracture has remained stable in recent years. The risk of prophylactic re-replacement continues to exceed the risk of fatal strut fracture. Strut fracture usually presents with sudden onset of rapidly progressive dyspnea, chest pain, impairment or loss of consciousness, or cardiac arrhythmia. Prosthetic sounds may have changed or become absent. A murmur may not be present. The patients are invariably hypotensive and have pulmonary edema. Diagnosis may be established by overpenetrated chest radiographs. This may reveal absence of a strut or disc in the proper location or presence of a strut or disc in another location within the heart or aorta. The clinical setting and abnormal chest x-rays indicate prompt reoperation without delay. Approximately two-thirds of patients with strut fracture have died. The risk of death before emergent reoperation seems to be higher in the aortic position. These events have received much attention in the media. In a letter of November 1990 distributed to physicians, Shiley Incorporated has sought to enroll all patients with the 60° Convexo-Concave B-S valve in Medic Alert's International Implant Registry to allow them to receive the identifying bracelet, as a means of contacting patients to disseminate accurate and timely information on the valve, and to enhance the chances for successful management of strut fracture should it occur.[80] Based upon fractures that have been reported to Shiley, the company outlined the linearized rates of fractures for 60° Convexo-Concave B-S valves through August 31, 1990 to be:

All 21 to 27 mm valves	2.0 per 10,000 per year (0.020% per year or $\frac{1}{5000}$ per year)
29 to 33 mm valves manufactured before February 1, 1981	5.3 per 10,000 per year (0.053% per year or $\frac{1}{1887}$ per year)
29 to 33 mm valves manufactured between February 1, 1981 and June 30, 1982	29.1 per 10,000 per year (0.291% per year or $\frac{1}{344}$ per year)
29 to 33 mm valves manufactured after June 30, 1982	9.2 per 10,000 per year (0.092% per year or $\frac{1}{1087}$ per year)

Convexo-Concave valves may be identified by the letters in the serial number. The alpha portion of 60° Convexo-Concave valve serial numbers ends in the letter, "C", "CM," or "CT" (e.g., 27MBRC12345 or 29AGVCM3579). Patients receive information about the specific risk of strut fracture for a particular valve when they provide the serial number to the International Implant Registry. *Any valve without a "C" in the serial number is not a Convexo-Concave valve.*

The *70° Convexo-Concave B-S* valve increased the opening angle from 60° to 70° opening angle. This further improved the valve's hemodynamic performance. The 70° Convexo-Concave B-S valve, distributed between 1980 and 1983, *was not used in the United States* and was also withdrawn from the market because of out-flow strut fractures. This occurred in 4 of 400 aortic and 9 of 172 mitral valves in the Karolinska Hospital series.[77] Lindblom and associates[81] have discussed mechanical failure of the Björk-Shiley valves in detail.

The most recently developed Björk-Shiley valve is the *Monostrut* valve, which has been widely distributed since 1982 outside the United States. Strut welds were eliminated by machining the valve from a single piece of Haynes 25 alloy. The single integral outflow strut is engineered to have a 10-fold increase in strength.[77] The Pyrolite convexo-concave disc has a maximal opening angle of 70°. Structural failure of this valve has not been reported. The PMA by the FDA is pending for the B-S Monostrut valve.

Hall, responding to concerns of the limitations of caged ball valves in small aortic roots and problems of high profile in the mitral position, began to evaluate tilting disc prostheses. He performed a randomized comparison of the L-K valve and the Standard B-S valve in the aortic position.[82] He preferred the hemodynamic performance of the B-S valve despite the larger maximal opening angle of the L-K. The problem of valve thrombosis and thromboembolism prompted Hall to team with Kaster and Woin to produce a new valve combining the best features of these two valves.[83,84] The *Hall-Kaster* valve, renamed the *Medtronic-Hall* valve with corporate acquisition, strived to improve the tilting disc concept by:

1. Moving the disc pivot point centrally to enlarge the minor orifice to improve hemodynamic and avoid stasis and valve thrombosis.
2. Introducing a sliding motion of the doughnut-shaped disc away from the tapered guide rod housing in full opening to wash away any potential platelet aggregates on the disc or struts.
3. Combining a Pyrolite disc with a titanium housing incorporating no welds to enhance durability.
4. Using a Teflon sewing ring to reduce fibrous overgrowth or pannus formation at the sewing ring valve interface.
5. Using a nonocclusive, nonoverlapping disc to allow for maximum orifice area.

The maximum opening angle is 75° in the aortic and 70° in the mitral position. Clinical implantation began in June, 1977. The Medtronic-Hall valve has not undergone any subsequent design modifications. There have been no reported structural failures.

BILEAFLET VALVES

Table 11–4 lists the bileaflet valves developed to date. Young and colleagues[85] reported the first experience with a hinged bileaflet valve that demonstrated improved hemodynamics by improving the orifice to tissue anulus ratio compared with the caged ball valves in small sizes. The valve was first implanted in 1961, but its clinical utility was limited by the tendency for thrombosis of the flexible Silastic

Table 11–4. Bileaflet
Mechanical Prostheses

Gott-Daggett
Kalke-Lillehei
St. Jude Medical
Duromedics
CarboMedics

vulcanized Teflon leaflets. The *Gott-Daggett* valve employed a graphite-benzalko-nium-heparin coated polycarbonate plastic housing.

The creative atmosphere at the University of Minnesota under the leadership of Lillehei and Kaster spawned the Lillehei-Kaster and Lillehei-Nakib Toroidal disc valve, described earlier, and the rigid bileaflet of *Kalke-Lillehei.*[60] The Kalke valve was a low profile, central flow, hingeless, double-leaflet valve. The valve was constructed entirely of titanium. *In vitro* testing supported improved hemodynamics with the 60° opening angle of each leaflet.[86] The Kalke valve was only implanted clinically once in 1968 owing to problems with thrombosis.

St. Jude Medical Inc. was founded in July 1976 as a remarkable entrepreneurial venture simply to develop a new cardiac valve prosthesis. The objectives of the *St. Jude Medical* (SJM) valve were a central flow, all pyrolytic carbon, bileaflet valve.[87] As described by Wang[88] in his article:

> The key design features of this valve included an orifice ring with integral pivot guards that housed spherically radiused "butterfly" pivotal areas and two leaflets with integral retention "ears." The orifice pivot guards were positioned upstream of the orifice throat. The leaflets were allowed to rotate or pivot within the butterfly cavities via the ears. The unique pivot design permitted leaflet retention and control of leaflet opening and closing angles without the use of pins or struts, allowed for central opening and permitted complete washing around all exposed leaflet surfaces.

Initial prototypes were constructed in September 1976 and the final design was completed in November 1976. The first all carbon 26-mm prototype was completed in May 1977. After *in vitro* testing and animal testing were completed, the first clinical implant was performed in October 1977 at the University of Minnesota.[87] Each leaflet opens to an 85° maximum angle. In the closed position, the valve leaflets reside at a 25 to 30° angle. The sewing cuff is a double velour Dacron. The SJM valve has undergone no design modifications. SJM leaflet escape has been reported.[89] The following is summarized from information on leaflet escape supplied by St. Jude Medical Inc.[90] In more than 320,000 implants performed during 13 years, 10 cases of leaflet escape have been reported to St. Jude Medical Inc. Of 10 patients, 9 underwent reoperation with 7 survivors. Seven leaflets were recovered for examination. Five exhibited signs of extrinsic damage, possibly related to intraoperative instrument trauma. One patient experienced the leaflet escape after severe chest compression during sports. One valve manufactured in 1977 demonstrated a flaw in the surface coating of the carbon leaflet that may have been responsible for the leaflet escape. Additional inspection and testing steps were instituted to minimize the possibility of such incidents for the future. As of December 31, 1990, 82 intraoperative leaflet breakages or dislodgements had been reported. These usually have been caused by use of clamps to position the valve or passage of rigid suction catheters or other instruments through the valve. These observations underscore the importance of extreme care in handling all cardiac prostheses during implantation.

Two additional bileaflet prostheses have been developed. These include the *Duromedics-Edwards* valve and the *CarboMedics* valve. The Duromedics valve was initially developed by the Hemex corporation and subsequently sold to Baxter Edwards. The Duromedics-Edwards valve is an all carbon valve with leaflet opening angles of 73° and closing angles of 2°. The leaflets are curved rather than flat and thicker than the SJM leaflets. The Duromedics-Edwards valve was withdrawn from the market after 12 leaflet escapes were reported in 20,000 implants.[91] The valve had received FDA PMA in 1986. Published data are not available to guide decisions regarding explantation. Clinical presentation of leaflet escape is similar to valve thrombosis. The differential diagnosis may be established with fluoroscopy.[92] Prompt reoperation is of course indicated.

CarboMedics Inc. has been the major manufacturer for Pyrolite carbon valve components for a number of years, and until recently was the only FDA-approved producer. Other manufacturers include Sorin in Italy and St. Jude Medical Inc., which received FDA approval for manufacture of SJM valve components in May 1991. The *CarboMedics* valve is manufactured by Carbomedics, Inc. The valve offers a rotatable valve with a carbon-coated Dacron sewing ring conceived to reduce tissue ingrowth and pannus formation. A titanium stiffening ring incorporated into the housing and increased tungsten content of the Pyrolyte leaflets enhance the radiolucency compared with other all carbon valves.[93] CarboMedics leaflet opening angle is 78° and closing angle 25°. CarboMedics valve implantation began in 1986. The company reports more than 25,000 implants outside the United States.[94] Only limited published information is available on this valve.[95,96]

CHOOSING A PROSTHESIS

In some ways, the choice of a mechanical prosthesis in the current era is more straightforward than in the past. This is particularly true for surgeons in the United States. The options are much more limited under FDA approval (Table 11–5). We have come to expect survival, symptom relief, and valve durability for appropriately selected patients undergoing valve replacement. This objective can be achieved with any of the FDA-approved valves now available and probably with the other well-studied options. Each valve has special characteristics that a surgeon should be aware of before implanting for the first time. These include considerations for suture techniques to avoid entrapment, appropriate valve sizing and orientation to optimize hemodynamic performance and avoid poppet interference, hemodynamic performance for various valve sizes, sewing ring options and characteristics, and so on.[97,98] Each valve is available in an adequate range of sizes in both the aortic and mitral position for most patients. Usually a selection of sewing ring options are available to meet special clinical needs and surgeon preference. In the United States, SJM and Medtronic-Hall supply composite valved conduits for combined ascending aorta and aortic valve replacement.

Table 11–5. Mechanical
Heart Valves Currently on
the Market, 1991

Caged Ball
Starr-Edwards
Tilting Disc
*Björk-Shiley Monostrut
Omniscience II
*Omnicarbon
Medtronic-Hall
*Sorin Biomedica
*Bicer valve
Bileaflet
St. Jude Medical
*Duromedics
*CarboMedics

*Not available in the United States.

HEMODYNAMIC PERFORMANCE

Detailed *in vitro* hemodynamic comparisons between valves are usually done on 27-mm valves by FDA convention.[99,100] Steady and pulsatile pressure drops, flow visualization, measurement of energy losses in systole and diastole, regurgitant volumes and calculation of shear stresses may all be helpful in comparing different valves but not always highly correlated with clinical events such as symptomatic improvement, thromboembolism, and hemolysis. Extrapolation of performance to smaller valve sizes may be misleading inasmuch as the events of hemodynamic performance are not linearly related to valve size. Performance index (PI) is the ratio of effective orifice area to valve sewing ring area and is one measure of how well a valve uses its *in vivo* anulus area in systole. Larger PI implies better valve performance. Yoganathan and associates[100] reported the following values for 27-mm valves: OS = 0.72, SJM = 0.71, Medtronic-Hall = 0.64, Convexo-Concave B-S = 0.45, S-C = 0.36, Starr-Edwards = 0.30. For 21-mm valves they observed: SJM = 0.60, Omniscience = 0.53, Medtronic-Hall = 0.53, Convexo-Concave B-S = 0.45. Knott and coworkers[99] have reported extensive *in vitro* comparisons of currently marketed valves. Comparison of *in vivo* valve performance is best done with calculation of effective valve areas for comparable size valves rather than simple gradients (either measured at cardiac catheterization or estimated by Doppler). Horstkotte and Dorfer,[101] in a single institutional study, compiled data comparing the Standard B-S, L-K, Starr-Edwards, Medtronic-Hall, and SJM at rest and during exercise. In 29-mm mitral valves, effective orifice areas at rest and exercise respectively in cm^2 were: SJM = 3.1 ± 0.8 and 3.4 ± 0.7; B-S = 2.2 ± 0.5 and 2.8 ± 0.6; Medtronic-Hall = 1.9 ± 0.5 and 2.3 ± 0.6; L-K = 1.7 ± 0.3 and 2.2 ± 0.4; Starr-Edwards = 1.8 ± 0.4 and 2.0 ± 0.4. In the aortic position, they reported for 23-mm valves the effective orifice areas in cm^2 at rest and exercise, respectively: SJM = 2.2 ± 0.3 and 2.5 ± 0.3; B-S = 1.5 ± 0.3 and 1.9 ± 0.3; L-K = 1.3 ± 0.1 and 1.6 ± 0.2; Starr-Edwards (24 mm) = 1.4 ± 0.2 and 1.7 ± 0.2. Similar patterns were reported for 25-mm aortic valves. They concluded that the SJM is a superior valve from a hemodynamic standpoint. Tatineni and colleagues[102] also have compared the SJM and Medtronic-Hall valves in both positions at rest and exercise. They reported no important differences between the valves in aortic sizes 21 to 31 and mitral sizes 25 to 33 for valve area at rest or during exercise. Comparable functional improvement was achieved with both valves. Other published clinical data also document satisfactory hemodynamic performance based on functional improvement and objective valve performance data for the other tilting disc valves on the market and larger sized Starr-Edwards valves. Limited information exists to compare the performance in the smaller valve sizes (19 mm SJM, 17 mm and 19 mm B-S, 19 mm Omniscience, 20 mm Medtronic-Hall).[103]

Some regurgitation is expected during valve closure and leakage in diastole. Some valve designs depend on this small amount of leakage to cleanse valve surfaces. Regurgitation tends to increase with slower heart rates and larger valve sizes and decrease as a percentage of cardiac output as output increases. The Starr-Edwards valve has the lowest regurgitant volume.[100] Disc valves with larger opening angles tend to close more slowly and hence have more closing regurgitation (Omniscience, Omnicarbon, Medtronic-Hall, B-S Monostrut). The SJM is intermediate owing to a shorter travel arc (55° − 60° vs. 70° − 75° Medtronic-Hall, Omniscience, and Omnicarbon). Leakage in diastole is higher for the SJM, Medtronic-Hall, Convexo-Concave B-S than for the B-S Monstrut, Omniscience, Omnicarbon, Duromedics that are designed with overlap between disc and housing.[99] Quantitation of regurgitation *in vivo* is problematic. No clinically important differences are generally observed in hemolysis despite differences in shear stresses demonstrated *in vitro*. Elevated LDH, reticulocyte counts, and decreased haptoglobins can be documented for most prostheses. This low-grade hemolysis is normally well compensated by increased erythropoiesis. The major factor in avoiding severe hemolysis is to avoid paravalvular leaks.

THROMBOEMBOLISM AND THROMBOSIS

Comparison of valves for thrombosis and thromboembolic events and anticoagulant-related bleeding complications is difficult because of lack of standardized methods of reporting. Institutional factors, which reflect differences in patient population and methods of anticoagulation surveillance, may also contribute to the observed variability. Linearized rates in events/100 valve-years (%/pt-yr) should be sought. Complications should be categorized as either fatal or nonfatal and permanent or transient for embolic complications. Two review articles are helpful in this regard.[104,105]

Some general conclusions can be inferred. No mechanical valve can be reliably managed without systemic anticoagulation with warfarin. Some controversy about this matter exists in the pediatric population.[106−109] Warfarin is used in all age groups. Thromboembolic and thrombotic events are more prevalent in the mitral position than in the aortic (3% to 4%/pt-yr vs. 1% to 2%/pt-yr). Early tilting disc valves (Standard B-S, Convexo-Concave B-S, OS-I) carry the highest risk of valve thrombosis. Thrombosis has been reported in all currently available mechanical prostheses. It most frequently is a sequela of a recent previous interval of inadequate anticoagulation. This complication requires prompt recognition and intervention. We recommend prompt reoperation for left-sided valves.[110] Thrombolytic therapy may be successful for right-sided prostheses but carries the hazard of systemic embolus for left-sided valves.[111,112] Valve thrombosis is usually marked by rapid onset of heart failure, shock, and diminished or absent prosthetic sounds.

Diagnosis can be confirmed by echocardiography or cinefluoroscopy. The caged ball valves tend to have higher rates of thromboembolism but lower rates of thrombosis. SJM and the later-generation tilting disc valves have comparably lower rates of thromboembolism and thrombosis compared with earlier generation valves. Most valves have the highest risk of events in the first year after implantation. Previous embolic events and prosthetic valve endocarditis are strong risk factors for future embolic events.

HEMORRHAGIC COMPLICATIONS

Bleeding complications occur at 1% to 2%/pt-yr in anticoagulated patients. Approximately 5% are fatal. We recommend anticoagulation control by using the International Normalized Ratio (INR) for surveillance.[113] An INR range of 3.0 to 4.5 (3.5 target) corresponds to a prothrombin time ratio of 1.5 to 2.0 and a prothrombin activity of 25% to 30%.[114] The combination of warfarin and aspirin is particularly likely to be complicated by bleeding. We believe patient education on the details of anticoagulation and its limitations helps to minimize errors that may result in complications.

SUMMARY

The four mechanical valve prostheses currently available on the U.S. market have evolved from a field of more than 50 valves produced for human implantation since the early 1950s (Tables 11-1 to 11-4). This literature establishes that good results can be achieved with a number of cardiac prostheses if properly used and monitored after implant. The current generation of valves have demonstrated ease of implantation, improved durability, good hemodynamic performance, and reduced thromboembolism and thrombosis with proper anticoagulation. The cost and complexity of completing PMA by the FDA, concern over product liability, and patent rights on design and raw materials have narrowed the choice of devices for surgeons in the United States and slowed the pace of new market entries. The evolution of mechanical valves has been reviewed and modes of valve failure reviewed when pertinent. Clinical expectations for earlier generation devices and present valves also are reviewed. Prostheses under evaluation are discussed along with considerations for valve implantation, surveillance, and anticoagulation.

We have employed the SJM valve since about 1985. The proven good hemodynamic performance in small sizes and low profile have made its application well suited to the pediatric population and for smaller aortic roots. The well-guarded hinge mechanism and low probability for disc entrapment have facilitated its use in chordal sparing mitral replacements in our experience. Application in the tricuspid position also has been successful but requires close attention to anticoagulation.

REFERENCES

1. Merendino, KA (ed): Prosthetic Valves for Cardiac Surgery. Charles C. Thomas, Publisher, Springfield, Ill., 1961.
2. Brewer, LA (ed): Prosthetic Heart Valves. Charles C. Thomas, Publisher, Springfield, Ill., 1969.
3. Lefrak, EA and Starr, A (eds): Cardiac Valve Prostheses. Appleton-Century-Crofts, New York, 1979.

4. Proceedings of World Congress on Heart Valve Replacement, January 15–18, 1989. Ann Thorac Surg 48:1989.

5. Crawford, FA (ed): State of the Art Reviews: Cardiac Surgery. Current Heart Valve Prostheses, Hanley & Belfus, Inc., Publishers, Philadelphia, 1987.

6. DeBakey, ME (ed): Advances in Cardiac Valves. Clinical Perspectives. Yorke Medical Books, 1983.

7. Harken, DE: Heart valves: Ten commandments and still counting. Ann Thorac Surg 48:518, 1989.

8. Williams, JB: US Patent No 19323, February 9, 1858.

9. Campbell, JM: An artificial aortic valve. J Thorac Cardiovasc Surg 19:312, 1950.

10. Hufnagel, CA: Aortic plastic valvular prosthesis. Bull Georgetown Univ Med Center 4:128, 1951.

11. Harken, DE, Soroff, HS, Taylor, WJ, et al: Partial and complete prosthesis in aortic insufficiency. J Thorac Cardiovasc Surg 40:744, 1960.

12. Starr, A and Edwards, ML: Mitral replacement: Clinical experience with a ball-valve prosthesis. Ann Surg 154:726, 1961.

13. Lefrak, EA and Starr, A: Caged-ball valves. In Lefrak, EA and Starr, A (eds): Cardiac Valve Prostheses. Appleton-Century-Crofts, New York, 1979, p 76.

14. Lefrak, EA and Grunkemeier, GL: Data base and methodology. In Lefrak, EA and Starr, A (eds): Cardiac Valve Prostheses, Appleton-Century-Crofts, New York, 1979, p 38.

15. Lefrak, EA and Starr, A: Starr-Edwards ball valve. In Lefrak, EA and Starr, A (eds): Cardiac Valve Prostheses. Appleton-Century-Crofts, New York, 1979, p 87.

16. Lefrak, EA and Starr, A: Magovern-Cromie valve. In Lefrak, EA and Starr, A (eds): Cardiac Valve Prostheses. Appleton-Century-Crofts, New York, 1979, p 133.

17. Magovern, GJ, Liebler, GA, Park, SB, et al: Twenty-five-year review of the Magovern-Cromie sutureless aortic valve. Ann Thorac Surg (Suppl)48:S33, 1989.

18. Lefrak, EA and Starr, A: DeBakey-Surgitool valve. In Lefrak, EA and Starr, A (eds): Cardiac Valve Prostheses. Appleton-Century-Crofts, New York, 1979, p 160.

19. Takashi, R, Kiso, I, Hirotani, T, et al: A case report of ball variance of Smeloff-Cutter prosthetic valve. Kyobu Geka 43:988, 1990.

20. Harlan, BJ, Smeloff, EA, Miller, GE, et al: Performance of the Smeloff aortic valve beyond ten years. J Thorac Cardiovasc Surg 91:86, 1986.

21. Kalke, B, Korns, ME, Goott, B, et al: Engagement of ventricular myocardium by open-cage atrioventricular valvular prosthesis. J Thorac Cardiovasc Surg 58:92, 1969.

22. Ibarra-Perez, C, Rodriguez-Trujillo, F, and Perez-Redondo, H: Engagement of ventricular myocardium by struts of mitral prosthesis: Fatal complication of use of open-cage cardiac valves. J Thorac Cardiovasc Surg 61:403, 1974.

23. Lefrak, EA and Starr, A: Smeloff-Cutter valve. In Lefrak, EA and Starr, A (eds): Cardiac Valve Prostheses. Appleton-Century-Crofts, New York, 1979, p 122.

24. Bull, BS, Fuchs, CAJ, and Braunwald, NS: Mechanism of formation of tissue layers on the fabric lattice covering intravascular prosthetic devices. Surgery 65:640, 1969.

25. Braunwald, NS and Bull, BS: Factors controlling the development of tissue layers on fabrics. In Brewer, LA, III (ed): Prosthetic Heart Valves. Charles C. Thomas, Publisher, Springfield, Ill. 1969, p 228.

26. Braunwald, NS and Morrow, AG: Tissue ingrowth and the rigid heart valve: Review of clinical and experimental experience during the past year. J Thorac Cardiovasc Surg 56:307, 1968.

27. Karp, RB, Kirklin, JW, Kouchoukos, NT, et al: Comparison of three devices to replace the aortic valve. Circulation 49(Suppl II):163, 1974.

28. Lefrak, EA and Starr, A: Braunwald-Cutter valve. In Lefrak, EA and Starr, A (eds): Cardiac Valve Prostheses. Appleton-Century-Crofts, New York, 1979, p 145.

29. Abdulali, SA, Silverton, NP, Schoen, FJ, et al: Late outcome of patients with Braunwald-Cutter mitral valve replacement. Ann Thorac Surg 38:579, 1984.

30. Jonas, RA, Barratt-Boyes, BG, Kerr, AR, et al: Late follow-up of the Braunwald-Cutter valve. Ann Thorac Surg 33:554, 1982.

31. Milam, JD, Bloodwell, RD, Hallman, GL, et al: Evaluation of hemolysis in patients with cardiac valve prostheses: A comparative study. In Brewer, LA, III (ed): Prosthetic Heart Valves. Charles C. Thomas, Publisher, Springfield, Ill. 1969, p 663.

32. Lefrak, EA and Starr, A: Kay-Shiley valve. In Lefrak, LA and Starr, A (eds): Cardiac Valve Prostheses. Appleton-Century-Crofts, New York, 1979, p 167.

33. Lefrak, EA and Starr, A: Kay-Shiley valve. In Lefrak, EA and Starr, A (eds): Cardiac Valve Prostheses. Appleton-Century-Crofts, New York, 1979, p 167.

34. Kitamura, S, Johnson, JL, Redington, JV, et al: Surgery for Ebstein's anomaly. Ann Thorac Surg 11:320, 1967.
35. Kay, JH, Tsuji, HK, Redington, JV, et al: The surgical treatment of Ebstein's malformation with right ventricular aneurysmorrhaphy and replacement of the tricuspid valve with a disc valve. Dis Chest 51:537, 1967.
36. Kay, JH, Tsuji, HK, Redington, JV, et al: Experiences with the Kay-Shiley disk valve. In Brewer, LA III, (ed): Prosthetic Heart Valves. Charles C. Thomas, Publisher, Springfield, Ill., 1696, p 609.
37. Brown, JW, Myerowitz, PD, Cann, MS, et al: Clinical and hemodynamic comparisons of Kay-Shiley, Starr-Edwards No. 6520, and Reis-Hancock porcine xenograft mitral valves. Surgery 76:983, 1974.
38. Paton, BC, Vogel, JHK, Ovary, H, et al: Follow-up results on the Kay-Shiley valve. In Brewer, LA, III (ed): Prosthetic Heart Valves. Charles C. Thomas, Publisher, Springfield, Ill., 1969, p 598.
39. Mulder, DG, Kattus, A, and Drinkwater, DC: Long-term survival after triple-valve replacement. Department of Cardiothoracic Surgery, University of California, School of Medicine, Los Angeles. Ann Thorac Surg 48:289, 1989.
40. Shigenobu, M, Mendez, MA, Zubiate, P, et al: Thirteen years' experience with the Kay-Shiley disc valve for tricuspid replacement in Ebstein's anomaly. Ann Thorac Surg 29:423, 1980.
41. Jugdutt, BI, Fraser, RS, Lee, SJ, et al: Long-term survival after tricuspid valve replacement. Results with seven different prostheses. J Thorac Cardiovasc Surg 74:20, 1977.
42. Wellons, HA, Jr, Strauch, RS, Nolan, SP, et al: Isolated mitral valve replacement with the Kay-Shiley disc valve. Acturial analysis of the long term results. J Thorac Cardiovasc Surg 70:862, 1975.
43. Rubin, JW, Ellison, RG, Moore, HV, et al: Twelve-year experience with mitral valve replacement. Ann Thorac Surg 19:659, 1975.
44. Edmiston, WA, Harrison, EC, Batista, E, et al: Clinical experience with the Kay-Shiley mitral valve prosthesis: An eleven-year follow-up study. Scand J Thorac Cardiovasc Surg 14:241, 1980.
45. Bowen, TE, Zajtchuk, R, Brott, WH, et al: Isolated mitral valve replacement with the Kay-Shiley prosthesis. Long-term follow-up and recommendations. J Thorac Cardiovasc Surg 80:45, 1980.
46. Clark, RE, Swanson, WM, Kardos, JL, et al: Durability of prosthetic heart valves. Ann Thorac Surg 26:323, 1978.
47. Nathan, MJ; Strut fracture: A late complication of Beall mitral valve replacement. Ann Thorac Surg 16:610, 1973.
48. Gold, H and Hertz, L: Death caused by fracture of Beall mitral prosthesis: Report of a case. Am J Cardiol 34:371, 1974.
49. Beall, AC, Morris, GC, Howell, JF, et al: Clinical experience with an improved mitral valve prosthesis. Ann Thorac Surg 15:601, 1973.
50. Saad, RM and Wolfe, MW: Progressive hemolytic anemia due to delayed recognition of a Beall mitral valve prosthesis. Chest 99:496, 1991.
51. Hill, RC, Sethi, GK, Scott, SM, et al: Disc embolization from a Beall mitral valve prosthesis. J Cardiovasc Surg (Torino) 30:384, 1989.
52. Silver, MD, Torok, PR, Slinger, RP, et al: Late strut fracture of the Beall model 105 disc valve prosthesis. J Thorac Cardiovasc Surg 96:448, 1988.
53. Conti, VR, Nishimura, A, Coughlin, TR, et al: Indications for replacement of the Beall 103 and 104 disc valves. Ann Thorac Surg 42:315, 1986.
54. Stross, JK, Willis, PW, and Kahn, DR: Diagnostic features of malfunction of disk mitral valve prostheses. J Am Med Assoc 217:305, 1971.
55. Lefrak, EA and Starr, A: Starr-Edwards disc valve. In Lefrak, EA and Starr, A (eds): Cardiac Valve Prostheses. Appleton-Century-Crofts, New York, 1979, p 197,
56. Lefrak, EA and Starr, A: Cooley-Cutter valve. In Lefrak, EA and Starr, A (eds): Cardiac Valve Prostheses. Appleton-Century-Crofts, New York, 1979, p 209.
57. Wright, JTM: Flow dynamics in prosthetic valves—An assessment of hydrodynamic performance. In Kalmanson, D (ed): The Mitral Valve: A Pluri-disciplinary Approach. Publishing Sciences Group, Acton, Mass., 1976, p 271.
58. Lefrak Chapter 11 Cooley-Cutter Valve p 211.
59. Wukasch, DC, Unger, F, Reul, GJ, et al: Long-term results in cardiac valve replacements: Comparison of 6,335 various type prostheses. In Davila, JC (ed): Second Henry Ford Hospital International Symposium on Cardiac Surgery. Appleton-Century-Crofts, New York, 1977, p 510.

60. Lillehei, CW, Nakib, A, Kaster, RL, et al: The origin and development of three new mechanical valve designs: Toroidal disc, pivoting disc, and rigid bileaflet cardiac prostheses. Ann Thorac Surg 48:S35, 1989.

61. Pierce, WS, Behrendt, DM, and Morrow, AG: A hinged prosthetic cardiac valve fabricated of rigid components. J Thorac Cardiovasc Surg 56:229, 1968.

62. Wada, J, Komatsu, S, and Kazui, T: Wada-Cutter heart valve: Overall experience at the Sapporo Medical College. Ann Thorac Surg 48:S38, 1989.

63. Cruz, AB, Kaster, RL, Simmons, L, et al: Flow characteristics of the meniscus prosthetic heart valve. J Thorac Cardiovasc Surg 49:813, 1965.

64. Personal communication, Medical Incorporated, April 1991.

65. Pilichowski, P, Gaudin, P, Brichon, Y, et al: Fracture and embolization of a Lillehei-Kaster mitral valve prosthesis disc: One case successfully operated. J Thorac Cardiovasc Surg 35:385, 1987.

66. Starek, PJK, Wilcox, BR, and Murray, GF: Hemodynamic evaluation of the Lillehei-Kaster pivoting disc valve in patients. J Thorac Cardiovasc Surg 71:123, 1976.

67. Forman, R, Gersh, BJ, Fraser, R, et al: Hemodynamic assessment of Lillehei-Kaster pivoting disc aortic and mitral prostheses. J Thorac Cardiovasc Surg 74:595, 1978.

68. Nitter-Hauge, S, Froysaker, T, and Hall, KV: Clinical and haemodynamic results following mitral valve replacement with the new Lillehei-Kaster disc valve prosthesis. Scand J Thorac Cardiovasc Surg 11:15, 1977.

69. Mikhail, AA, Ellis, R, and Johnson, S: Eighteen-year evolution from the Lillehei-Kaster valve to the Omni design. Ann Thorac Surg 48:S61, 1989.

70. Fananapazir, L, Clark, DB, Dark, FJ, et al: Results of valve replacement with the Omniscience prosthesis. J Thorac Cardiovasc Surg 86:621, 1983.

71. Rabago, G, Martinelli, J, Fraile, J, et al: Results and complications with the Omniscience prosthesis. J Thorac Cardiovasc Surg 87:136, 1984.

72. DeWall, RA: Mitral valve replacement with the Omniscience prosthesis. Evaluation of prosthesis orientation. Thai J Surg 8:217, 1987.

73. Lillehei, CW: Heart valve replacement with the pivoting disc prosthesis: Appraisal of results and description of a new all-carbon model. Med Instrum 11(2):85, 1977.

74. DeWall, RA, et al: The Omni design: Evolution of a valve. J Thorac Cardiovasc Surg 98:999, 1989.

75. Caffarena, R, et al: Three year results of the Omnicarbon prosthesis in 248 patients. J Cardiovasc Surg 29:22, 1988.

76. Thevenet, A, et al: Clinical experience with the Omnicarbon cardiac valve prosthesis. J Cardiovasc Surg 29:22, 1988.

77. Björk, VO: The Björk-Shiley tilting disc valve: past, present and future. In Crawford, FA (ed): State of the Art Reviews: Cardiac Surgery. Current Heart Valve Prostheses, Hanley & Belfus, Inc., Publishers, Philadelphia, 1987, p 183.

78. Björk, VO: Delrin as implant material for valve occluders. Scand J Thorac Cardiovasc Surg 6:103, 1973.

79. Hiratzka, LF, Kouchoukos, NT, Grunkemeier, GL, et al: Outlet strut fracture of the Björk-Shiley 60 deg. Convexo-Concave valve: Current information and recommendations for patient care. J Am Coll Cardiol 11:1130, 1988.

80. Shiley Inc. letter, dated November 1990.

81. Lindblom, D, Rodriguez, L, and Björk, VO: Mechanical failure of the Björk-Shiley valve. Updated follow-up and considerations on prophylactic rereplacement. J Thorac Cardiovasc Surg 97:95, 1989.

82. Levang, OW, Nitter-Hauge, S, Levorstad, K, et al: Aortic valve replacement: A randomized study comparing the Björk-Shiley and Lillehei-Kaster disc valves. Late hemodynamics related to clinical results. Scand J Thorac Cardiovasc Surg 13:199, 1979.

83. Hall, KV: The Medtronic Hall heart valve: Background, latest results, and future work. Ann Thorac Surg 48:S47, 1989.

84. Starek, PJK, Beaudet, RL, Hall, K-V: The Medtronic-Hall valve: Development and clinical experience. In Crawford, FA (ed): State of the Art Reviews: Cardiac Surgery. Current Heart Valve Prostheses, Hanley & Belfus, Inc., Publishers, Philadelphia, 1987, p 223.

85. Young, WP, Daggett, RL, and Gott, VL: Long-term follow-up of patients with a hinged leaflet prosthetic heart valve. In Brewer, LA (ed): Prosthetic Heart Valves. Charles C. Thomas, Publisher, Springfield, Ill. 1969, p 622.

86. Kalke, BR, Mantini, EL, Kaster, RL, et al: Hemodynamic features of a double-leaflet prosthetic heart valve of new design. Trans Am Soc Artif Intern Organs 13:105, 1967.

87. Villafana, MA: "It will never work!"—The St. Jude Valve. Ann Thorac Surg 48:S53, 1989.

88. Wang, JH: The design simplicity and clinical elegance of the St. Jude Medical heart valve. Ann Thorac Surg 48:S55, 1989.
89. Odell, JA, Durandt, J, Shama, DM, et al: Spontaneous embolization of a St. Jude prosthetic mitral valve leaflet. Ann Thorac Surg 39:569, 1985.
90. Personal communication, St. Jude Medical Incorporated, April 1991.
91. Moritz, A, Klepetko, W, Khunl-Brady, G, et al: Four year follow-up of the Duromedics Edwards bileaflet valve prostheses. J Cardiovasc Surg (Torino) 31:274, 1990.
92. Deuvaert, FE, Dumont, N, and Primo, GC: Fluoroscopic differentiation between leaflet escape (LE) and valve thrombosis (VT) of the Edwards-Duromedics mitral valve. Acta Cardiol 44(3):221, 1989.
93. Bortolotti, U, Guerra, F, Milano, A, et al: Radiographic identification of the CarboMedics prosthetic valve. The Clinical Report 2: 1, 1990.
94. Personal communication, CarboMedics Inc., March 1991.
95. Chard, RB and Cartmill, T: Thrombosed CarboMedics mitral valve prosthesis. J Thorac Cardiovasc Surg 100(5):800, 1990.
96. Subotic, S, Petrovic, P, Boskovic, D, et al: Clinical and functional evaluation of the CarboMedics prosthetic heart valve in the mitral position. Preliminary results. J Cardiovasc Surg (Torino) 31(4):509, 1990.
97. Roe, BB: Iatrogenic factors in cardiac valve evaluation. Ann Thorac Surg 48:S65, 1989.
98. Starek, PJK: Immobilization of disc heart valves by unraveled sutures. Ann Thorac Surg 31:66, 1981.
99. Knott, E, Reul, H, Knoch, M, et al: In vitro comparison of aortic heart valve prostheses: Part I: Mechanical valves. J Thorac Cardiovasc Surg 96:952, 1988.
100. Yoganathan, AP, Woo J-R, and Williams, FP: In vitro hydrodynamic characteristics of the St. Jude bileaflet aortic prosthesis. In DeBakey, ME (ed): Advances in Cardiac Valves. Clinical Perspectives. Yorke Medical Books, 1983, p 229.
101. Horstkotte, D and Korfer, R: The influence of prosthetic valve replacement on the natural history of severe acquired heart valve lesions: A comparison of complications and clinical and hemodynamic findings after implantation of Björk-Shiley, St. Jude Medical, and other heart valve prostheses. In DeBakey, ME (ed): Advances in Cardiac Valves. Yorke Medical Books, 1983, p 47.
102. Tatineni, S, Barner, HG, Pearson, AC, et al: Rest and exercise evaluation of St. Jude Medical and Medtronic Hall prostheses. Influence of primary lesion, valvular type, valvular size, and left ventricular function. Circulation (Suppl I) 80:I-16, 1980.
103. Foster, AH, Tracy, CM, Greenberg, GJ, et al: Valve replacement in narrow aortic roots: Serial hemodynamics and long-term clinical outcome. Ann Thorac Surg 42:506, 1986.
104. Edmunds, LH: Thrombotic and bleeding complications of prosthetic heart valves. Ann Thorac Surg 44:430, 1987.
105. Grunkemeier, GL: Artificial heart valves. Annu Rev Med 41:251, 1990.
106. Rao, PS, Solymar, L, Mardini, MK, et al: Anticoagulant therapy in children with prosthetic valves. Ann Thorac Surg 47:589, 1989.
107. Stewart, S, Cianciotta, D, Alexson, C, et al: The long-term risk of warfarin sodium therapy and the incidence of thromboembolism in children after prosthetic cardiac valve replacement. J Thorac Cardiovasc Surg 93:551, 1987.
108. Schaffer, MS, Clarke, DR, Campbell, DN, et al: The St. Jude Medical cardiac valve in infants and children: Role of anticoagulant therapy. J Am Coll Cardiol 9:235, 1987.
109. Verrier, ED, Tranbaugh, RF, Soifer, SJ, et al: Aspirin anticoagulation in children with mechanical aortic valves. J Thorac Cardiovasc Surg 92:1013, 1986.
110. Wright, JO, Hiratzka, LF, Brandt, B, et al: Thrombosis of the Björk-Shiley prosthesis. Illustrative cases and review of the literature. J Thorac Cardiovasc Surg 84:138, 1982.
111. Boskovic, D, Elozovic, I, Boskovic, D, et al: Late thrombosis of the Björk-Shiley tilting disc valve in the tricuspid position. J Thorac Cardiovasc Surg 91:1, 1986.
112. Ledain, LD, Ohayon, JP, Colle, JP, et al: Acute thrombotic obstruction with disc valve prostheses: Diagnostic considerations and fibrinolytic treatment. J Am Coll Cardiol 7:743, 1986.
113. Hirsh, J and Levin, M: Conclusion over the therapeutic range for monitoring oral anticoagulant therapy in North America. Thromb Haemost 59:129, 1988.
114. Koepke, JA: Coagulation testing systems. In Koepke, JA (ed): Laboratory Hematology. Churchill Livingstone, New York, 1984.

CHAPTER 12

Mitral Valve Reconstruction

Michael D. Strong III, M.D.
Stanley K. Brockman, M.D.

The present day operative procedure for the reconstruction of the mitral valve has a distinct place in the history of cardiac surgery. The first suggestion of opening the stenotic mitral valve by operative means was made by Brunton[1] in 1902. Cutler and Levine[2] in 1923 did experimental work relating to the surgical treatment of mitral stenosis. In 1925, Souttar[3] in England digitally opened a stenotic mitral valve through the left atrium with a brilliant result. Unfortunately, he was never referred another patient. In 1947, Bailey[4] in Philadelphia did the first successful mitral commissurotomy in the United States. Harken and coworkers in Boston[5] followed Bailey's success within a few weeks and untold numbers of mitral commissurotomies were performed subsequently. Despite advances in techniques, closed mitral commissurotomy had a distinct recurrence rate and was eventually replaced by open mitral commissurotomy using cardiopulmonary bypass (CPB). Lillehei and associates[6] was the first to successfully correct mitral insufficiency by narrowing the anulus under direct vision using CPB. Long-term results were poor and technical modifications were required. Superior long-term results were achieved by posteromedial anuloplasty described by Merendino,[7] Kay,[8] Wooler,[9] and Reed[10] and their respective colleagues. The results of asymmetric posteromedial anuloplasty achieved better results but eventually also led to recurrent mitral insufficiency. McGoon[11] in 1960 described, and had success with, the repair of mitral insufficiency secondary to ruptured chordae tendineae. In 1961, Starr and Edwards[12] reported the first successful mitral replacement using a prosthetic ball valve in the anatomic position. During the next 10 to 15 years, mitral valve replacement became the treatment of choice for symptomatic mitral insufficiency. Carpentier in Paris, France[13–18] has become the father of modern techniques of mitral valve reconstruction. Carpentier has analyzed the anatomic, functional, and pathologic aspects of mitral insufficiency and has developed a series of brilliant technical operations for mitral valve reconstruction. The older techniques of mitral anuloplasty have been abandoned, and Carpentier's methods of mitral valve reconstruction are being used with greater frequency in the United States.

ANATOMIC, PATHOLOGIC, AND FUNCTIONAL ASPECTS OF THE MITRAL VALVE

The mitral valve and its entire complex consists of anterior and posterior leaflets, the atrial wall, the left ventricular wall, the anulus, the chordae tendinae, and the papillary muscles. A patient with poor left atrial compliance will tolerate residual mitral stenosis or insufficiency poorly. When there is poor left ventricular contractility, the left ventricle will function better if the chordal attachments are preserved. The mitral anulus changes its size and shape during the cardiac cycle and is a fibrous structure. There are two areas of mitral anulus, an anterior and a posterior portion. The anterior portion is attached to the right and left fibrous trigones of the cardiac skeleton and is in fibrous continuity with the adjacent parts of the posterior and left aortic valve cusps. The anterior portion of the mitral anulus is relatively fixed by virtue of its attachments and plays little or no role in dilation of the mitral valve. The posterior portion of the anulus includes both commissures and has the posterior mitral leaflet attached to it. The stretching of the posterior portion of the mitral anulus is a major factor in mitral regurgitation (MR). There are primary, secondary, and tertiary chordae tendinae, which insert from the free edge to the base of the ventricular side of the mitral leaflets, respectively. There are two papillary muscles, an anteromedial and a posterolateral. The chordae fan out from the papillary muscles to insert on each leaflet. Pathologic changes on any one or all components of the mitral valve apparatus can cause mitral insufficiency.

Carpentier[17] defined three types of MR characterized by normal leaflet motion, leaflet prolapse, and restricted leaflet motion as shown in Figure 12–1. Mitral regurgitation with normal leaflet motion is caused by anular dilation, which is usually secondary to ventricular dilation or to leaflet perforation secondary to endocarditis. Mitral regurgitation with leaflet prolapse is usually due to prolapse of the mitral valve and coronary artery disease, which is associated with chordal rupture and elongation or papillary muscle rupture and elongation. Mitral regurgitation with restricted leaflet motion usually follows rheumatic heart disease and involves commissural fusion, leaflet thickening, chordal fusion, and chordal thickening. Rheumatic valvulitis (49%) and degenerative disease (40%) were the two most common etiologies of mitral valve disease at the Cleveland Clinic[19] from 1985 through 1988. Other etiologies included endocarditis (3%), ischemic heart disease (4%), and mis-

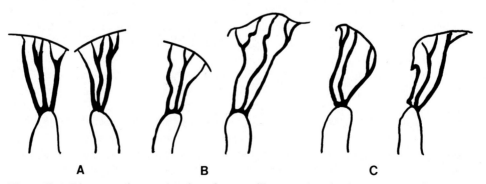

Figure 12–1. Diagrammatic representation of two papillary muscles, chordae, and two leaflets in (A) normal leaflet motion, (B) leaflet prolapse, and (C) restricted leaflet motion.

cellaneous (4%). With rheumatic valvulitis decreasing in the United States, degenerative disease will probably dominate in future years.[20]

Preoperative valve analysis is aimed at determining whether the leaflet motion is normal, prolapsed, or restricted. This evaluation is done by cardiac catheterization and Doppler echocardiography preoperatively and by transesophageal echocardiography and direct inspection in the operating room. In most instances, transesophageal Doppler echocardiography can identify leaflet prolapse, central or lateral regurgitation, and papillary muscle rupture. Generally, preoperative studies will differentiate rheumatic, degenerative, ischemic, or infective etiologies. At operation, the atrium is evaluated for compliance and for the presence of a jet lesion suggesting prolapse of the opposite leaflet. The anulus is evaluated for dilation. A blunt nerve hook is used to evaluate leaflet pliability, prolapse, or restriction. The presence of fibrosis and calcification of leaflets and posterior anulus is determined. The degree of prolapse is evaluated by direct vision and the forceful injection of saline into the left ventricle. The latter is helpful in evaluating which of the scalloped areas of the posterior leaflet has the most prolapse. The presence of leaflet prolapse, vegetations, fibrosis, and calcification are carefully evaluated.

In the Cleveland Clinic study,[19] the pathologic anatomy of degenerative disease revealed posterior chordal rupture in 41%, anterior chordal rupture in 10%, dilated anulus in 15%, anterior and posterior chordal rupture in 4%, and elongated chordae in 30%. When chordal rupture requires resection of more than one-fourth of the leaflet, mitral valve replacement rather than repair is required.[16] When the valve leaflets are not pliable and have significant fibrosis and calcification, the potential for valve repair is poor. When the subvalvular apparatus has significant deformity and fibrosis, the potential for valve repair is also poor. Older patients with calcified and fibrotic rheumatic valves are usually not candidates for repair. Approximately 69% of all patients with mitral insufficiency can undergo valve repair.[19]

SURGICAL PRINCIPLES

Standard techniques of cardiopulmonary bypass are used. After the pericardium is divided in the midline, the right side of the pericardium is sutured under tension allowing the apex of the heart to drop down. Any adhesions preventing this are divided. The inferior and superior vena cava are mobilized. The left atrium is opened parallel to the intra-atrial groove. A self-retaining retractor using two or three blades is placed to afford wide exposure. Finally, excellent exposure of the mitral valve is obtained by rotating the operating table away from the surgeon.

COMMISSUROTOMY

Commissurotomy has been the most frequent technique of repair in the past and has been performed almost exclusively for rheumatic valvulitis. The commissures are separated by sharp dissection. Separation or resection of chordae and splitting of the papillary muscle may be required. Areas of fibrous tissue may be resected. Any of the techniques described by Carpentier may be applied. It is outside the scope of this report to discuss the repair of rheumatic valve disease in-depth; rather the reconstruction of degenerative valve disease is emphasized.

ANULOPLASTY

The use of a prosthetic ring to correct dilation of the mitral anulus, primarily by shortening the posterior anulus, is an integral part of correction of mitral insufficiency in almost all cases. There are two types of mitral rings, one rigid and one flexible. The rigid ring was developed by Carpentier[13–17] and was designed to shorten the length of the posterior anulus and to remodel the mitral orifice to regain its normal shape and configuration. Selection of ring size is made with a sizing obturator. Interrupted mattress sutures are used to fix the ring in place. Two flexible rings, the Duran ring[21] and the Puig Massana ring,[22] are available. The Duran ring is 3 mm thick and is thought to be able to adapt to any deformation or configuration of the mitral anulus. The ring, which is available in many sizes, is inserted in the same fashion as the Carpentier ring. The Puig Massana ring is a similar flexible ring but has a Dacron suture threaded through its center with each end protruding. This suture can be snugged down and tied to tailor the reduction in the mitral orifice. Thus the Puig Massana ring has only two sizes, which can accommodate all sizes of the mitral orifice. Figure 12–2 depicts a flexible Puig Massana ring fixed in place with continuous suture with the ends of the central suture protruding and ready to be snugged down to the desired degree and tied.

Prosthetic ring anuloplasty alone may suffice when there is normal leaflet motion and a dilated mitral orifice. Ring anuloplasty is almost always performed along with all other types of repair to avoid recurrence. Fixation of the mitral anulus with a rigid ring may impair left ventricular function. David and coworkers[23] indicated that a flexible ring resulted in better left ventricular function than a rigid ring. The rigid Carpentier ring has caused left ventricular outflow tract obstruction secondary to systolic anterior motion of the mitral valve.[24,25] The main obstructing factor was the excess posterior leaflet tissue. Carpentier[18] described an operative technique to eliminate this complication in which the amount of posterior leaflet tissue is reduced by his "sliding leaflet" technique as shown in Figure 12–3. In any case, by 1 year after mitral valve repair, maximal improvement of left ventricular function will occur whether a rigid or flexible anuloplasty ring is used.[26]

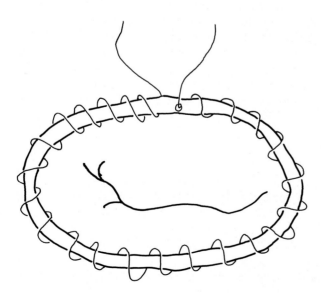

Figure 12–2. Puig Massana flexible anuloplasty ring fixed in place with continuous suture. The ends of the central suture are ready to be snugged and tied.

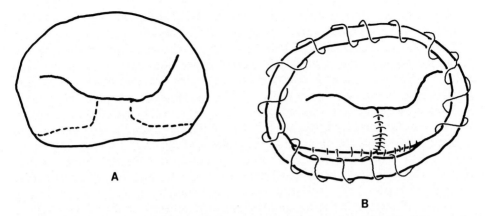

Figure 12–3. The sliding leaflet technique of Carpentier employed to reduce the height of the posterior leaflet. (A) Shows the dotted line of resection and (B) the completed repair with anuloplasty ring.

SURGICAL TECHNIQUE

As already noted, complete evaluation of the anatomy and pathology of the mitral mechanism along with excellent operative exposure are the basic requirements for mitral valve reconstruction. Chordal rupture of the anterior leaflet is less common than the posterior leaflet. The anterior leaflet is larger and more important to the valvular mechanism. When only the central chordae are ruptured and when the main chordae supporting each half of the anterior leaflet are intact, a limited central triangular resection can be accomplished as shown in Figure 12–4A and B.

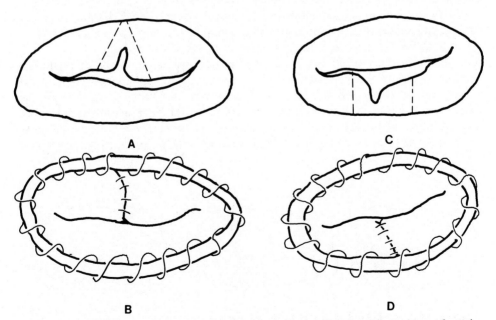

Figure 12–4. Repair of chordal rupture. (A) Small triangular resection of unsupported area of anterior leaflet. (B) Repair of anterior leaflet with 5-0 suture and insertion of anuloplasty ring. (C) Quadrangular resection of central scollop of unsupported posterior leaflet with (D) suture repair of posterior leaflet and insertion of anuloplasty ring.

The defect in the valve leaflet is repaired with 5-0 suture, and a prosthetic anulo-plasty ring is fixed in place. Larger resections of the anterior leaflet usually result in recurrent mitral insufficiency. Chordal transfer is another operation that may be performed when a larger segment of anterior leaflet requires support. A quadrangular resection of a segment of posterior leaflet with intact chordae opposite the unsupported anterior leaflet can be transferred and sutured to the affected segment of the anterior leaflet as shown in Figure 12–5. The defect in the posterior leaflet is sutured to avoid compromise of the function in the leaflet, and an anuloplasty ring is inserted. The most common chordal rupture is of the central scallop of the posterior leaflet. A quadrangular resection of the posterior leaflet and anulus is performed. The leaflet is approximated with suture and an anuloplasty ring inserted as shown in Figure 12–4. The most common technique for elongated chordae is shortening of the chordae, although resection such as described for chordal rupture or chordal transfer may be performed in selected cases. Chordal shortening is performed by incising the papillary muscle adjacent to the elongated chordae creating a trench as shown in Figure 12–6. A suture is passed through the papillary muscle, around the elongated chord, and through the other side of the papillary muscle. Felt pledgets are used to prevent tissue damage or disruption. When the suture is tied down, the chord is shortened by twice the depth of the trench in the papillary muscle. The suturing must be done carefully to avoid any damage or necrosis of the papillary muscle. As with other types of repair, chordal shortening is accompanied by insertion of an anuloplasty ring.

In patients with ischemic MR with normal leaflets and fibrosis of the papillary muscle and adjacent left ventricular wall, a prosthetic anuloplasty ring alone may suffice. When ischemic mitral insufficiency is mild or mitral insufficiency occurs only at times of ischemia, aortocoronary bypass will usually suffice. When there is papillary muscle rupture, emergency operation is required. When the papillary muscle and adjacent left ventricular wall are involved in massive infarction, repair is not possible and the valve must be replaced. In the absence of massive infarction and when the adjacent left ventricular wall is still healthy enough to hold sutures, reimplantation of the papillary muscle may be considered. Pledgetted mattress sutures appropriately placed have had a few successes.[27,28] When there is no muscle invasion or significant areas of active infection, mitral valve insufficiency due to endocarditis may be repaired. Involved areas of leaflet may be removed and repair undertaken as previously described. Fenestrations may be corrected by pericardial

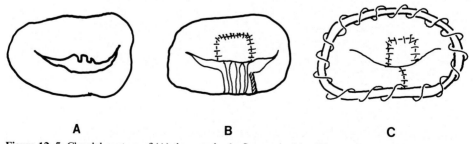

A   **B**   **C**

Figure 12–5. Chordal rupture of (A) the anterior leaflet repaired by (B) transfer and suture of a quadrangular segment of the posterior leaflet opposite the chordal rupture with (C) suture repair of the posterior leaflet and insertion of a prosthetic anuloplasty ring.

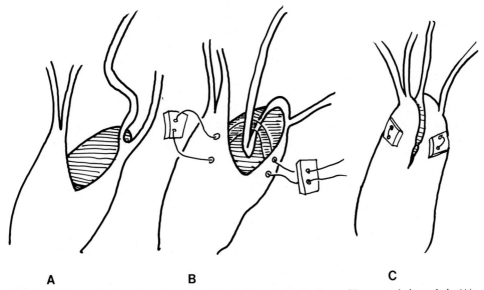

Figure 12–6. Chordal shortening. An incision creating a trench in the papillary muscle is made in (A). A pledgetted suture is placed through each side of the papillary muscle and around the elongated chord in (B). When the suture is tied in (C), the chord is shortened by twice the length of the trench.

patches. Any or all of the techniques already described may be applied to repair the mitral valve with endocarditis.

COMPLICATIONS

The major complications of mitral valve repair are residual regurgitation and prosthetic ring dehiscence. With the use of operative Doppler transesophageal echocardiography, residual significant insufficiency should prompt reinstitution of extracorporeal circulation and correction by further valve repair or crossover to valve replacement.

RESULTS

Carpentier[18] reported a 10-year actuarial survival rate of 90%. There was a 15-year probability of survival of 72.5%. Freedom from reoperation was 92%. Freedom from thromboembolism, anticoagulant-related hemorrhage, and endocarditis was between 93% and 97%. The Cleveland Clinic study[19,29] reported similar results, and 68% of their patients with degenerative mitral valve insufficiency were able to undergo valve repair. Numerous other workers are reporting similar successes.

COMMENT

Closed mitral commissurotomy was the first successful mitral valve repair procedure and was widely used in the 1950s and 1960s. With the advent of extracorporeal circulation, open mitral commissurotomy under direct vision replaced the closed procedure. The open procedure still remains somewhat unsatisfactory because of its tendency toward continued fibrosis and calcification in patients with rheumatic valvulitis. The year 1961 heralded the first total prosthetic replacement of the mitral valve. Mitral valve replacement remains the procedure of choice in fibrotic and calcified mitral valves and all other valves in which repair is not possible.

Carpentier, during the last two decades, has distinguished himself as the father of modern mitral valve repair. Carpentier's best results are in patients with degenerative valve disease.[18] The basic principles of Carpentier's repairs begin with total knowledge of the anatomy and pathology of the mitral valve in each patient. The basic operation includes insertion of a prosthetic anuloplasty ring in almost all operations, leaflet resection for ruptured chordae, chordal transfer, chordal shortening, and other procedures. Each of these procedures has been described in this communication. Other workers have substituted a flexible anuloplasty ring for Carpentier's rigid ring, and these appear equally good and possibly superior. The lack of thromboembolism and lack of bleeding speak strongly in favor of valve repair rather than replacement. Improved postoperative ventricular function with repair results from leaving the subvalvular mechanism intact, and there are many experimental and clinical studies to support this. There has been a general lack of reoperation in mitral valve repair indicating excellent long-term results.

Mitral valve repair requires a longer period of cardiopulmonary bypass than valve replacement. Fastidious operative ventricular protection is necessary. There may be an occasional critical patient in whom mitral valve replacement with a short bypass time would reduce the mortality rate. Although the long-term results of valve repair are proving to be superior, valve replacement in some studies appears to offer essentially the same. In a recent study, Craver and associates[30] compared a closely matched population and showed that mitral valve repair yielded results comparable to valve replacement. These workers emphasized that the benefits of repair are becoming more apparent with longer follow-up.

Although the use of mitral valve repair has lagged in the United States, it is becoming progressively popular. Degenerative valve disease has increased 23% to 60% during the past three decades in the United States, primarily as a result of the decrease in rheumatic heart disease.[31] It is important to compare the type of material available to Carpentier in Europe with that in the United States.[18,19,32] Carpentier[32] reported 206 consecutive patients having mitral valve repair during a 7-year period. Degenerative disease was present in 58%, rheumatic valvulitis in 38%, and other conditions, such as endocarditis and ischemic disease, comprised 4%. Atrial fibrillation was present in 48%. The mean age was 46.7 years and the follow-up averaged 13.2 years. An anuloplasty ring was placed in 95.5% of the patients, leaflet resection in 80.9%, chordal shortening in 45.6%, leaflet transfer in 5.4%, commissurotomy in 5.2%, and papillary muscle reimplantation in 1.1%. There were slightly more men than women. In the United States, the Cleveland Clinic group[32] reported on 520 patients who underwent mitral valve operations in a 2-year period. There were more women than men. The mean age was 60 years. There were 269 (52%) patients with pure regurgitation. Rheumatic valvulitis was present in 286 (55%) patients. Degenerative valve disease was found in 168 patients, which was 33% of the entire group and 63% of the group having pure MR. The remaining patients with pure mitral insufficiency had ischemic heart disease (14%), rheumatic heart disease (13%), endocarditis (6%), and congenital anomalies (4%). In a more recent report,[19] the Cleveland Clinic group reported the causes of MR to be rheumatic

49%, degenerative 40%, and all others 11%. In comparing the Cleveland Clinic group with Carpentier's study, the mean age was greater and the incidence of rheumatic heart disease higher in the Cleveland Clinic study.[32] The details of mitral valve repair and ischemic heart disease and endocarditis were scanty. The patient referral pattern to these institutions is from a very wide area and even transcends continents.

At Hahnemann University Hospital, we performed 167 mitral valve procedures in the 2-year period 1989 to 1991. The mean age was 66.7 years and there were more females. Sixty-eight percent of the patients ranged from 60 to 88 years. The etiology was rheumatic heart disease in 65%, degenerative valve disease in 20%, and ischemic heart disease and endocarditis in 15%. Of the 167 patients, 28% were "redo" procedures. Thirty percent of the patients had additional procedures. Only 16 patients (10%) had mitral valve repair according to the principles established by Carpentier. The remaining patients with degenerative valve disease were not candidates for valve repair. Atrial fibrillation was present in 146 (88%) patients. Only one of the patients with mitral valve repair died. During the past 7 years, we have undertaken valve repair in only 52 patients. At Hahnemann University Hospital, our patient referral pattern is essentially from a 100-mile radius to an inner-city university hospital and differs strikingly from the other two institutions analyzed. Our average age is considerably higher, and "redo" procedures are frequent, suggesting an increased severity of disease. Our incidence of rheumatic disease is much higher, and the incidence of degenerative disease much lower. There were no mitral valve repairs in very old patients with rheumatic valvulitis. With the very high incidence of atrial fibrillation, anticoagulants are required in most patients. Only a small group of patients with degenerative disease and sinus rhythm did not require anticoagulation. We would caution those in the early phase of the mitral valve experience to be aware of their learning curve and to be very cautious of overzealousness in trying to repair a valve that should be replaced.

REFERENCES

1. Brunton, L: Preliminary note on the possibility of treating stenosis by surgical methods. Lancet 1:461, 1902.
2. Cutler, EC and Levine, SA: Cardiotomy and valvulotomy for mitral stenosis: Experimental observations and clinical notes concerning an operated case with recovery. Boston Med Surg J 188:1023, 1923.
3. Souttar, HS: The surgical treatment of mitral stenosis. Br Med J 2:603, 1925.
4. Bailey, EP: The surgical treatment of mitral stenosis (commissurotomy). Chest 15:377, 1949.
5. Harken, DE, Ellis, LB, Ware, PF, et al: The surgical treatment of mitral stenosis. I. Valvuloplasty. N Engl J Med 239:801, 1948.
6. Lillehei, CW, Gott, VL, De Wall, RA, et al: Surgical correction of mitral insufficiency by annuloplasty under direct vision. Lancet 77:446, 1957.
7. Merendino, KA, Thomas, GI, Jesseph, JE, et al: The open correction of rheumatic mitral regurgitation and/or stenosis: With special reference to regurgitation treated by posteromedial annuloplasty using a pump-oxygenator. Ann Surg 150:5, 1959.
8. Kay, JH, Magidson, O, and Meihaus, JE: The surgical treatment of mitral insufficiency and combined mitral stenosis and insufficiency using the heart-lung machine. Am J Cardiol 9:300, 1962.
9. Wooler, GH, Nixon, PGF, Grimshaw, VA, et al: Experiences with the repair of the mitral valve in mitral incompetence. Thorax 17:49, 1962.
10. Reed, GE, Tice, DA, and Clauss, RH: Asymmetric exaggerated mitral annuloplasty: Repair of mitral insufficiency with hemodynamic predictability. J Thorac Cardiovasc Surg 49:752, 1965.

11. McGoon, DC: Repair of mitral insufficiency due to ruptured chordae tendineae. J Thorac Cardio-vasc Surg 39:357, 1960.

12. Starr, A and Edwards, ML: Mitral replacement: Clinical experience with a ball valve prosthesis. Ann Surg 154:726, 1961.

13. Carpentier, A: La valvuloplastie reconstitutive. Une nouvelle technique de valvuloplastie mitrale. Presse Méd. 77:25, 1969.

14. Carpentier, A, Deloche, A, Dauptain, J, et al: A new reconstructive operation for correction of mitral and tricuspid insufficiency. J Thorac Cardiovasc Surg 61:1, 1971.

15. Carpentier, A, Relland, J, Deloche, A, et al: Ann Thorac Surg 26:294, 1978.

16. Carpentier, A, Chauvaud, S, Fabiani, J, et al: Reconstructive surgery of mitral valve incompetence. Ten-year appraisal. J Thorac Cardiovasc Surg 79:338, 1980.

17. Carpentier, A: Cardiac valve surgery—The "french correction." J Thorac Cardiovasc Surg 86:323, 1983.

18. Deloche, A, Jebara, V, Relland, J, et al: Valve repair with Carpentier techniques: The second dec-ade. J Thorac Cardiovasc Surg 99:990, 1990.

19. Cosgrove, DM: Surgery for degenerative valve disease. Semin Thorac Cardiovasc Surg 1:183, 1989.

20. Gordie, L: The virtual disappearance of rheumatic fever in the United States: Lessons in the rise and fall of disease. Circulation 72:1155, 1985.

21. Duran, CB, and Ubago, JLM: Clinical and hemodynamic performance of a totally flexible pros-thetic ring for atrioventricular valve reconstruction. Ann Thorac Surg 22:458, 1976.

22. Puig Massana, M, Calbert, JM, and Castells, D: Conservative surgery of the mitral valve: Annulo-plasty on a new adjustable ring: In Burks, W, Ostermeyer, J, and Schults, HD (eds): Proceedings of the 29th International Congress of the European Society of Cardiovascular Surgery. Springer-Verlag, New York, 1981, pp 30–37.

23. David, TE, Komeda, M, Pollick, C, et al: Mitral valve annuloplasty: The effect of the type on left ventricular function. Ann Thorac Surg 47:524, 1989.

24. Schiavone, WA, Cosgrove, DM, Lever, HM, et al: Long-term follow-up of patients with left ven-tricular outflow tract obstruction after Carpentier ring mitral valvuloplasty. Circulation 78(Suppl I):60, 1988.

25. Kreindel, MS, Schiavone, WA, Lever, HM, et al: Systolic anterior motion of the mitral valve after Carpentier ring valvuloplasty for mitral valve prolapse. Am J Cardiol 57:408, 1986.

26. David, TE: Effect of mitral annuloplasty ring in left ventricular function. Semin Thorac Cardiovasc Surg 1:144, 1989.

27. Gula, G and Yacoub, MH: Surgical correction of complete rupture of the anterior papillary muscle. Ann Thorac Surg 32:88, 1981.

28. Carpentier, A and Didier, L: Surgical anatomy and management of ischemic mitral valve incom-petence. Circulation 76(Suppl.): 1776, 1987.

29. Loop, FD: Long-term results of mitral valve repair. Semin Thorac Cardiovasc Surg 1:203, 1989.

30. Craver, JM, Cohen, C, and Weintraub, WS: Case-matched comparison of mitral valve replacement and repair. Ann Thorac Surg 49:964, 1990.

31. Olsen, LJ, Subramauian, R, Ackerman, DM, et al: Surgical pathology of the mitral valve: A study of 712 cases spanning 21 years. Mayo Clin Proc 62:22, 1987.

32. Chavez, AM, Cosgrove, DM, Lytle, BW, et al: Applicability of mitral valvuloplasty techniques in a North American population. Am J Cardiol 62:253, 1988.

CHAPTER 13

Tricuspid Valve Surgery: Indications, Methods, and Results

Adnan Cobanoglu, M.D.
Gary Y. Ott, M.D.

Following the first successful replacement of the aortic and mitral valves by Harken and associates[1] and Starr[2], it quickly became apparent in patients with left-sided valvular heart disease that correction of associated tricuspid valve pathology added to improvement in cardiac performance. Despite the more than 2 decades that have passed since the first successful triple valve replacement,[3] the management of tricuspid valve disease remains controversial at best, and it frequently presents a diagnostic and therapeutic challenge for the cardiologist and the cardiac surgeon. However, progress in the areas of disease recognition, patient selection, and expanding options in surgical management promise continued improvement of results in the field of tricuspid valve surgery.

PATHOLOGY

Acquired tricuspid valve disease is classified as either functional or organic, indicating the underlying etiology. Rheumatic fever is the most common cause of organic disease, that is, intrinsic pathology of the valve apparatus. This is marked by cusp thickening, commissural fusion, or involvement of chordae and papillary muscles, resulting in valve stenosis or both stenosis and regurgitation. In pathology studies, tricuspid valve involvement is reported in 30% to 50% of patients with rheumatic heart disease.[4,5] Rheumatic tricuspid stenosis rarely occurs in isolation; concomitant involvement of the mitral or aortic valves is common. Other causes of organic disease include infective endocarditis, congenital anomaly (e.g., Ebstein's anomaly), trauma, cardiomyopathy, eosinophilic leukemia, diffuse collagen vascular disorders, and carcinoid syndrome. The incidence of organic tricuspid regurgitation has been reported at 16% to 50%.[5]

Most commonly, tricuspid regurgitation (TR) is functional, that is, secondary to left-sided pathology. Functional tricuspid insufficiency occurs when the valve leaflets and subvalvular apparatus retain their anatomic integrity, and regurgitation results due to anular dilation. The degree of functional impairment is related to the severity and duration of accompanying aortic or mitral valve dysfunction, causing changes in pulmonary vascular resistance, pulmonary hypertension, and right ventricular dilation with poor coaptation of the valve leaflets.[6,7] Anular enlargement occurs principally along the major portion of the attachment of the anterior leaflet, the posterior leaflet, and the lateral third of the septal leaflet. Thus, the anulus is deformed with the anterior–posterior diameter greater than the transverse diameter, contrary to normal.[8]

ASSESSMENT OF TRICUSPID VALVE DISEASE

Tricuspid valve disease is commonly insidious in onset and well tolerated for years. Frequently, the prominent symptoms and findings are related to the left-sided valve pathology, and delineation of tricuspid valve involvement necessitates specific suspicion and attention. Despite meticulous search, up to 30% of patients who undergo surgery for rheumatic aortic and mitral valve disease may have severe TR that is not evident by clinical examination or by hemodynamic study.[9]

Tricuspid stenosis, usually associated with a gradient of 5 mm Hg or more, causes right heart failure with jugular venous distension, hepatosplenomegaly, ascites, and peripheral edema. As indicated earlier, isolated tricuspid stenosis is rare, and most patients with tricuspid valve disease present with either functional or organic TR.

Typical findings in TR include prominent jugular venous V waves with rapid Y descent, and a holosystolic murmur over the left lower sternal border that increases with inspiration (Carvallo's sign). This murmur increases with exercise, but it is noteworthy that the intensity of the murmur does not correlate with the severity of regurgitation. Carvallo's sign may be absent in up to 30% of patients with severe TR. Pulsatile hepatomegaly is usually found, but in longstanding cases, the liver may be firm and without pulsations. A chest x-ray may show right atrial enlargement, but this finding is not specific for TR. The electrocardiogram (ECG) frequently shows atrial fibrillation and right atrial or right ventricular hypertrophy.

Two-dimensional (2-D) echocardiography provides complementary information to cardiac catheterization in evaluating tricuspid valve disease. It can, for example, delineate structural involvement by the rheumatic process. Daniels and coworkers[10] in a study of 372 patients with 2-D echocardiographic features of rheumatic mitral valve disease accurately showed features of rheumatic tricuspid valve disease in 6.2%. Thickening of the leaflets, restriction of leaflet motion, and diastolic doming were detected in patients with tricuspid stenosis. The size of the tricuspid anulus can be determined, and, if TR is present, the percentage of systolic shortening of anular size is reduced. Estimates of transvalvular flow velocities and gradients also may be obtained.

Cardiac catheterization usually reveals hemodynamic criteria specific for TR. The right atrial pressure contour shows a ventricularization pattern with similar but lower amplitude; prominent V waves with steep Y descents are characteristic. The right ventricular end-diastolic pressure may be normal or elevated with volume overload. If the right ventricular and pulmonary artery systolic pressures are high (>50 to 60 mm Hg), the TR is most likely secondary; with lesser pressures and severe regurgitation, the likelihood of organic tricuspid disease increases. Right ventriculography demonstrates regurgitation of dye into the right atrium, with opacification of both cava and hepatic veins in severe cases. Recently, preshaped catheters have been developed to overcome the frequent problem of iatrogenic regurgitation caused by the catheter traversing the tricuspid leaflets.[11] Although all these sophisticated studies are available, emphasis should be placed on a good history from the patient and the referring cardiologist. Clinical history gives a prolonged account of the problem, and the diagnosis is usually confirmed by careful physical examination.

INDICATIONS FOR OPERATION

In preoperative assessment, the degree of TR may be influenced by attentive medical treatment, including restriction of fluid intake and diuretic and vasodilator drug administration, thus underscoring the importance of a careful search for signs and symptoms of tricuspid valve disease. A common mistake is to underestimate the degree of TR due to the very intense medical regimen that these patients undergo immediately before surgical consultation. A definite history of tricuspid valve-related signs and symptoms should prompt tricuspid valve exploration and direct visualization at the time of left-sided heart surgery, regardless of the immediate preoperative physical and hemodynamic findings.

If the preoperative findings indicative of secondary tricuspid involvement are not clear, intraoperative digital exploration of the valve should be performed. The presence of a significant regurgitant jet requires visual assessment of valve pathology. A useful adjunct to evaluation of the tricuspid valve has been application of intraoperative color and contrast Doppler echocardiography. These techniques have allowed quantification of residual tricuspid insufficiency immediately following termination of bypass in left heart operations.[12] Although conservative management of TR after left-sided valve correction has been advocated by some,[13] ignoring significant tricuspid disease may compromise both immediate and long-term outcome.[9,14] In our experience, the postoperative course has been smoother in those patients with repaired and competent tricuspid valves. In addition, reoperation for residual tricuspid insufficiency after left-sided valve replacement has carried a high operative mortality.[14]

In secondary or functional TR, the valve should be preserved if at all possible. Measurement of pulmonary artery systolic pressures alone can accurately separate anatomically normal valves from abnormal regurgitant valves in a majority of cases.[15] Functional regurgitation is almost always reversible if the preoperative pulmonary artery pressure is high and the evidence of tricuspid insufficiency is of brief duration. Functional regurgitation is likely to be irreversible if it has been present for a long time or the pulmonary artery pressure is lower than that expected with severe left-sided disease.

If organic tricuspid disease is present and the valve is found at inspection to be irreversibly damaged structurally with significant chordal or leaflet pathology, the valve is replaced with a prosthesis. Replacement also may be necessary to ensure valve competence in those cases in which the underlying problem is not amenable to surgical repair, such as cardiomyopathy, large right ventricular infarction, or extensive right ventricular fibrosis. Bioprostheses are preferred for use in the tricuspid position.

SELECTION OF A PROSTHESIS

A great variety of prostheses have been used in the triscuspid position. Extensive experience has been acquired with the caged ball (Starr-Edwards), tilting disc (Björk-Shiley), and several xenograft bioprostheses. The use of mechanical valves has been associated with an unacceptably high complication rate due to thrombosis. In the case of tilting disc valves, the incidence of valve thrombosis has been reported in the 20% to 25% range despite systemic anticoagulation.[16,17] Thrombus formation begins at the sewing ring margin and progresses to involve the minor orifice and interfere with disc excursion leading to occlusion.

Better results are found with the ball valve, which has a much lower rate of thrombotic stenosis. Here, the thrombus characteristically begins in the right ventricle where the cage may penetrate into the interventricular septum. This is a relatively gradual process. In addition, Cobanoglu and Starr[17] have noted that when valve thrombosis occurred with the caged-ball prosthesis, it produced slow-onset congestive heart failure, whereas the failure mode has been catastrophic and often fatal with tilting-disc prostheses. The St. Jude valve has theoretical advantages that may make it well suited for tricuspid valve replacement. This bileaflet design allows for central flow and lower transvalvular gradients owing to large effective cross-sectional orifice and low profile. Early clinical results with this device are promising.[18] Current practice favors the use of bioprostheses in the tricuspid position owing to the lower incidence of valve complications, particularly late thrombosis.[19] In one series, follow-up of 151 patients with tricuspid bioprostheses for a mean of 50 months revealed that only 2 patients had suffered valve thrombosis (1.3% incidence).[20] Although an ultimate replacement may be contemplated, bioprosthetic degeneration and calcification is much less a concern than in left-sided valve replacement. Bioprostheses in the tricuspid position undergo much more extensive epithelialization compared with those in the mitral and aortic positions.[21] This may enhance the durability of right-sided bioprostheses. In children, bioprostheses in the right cardiac chambers have better survival than those in the left heart.[22]

TECHNIQUE OF OPERATION

TRICUSPID VALVE REPAIR

Repair of the tricuspid valve should be possible in most cases of left-sided valvular disease and secondary tricuspid insufficiency. The DeVega[23] and Carpentier[24] anuloplasty techniques have attained widespread popularity. A number of variations of these techniques also have been reported to have good results.[25–30] Use of the Carpentier ring is particularly suited to instances when the TR is of long duration and a remodeling of the anulus is required. This method also is indicated in mixed stenosis and insufficiency when extensive repair of the leaflets, including leaflet resection and shortening of the chordae, is necessary. The DeVega anuloplasty is useful and sufficient for all other reparable conditions.

Operations are performed through a median sternotomy, employing bi-caval and ascending aortic cannulation, and moderate hypothermia (26°C). Cold-blood potassium cardioplegia adds to the safety of the operation. The tricuspid valve is exposed last, that is, after the left-sided valve procedures are carried out. DeVega anuloplasty is carried out by starting a double-armed 2-0 monofilament (polypropylene) suture through a pledget at the junction of the anterior and the septal cusps.

Interrupted bites are taken throughout the anulus in a clockwise fashion until the commissure between the posterior and septal cusps is reached. The suture is passed through a Teflon pledget and carried around to its origin in a counterclockwise fashion 2 to 3 mm outside the previous suture line (Fig. 13–1). A prosthetic valve sizer appropriate for the patient's size (commonly 28 to 29 mm for a female and 30 to 31 mm for a male patient) is placed within the tricuspid anulus, and the suture is tied down over a pledget, reducing the anulus to the desired size. Valve competence is checked by filling the right ventricle with cold saline using a bulb syringe. Overcorrection is not necessary, because there is only anular dilation without any abnormality of the leaflets. This technique is both simple and effective.

Carpentier ring anuloplasty is carried out through a similar exposure. The anulus size is ascertained. The ring is manufactured incomplete in the area corresponding to the medial aspect of the septal leaflet and the bundle of His to avoid injury to the conduction system. Horizontal mattress passes are taken with double-armed 2-0 multifilament sutures into the anulus. After all sutures are placed into the anulus, they are passed into the ring, keeping the distance between the two bites, with the same stitch closer on the ring than the anulus (Fig. 13–2). The ring is seated and tied, thus reestablishing the ovoid shape of the tricuspid anulus. Valve competence is assessed by filling the right ventricle with cold saline via bulb syringe. The atriotomy is closed in the usual manner.

The Carpentier ring allows for a selective remodeling of the tricuspid anulus, including the septal area, which is not shortened in the DeVega technique. The

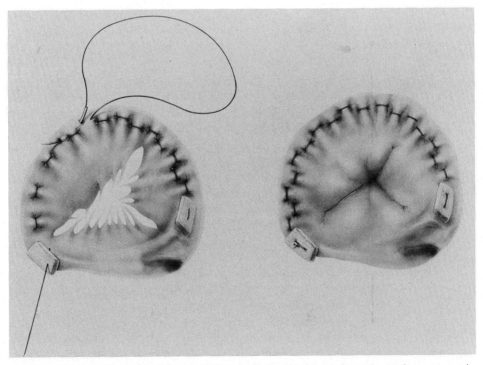

Figure 13–1. De Vega tricuspid anuloplasty. Suturing is done in the anterior and posterior cusp areas in order not to injure the conduction tissue. Note the coronary sinus orifice on bottom right-hand corner.

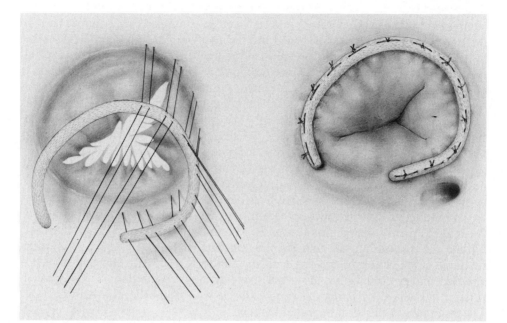

Figure 13–2. Carpentier ring anuloplasty. Bites are wider in the anulus than in the prosthesis. Again the gap in the ring is to avoid suturing the area of the bundle of His.

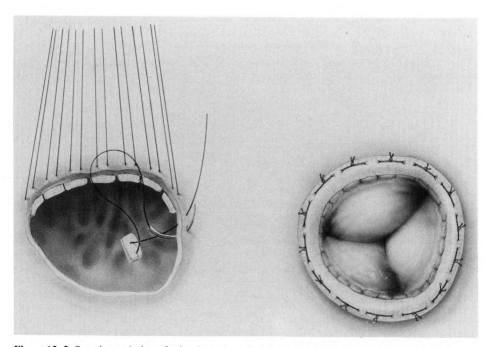

Figure 13–3. Suturing technique for implantation of a bioprosthesis. Note interrupted horizontal mattress sutures with pledgets on the ventricular side of the anulus.

analogous Duran ring is flexible and offers the theoretical advantage of preserving physiological shortening of the tricuspid anulus. However, a clear superiority in postoperative results in comparison of these two types of prostheses is not obviously demonstrated.[8]

TRICUSPID VALVE REPLACEMENT

Exposure is similar to that used in tricuspid valve repair. Native valve excision is carried out with attention given to leaving a 3 to 4 mm portion of the septal leaflet for safe placement of sutures in this particular portion of the anulus. Using pledgeted sutures of 2-0 multifilament braided material, horizontal mattress sutures are placed into the septal leaflet remnant and into the remainder of the anulus (Fig. 13–3). This technique prevents injury to the conduction system, particularly the bundle of His in this area of the interventricular septum. The pledgets are left on the ventricular side of the anulus. After all sutures are placed, they are passed through the sewing ring of the prosthesis, the valve is seated, and the sutures are tied.

OPERATIVE RESULTS

The majority of patients considered for tricuspid valve surgery have concomitant mitral and aortic valvular disease, and the operative results reflect the high surgical risk in this group with advanced multivalvular disease. McGrath and coworkers[20] have reported an overall operative mortality of 15% in a group of 530 patients undergoing tricuspid valve procedures of all types. Late deaths occurred in 40% of this series, mainly due to cardiac failure. Overall, the survival rate was only 20% at 15 years follow-up. Operative survivors continue to be at high risk for cardiac death, indicating progression of cardiomyopathy after valve repair or replacement. In an earlier report from the Oregon Health Sciences University, 37 operative deaths were found among a series of 214 patients undergoing tricuspid valve surgery of all types.[17] Operative repair vs. replacement did not have an effect on long-term outcome. Of those who had replacement, 59(+4)% and 23(+4)% were alive at 5 and 15 years, respectively, compared with 51(+7)% and 22(+8)% in those who had tricuspid valve repair. Again, the most common cause of late death was congestive heart failure.

The results of combined left-sided valve procedure with either Carpentier ring or DeVega anuloplasty have been good from a functional standpoint. Abe and associates[31] noted an improvement to New York Heart Association (NYHA) class I to II in 90% of their series of 110 DeVega anuloplasty patients. Actuarial survival was 86% at 10 years, and the actuarial freedom from reoperation on the tricuspid valve was 96.7%.[31]

Triple valve replacement is now less commonly employed owing to the widespread acceptance of valve-sparing procedures. Various reports have placed the operative mortality from 5% to 37%. Follow-up also has shown a better long-term survival in valve repair as opposed to valve replacement groups. This may be so because the patients with more severe degrees of pulmonary hypertension and right ventricular dilation tend to require valve replacement.[32] A low risk of valve-related events has been demonstrated with the use of a bioprosthesis in the tricuspid position.[20]

Consistent predictors of poor outcome have been identified as advanced age, reoperation, hepatic dysfunction, significant pulmonary artery hypertension, and preoperative NYHA class IV.[20,31-35] The outcome of tricuspid valve procedures is dependent upon the adequate repair of concomitant left-sided lesions, the reversibility of elevated pulmonary vascular resistance, and the severity of both left and right ventricular dysfunction.

SPECIAL PROBLEMS IN TRICUSPID VALVE SURGERY

INFECTIVE ENDOCARDITIS

Involvement of the tricuspid valve occurs in only 5% to 10% of patients with infective endocarditis; however, right-sided endocarditis has been on the rise in the last decade. An increase in parenteral drug abuse and the widespread use of chronic indwelling intravenous cannulae have contributed to this trend. Unlike the microorganisms found in left-sided endocarditis, pathogens isolated from tricuspid valve endocarditis are usually highly virulent and include *Staphylococcus aureus, Staphylococcus epidermidis,* streptococci, gram-negative bacteria (particularly Pseudomonas), and fungi. Nonetheless, right heart endocarditis less frequently requires surgical intervention (24%) and carries a more favorable prognosis (14% overall mortality) than left heart involvement.[36]

Operative intervention is undertaken when medical therapy is unsuccessful, that is, with resultant intractable infection, anular abscess formation, persistent bacteremia, recurrent pulmonary emboli, or development of progressive and severe congestive heart failure. The mere demonstration of vegetations on the tricuspid valve per se is not an indication for surgery. However, vegetation size >1 cm on echocardiographic studies suggests a higher incidence of medical treatment failure.[37] Operative therapy is rarely indicated for hemodynamic reasons alone.

The procedure of choice in right-sided infective endocarditis is a subject of controversy. Arbulu and Asfaw[38] reported on 61 patients who underwent tricuspid valve resection without prosthetic replacement, with 6% early and 8% late deaths, and with 86% survival at 10 years. Subsequent insertion of a prosthetic tricuspid valve was required in 18% of this group. Results of immediate tricuspid valve replacement have been reported by Stern and colleagues.[39] In drug-addicted patients, insertion of a prosthesis allowed each to be discharged free of infection or heart failure. However, late septic death occurred in three patients owing to the resumption of drug abuse.

The operative goal in reparative techniques must primarily be adequate debridement of vegetations and all involved tissues. Residual endocarditis has been associated with high operative mortality; sacrifice of entire leaflets and the subvalvular apparatus may be necessary.[40] In some instances, a truly polypoid vegetation is present and excision can be carried out with total preservation of the apparently normal valve. Involvement of a single major and minor leaflet alone usually allows debridement without complex reconstruction. If necessary, leaflet and chordal remodeling with autogenous pericardium is possible and has given encouraging early results in selected patients.[41,42]

To summarize, it appears that an attempt at valve repair is justified if the infection is localized and the anulus is not involved. Otherwise, our preference has been to replace the valve with a porcine bioprosthesis. Although there is no difference in susceptibility to infection between mechanical valves and bioprostheses, the latter, once infected, appear to be more easily sterilized.[43] Resection of the valve without replacement alone remains a viable option particularly in cases of ongoing acute infection in patients with normal left-sided cardiac function. Whichever approach is chosen, adequate debridement at surgery and avoidance of continued drug abuse are imperative to successful long-term outcome.

CARCINOID DISEASE

Tricuspid valve surgery may become necessary with progressive involvement of the tricuspid valve and right ventricle with the fibrotic process. The valve nearly always requires replacement, and early operation is recommended before progression of extensive fibrosis and severe right-sided heart failure occurs.[44]

PERMANENT PACEMAKER INSERTION

Passage of a transvenous pacemaker lead across a mechanical prosthesis could interfere with poppet or disc motion. With bioprostheses, leaflet tear, perforation, and pressure injury to the cusps might occur. In addition, thrombus formation may be facilitated. Therefore, those patients with a prosthetic tricuspid valve in place who require permanent cardiac pacing should have epicardial lead placement via thoracotomy or subxiphoid approach. An alternative procedure is placement of a transvenous lead into a tributary of the coronary sinus, that is, the middle cardiac or posterior left ventricular veins. Good results have been reported with this method.[45]

EBSTEIN'S ANOMALY

The optimal surgical approach for this condition has not been established, but surgery is considered for those with class 3 or 4 symptoms, moderate-to-severe cyanosis or paradoxic emboli, and some class 2 patients with a rapid increase in cardiac size, dyspnea, and cyanosis. Both valve repair and replacement have their proponents.[46,47] In a child in whom valve replacement is necessary, the anatomy of Ebstein's anomaly allows placement of a caged-ball valve without impingement of the struts.

ISCHEMIC TRICUSPID REGURGITATION

Tricuspid regurgitation may occur as a complication of inferior-wall right ventricular infarction and produce a significant detrimental effect on cardiac output. Although prosthetic valve replacement may occasionally be required,[48] repair is usually all that is necessary inasmuch as the leaflets are essentially normal.

CONCLUSIONS

Isolated tricuspid valve disease is an uncommon entity; most disease is related to dysfunction of the aortic or mitral valves. Earlier surgery for correction of left-sided valvular disease should decrease the incidence and severity of right ventricular dysfunction and functional tricuspid insufficiency. In spite of numerous sophisticated methods of evaluating the tricuspid valve preoperatively, a precise clinical history, physical examination, and intraoperative assessment are the most important elements in deciding on the appropriate course of treatment. If technically feasible, the simplicity and effectiveness of current anuloplasty methods make valve-sparing operations the procedure of choice. Such is the case in most instances of left-sided heart disease with secondary tricuspid valve involvement. With severe organic disease of the tricuspid valve, or with other primary disease that is not correctable, such as cardiomyopathy, the valve should be replaced. Bioprostheses are favored for use in the tricuspid position owing to a decreased risk of thromboembolism and better hemodynamic performance. Although good functional results have been attained following tricuspid valve procedures, this remains a high-risk subset of cardiac surgery, and the course of these patients remains dependent upon the underlying left-sided valvular and ventricular dysfunction.

REFERENCES

1. Harken, DE, Saroff, HS, Taylor, WJ, et al: Partial and complete prosthesis in aortic insufficiency. J Thorac Cardiovasc Surg 40:744, 1960.
2. Starr, A and Edwards, ML: Mitral replacement: Clinical experience with a ball-valve prosthesis. Ann Surg 154:726, 1961.
3. Starr, A, McCord, CW, Wood, J, et al: Surgery for multiple valve disease. Ann Surg 160:596, 1964.
4. Smith, JA and Levine, SA: The clinical features of tricuspid stenosis. Am Heart J 23:739, 1942.
5. Chopra, P and Tandou, HD: Pathology of chronic rheumatic heart disease with particular reference to tricuspid valve involvement. Acta Cardiol 32:423, 1975.
6. Tei, C, Pilgrim, JP, Shah, PM, et al: The tricuspid valve annulus: Study of size and motion in normal subjects and in patients with tricuspid regurgitation. Circulation 66:665, 1982.
7. Karp, RB: Acquired disease of the tricuspid valve. In Sabiston, DC and Spencer, FC (eds): Surgery of the Chest. WB Saunders, Philadelphia, 1990, p 1504.
8. Lambertz, H, Minale, C, Flachskampf, FA, et al: Long-term follow up after Carpentier tricuspid valvuloplasty. Am Heart J 117(3):615, 1989.
9. Starr, A, Herr, R, and Wood, J: Tricuspid replacement of acquired valve disease. Surg Gynecol Obstet 122:1295, 1966.
10. Daniels, SJ, Mintz, GS, and Kotler, MN: Rheumatic tricuspid disease: Two dimensional echocardiographic, hemodynamic and angiographic correlations. Am J Cardiol 51:492, 1983.
11. Ubago, JL, Figueroa, A, Colman, T, et al: Right ventriculography as a valid method for the diagnosis of tricuspid insufficiency. Cathet Cardiovasc Diagn 7:433, 1981.
12. Goldman, ME, Guarino, T, Fuster, V, et al: The necessity for tricuspid valve repair can be determined intraoperatively by two-dimensional echocardiography. J Thorac Cardiovasc Surg 94(4):542, 1987.
13. Braunwald, NS, Ross, J, and Morrow, A: Conservative management of tricuspid regurgitation in patients undergoing mitral valve replacement. Circulation 35-36:1, 1967.
14. King, RM, Schaff, HV, Danielson, GK, et al: Surgery for tricuspid regurgitation late after mitral valve replacement. Circulation 70(Pt 2):I193, 1984.
15. Waller, BF: Etiology of pure tricuspid regurgitation. Cardiovasc Clin 17(2):53, 1987.
16. Thorburn, CA, Morgan, J, Shanahan, M, et al: Long-term results of tricuspid valve replacement and the problem of prosthetic valve thrombosis. Am J Cardiol 51:1128, 1983.
17. Cobanoglu, MA and Starr, A: Tricuspid valve surgery: Indications, methods, results. In Brest, AN and Frankl, WS (eds): Valvular Heart Disease: Comprehensive Evaluation and Management. FA Davis, Philadelphia, 1985, p 375.
18. Singh, AK, Christian, DF, Williams, DO, et al: Follow-up assessment of the St. Jude Medical prosthetic valve in the tricuspid position: Clinical and hemodynamic results. Ann Thorac Surg 37:324, 1984.
19. Wellens, F and Jacques, G: Tricuspid valve replacement. Cardiovasc Clin 17(2):111, 1987.
20. McGrath, LB, Gonzalez-Lavin, L, Bailey, BM, et al: Tricuspid valve operations in 530 patients. Twenty five year assessment of early and late phase events. J Thorac Cardiovasc Surg 99(1):124, 1990.

21. Ishihara, O, Ferrans, VJ, Jones, M, et al: Occurrence and significance of endothelial cells in implanted porcine bioprosthetic valves. Am J Cardiol 48:443, 1981.
22. Dunn, J: Porcine valve durability in children. Ann Thorac Surg 32:357, 1981.
23. DeVega, NG: La anuloplastica selectiva, regulable y permanente. Rev Esp Cardiol 25:6, 1972.
24. Carpentier, A, Deloche, A, Hanania, G, et al: Surgical management of acquired tricuspid valve disease. J Thorac Cardiovasc Surg 67:53, 1974.
25. Duran, CG and Ubago, JL: Clinical and hemodynamic performance of a totally flexible ring for atrioventricular valve construction. Ann Thorac Surg 22:458, 1976.
26. Kay, JH, Mendez, AM, and Zubiate, P: A further look at tricuspid annuloplasty. Ann Thorac Surg 22:498, 1976.
27. Minale, C, Lambertz, H, and Messmer, BJ: New developments for reconstruction of the tricuspid valve. J Thorac Cardiovasc Surg 94(4):626, 1987.
28. Revuelta, JM and Garcia-Rinaldi, R: Segmental tricuspid anuloplasty: A new technique (letter). J. Thorac Cardiovasc Surg 97(5):799, 1989.
29. Kurlanski, PA, Rose, EA, and Malm, JR: Adjustable annuloplasty for tricuspid insufficiency (letter). Ann Thorac Surg 48(3):457, 1989.
30. Sutlic, Z, Schmid, C, and Borst, HG: Repair of flail anterior leaflets of tricuspid and mitral valves by cusp remodeling. Ann Thorac Surg 50(6):927, 1990.
31. Abe, T, Tukamoto, M, Yanagiya, M, et al: DeVega anuloplasty for acquired tricuspid disease: Early and late results in 110 patients. Ann Thorac Surg 48(5):670, 1989.
32. Rabago, G, Fraile, J, Martinelli, J, et al: Technique and results of tricuspid annuloplasty. J Cardiovasc Surg 1:247, 1986.
33. Mullany, CJ, Gersh, BJ, Orzulak, TA, et al: Repair of tricuspid valve insufficiency in patients undergoing double (aortic and mitral) valve replacement. Perioperative mortality and long-term (1–20 years) follow-up in 109 patients. J Thorac Cardiovasc Surg 94(5):740, 1987.
34. Coll-Mazzei, JV, Jegaden, O, Janody, P, et al: Results of triple valve replacement: Perioperative mortality and long-term results. J Cardiovasc Surg (Torino) 28(4):369, 1987.
35. Nakano, S, Kawashima, Y, Hirose, H, et al: Evaluation of long-term results of bicuspidalization annuloplasty for functional tricuspid regurgitation. A seventeen year experience with 133 consecutive patients. J Thorac Cardiovasc Surg 95(2):340, 1988.
36. Chan, P, Ogilby, JD, and Segal, B: Tricuspid valve endocarditis. Am Heart J 117(5):1140, 1989.
37. Robbins, MJ, Frayer, RWM, Soeiro, R, et al: Influence of vegetation size on clinical outcome of right-sided infective endocarditis. Am J Med 80:165, 1986.
38. Arbulu, A and Asfaw, I: Tricuspid valvulectomy without prosthetic replacement. J Thorac Cardiovasc Surg 82:684, 1981.
39. Stern, HJ, Sisto, DA, Strom, JA, et al: Immediate tricuspid valve replacement for endocarditis. Indications and results. J Thorac Cardiovasc Surg 91(2):163, 1986.
40. Chandraratna, PA, Reagan, RB, Imiazuni, T, et al: Infective endocarditis cured by resection of a tricuspid valve vegetation. Ann Intern Med 89:517, 1978.
41. Yee, ES and Ullyot, DJ: Reparative approach for right sided endocarditis. J Thorac Cardiovasc Surg 96:133, 1988.
42. Yee, ES and Khonsari, S: Right-sided infective endocarditis: Valvuloplasty, valvectomy or replacement. J Cardiovasc Surg (Torino) 30(5):744, 1989.
43. Rossiter, SJ, Stinson, EB, Oyer, PE, et al: Prosthetic valve endocarditis: Comparison of heterograft tissue valves and mechanical valves. J Thorac Cardiovasc Surg 76:795, 1978.
44. Miller, BR, Vohr, FH, Christian, FV, et al: Cardiac valvular replacement in carcinoid heart disease. Am J Med 75:896, 1983.
45. Lee, ME: Special considerations in ventricular pacing in patients with tricuspid valve disease. Ann Thorac Surg 36:89, 1983.
46. McFaul, R, Davis, Z, Giuliani E, et al: Ebstein's malformation. J Thorac Cardiovasc Surg 72:910, 1976.
47. Abe, T and Komatsu, S: Valve replacement for Ebstein's anomaly of the tricuspid valve. Chest 84:417, 1983.
48. Silverman, BD, Carabajal, NR, Chorches, MA, et al: Tricuspid regurgitation and acute myocardial infarction. Arch Intern Med 142:1394, 1982.

CHAPTER 14

Immediate Postoperative Management

Daniel M. Kolansky, M.D.
Lawrence S. Cohen, M.D.

The surgical treatment of patients with valvular heart disease has advanced dramatically in the past 3 decades. Perioperative medical management has kept pace through a better understanding of the pathophysiology of cardiac function after surgery and with improved pharmacologic and physiologic treatment methods. In approaching the patient after valvular surgery, a number of factors must be considered. The level of preoperative cardiac function is a major determinant of management and outcome. The perioperative stress imposed on the heart, as well as the cardiovascular adaptations to the altered hemodynamics of a new or reconstructed cardiac valve, is also important. Recovery of left ventricular function will not be the same for all valvular lesions and will depend upon the specific valvular and hemodynamic abnormalities that were present preoperatively. Additionally, specific postoperative complications can be anticipated and treated prophylactically or when they occur. These include arrhythmias, perioperative ischemia, and postoperative bleeding. Management also must include initiation of anticoagulation when appropriate and prophylaxis for endocarditis. This chapter will review these issues and indicate management problems related to specific valvular lesions.

CARDIOVASCULAR HEMODYNAMICS

HEMODYNAMIC ASSESSMENT

The most immediate consideration following open heart surgery is to determine whether or not the cardiac output is adequate to support the needs of the patient.[1] Both clinical examination and hemodynamic monitoring are used. Clinically, one needs to assess signs of perfusion including blood pressure, skin turgor, and urine output. Additionally, a pulmonary artery (Swan-Ganz) catheter during the first 24 hours postoperatively will help to identify causes of poor perfusion and hypotension and is used in all patients. Measurements from the Swan-Ganz catheter will include pulmonary capillary wedge pressure (PCWP), cardiac output, and calculation of systemic vascular resistance.

A number of circumstances can contribute to a low cardiac output and systemic hypotension. After surgery, the effects of cardiopulmonary bypass will often still be apparent. The heart may remain cool and may show effects of ischemia if myocardial protection was incomplete. In the patient with significant preexisting left ventricular dysfunction from mitral regurgitation (MR), aortic regurgitation (AR), or severe aortic stenosis (AS), improvement in myocardial mechanics may require more time than for patients with normal left ventricular function. Another frequent cause of hypotension is volume depletion. This is generally the result of blood loss and hemolysis during cardiopulmonary bypass and extravasation of fluids to the extravascular spaces during the operative period. Volume replacement with blood products to a hematocrit of 30% to 35% is generally indicated; once this is achieved, hypotension that is accompanied by a low PCWP is treated with colloid replacement such as 5% albumin.

The impact of the heart rate on cardiovascular function postoperatively also can be of considerable importance. Bradycardia related to the effects of cardiopulmonary bypass, hypokalemia, medications, or mechanical damage to the sinoatrial (SA) or atrioventricular (AV) node should be treated with temporary atrial or ventricular pacing. Sinus tachycardia and other supraventricular arrhythmias will lead to impaired ventricular filling and should be treated by correction of the underlying cause if possible and then with specific agents if needed, as will be discussed below.

LEFT VENTRICULAR DYSFUNCTION

Pharmacologic Support

Postoperative left ventricular function will be influenced by the preoperative function, the adaptation to new prosthetic valves, the effects of cardioplegia and myocardial protection, and by the volume status of the patient. Treatment may require both pharmacologic and mechanical support, although the latter is needed relatively infrequently.

Inotropic support is commonly required for weaning from cardiopulmonary bypass. Six intravenous agents, each with specific advantages and disadvantages, are frequently used in the first 24 hours (Table 14–1).[2] In general, sympathomi-

Table 14–1. Intravenous Agents for Inotropic Support after Cardiac Surgery

Agent	Dose Range	Comments
Epinephrine	0.01–0.1 μg/kg per minute	α, β_1 > β_2 activity; potent agent
Norepinephrine	0.02–0.2 μg/kg per minute	α, β_1 activity; no β_2 activity; potent agent, but may increase afterload
Isoproterenol	0.01–0.1 μg/kg per minute	β_1, β_2 activity; no α activity; may decrease afterload and cause hypotension
Dopamine	1–30 μg/kg per minute	α, β_1 > β_2 activity; potent agent; renal vasodilator at low doses
Dobutamine	1–30 μg/kg per minute	β_2 > β_1 > α activity; predominantly increases cardiac contractility; less effect on systemic blood pressure
Amrinone	0.75 mg/kg bolus; then 5– 10 μg/kg per minute	Nonsympathomimetic agent; both inotropic and vasodilatory effects

Source: Adapted from Elefteriades and Geha[56] 1985, p 87, and from Sonnenblick et al,[6] 1979, p. 17.

metic amines with potent effects on myocardial (β_1) adrenoreceptors are required. Epinephrine stimulates both α- and β-adrenergic receptors and is often a first agent for inotropic support, used at a dose of 0.01 to 0.1 μg/kg per minute. It raises blood pressure by increasing inotropy and heart rate, and by peripheral vasoconstriction. This latter action is often balanced by β_2-receptor effects, so that a net increase in vasoconstriction and afterload does not occur, with the overall effect being that of a strong inotrope.[1,3] Norepinephrine (0.02 to 0.2 μg/kg per minute) also stimulates α- and β_1-receptors and will support systemic blood pressure, but it has little effect on β_2-receptors.[3] Therefore, it has the disadvantage of markedly increasing afterload through peripheral α-receptor mediated vasoconstriction. Although it is not generally used as an initial inotropic agent, it may be specifically useful in a subgroup of patients with systemic vasodilation and decreased systemic vascular resistance often secondary to sepsis.

Isoproterenol (0.01 to 0.1 μg/kg per minute) has only β-agonist activity.[3] Although it will provide inotropic support to the failing ventricle, it also may contribute to systemic hypotension from its unopposed β_2 stimulatory effects, which cause peripheral vasodilation. Its use is also complicated by tachycardia and arrhythmias. One role for isoproterenol may be in reducing pulmonary vascular resistance in patients with pulmonary hypertension after mitral valve surgery,[2] although its effects are modest.

Two agents that have become quite useful and tend to cause less tachycardia and vascular effects are dopamine and dobutamine.[3,4] Dopamine, an endogenous catecholamine, exerts dose-dependent hemodynamic effects. At low doses (0.5 to 2 μg/kg per minute), there is mild stimulation of β_1-receptors in the myocardium, but the dopaminergic-receptor effects on the renal and splanchnic vasculature are more pronounced, with a resulting increase in renal blood flow. This "renal-dose" dopamine not only provides inotropic support but can produce a clinically important diuresis. At moderate doses (2 to 5 μg/kg per minute), cardiac output is enhanced by β_1 inotropic and chronotropic effects on the heart. This range is useful postoperatively for left ventricular dysfunction and congestive heart failure and is frequently used.[2,5] Higher doses (>5 to 10 μg/kg per minute) result in peripheral vasoconstriction with an increase in afterload, which can be detrimental to cardiac function.

Dobutamine (1 to 30 μg/kg per minute), a synthetic sympathomimetic agent, is also useful for increasing cardiac inotropy without marked tachycardia.[6] It does not dilate the renal bed. It may increase forward flow and decrease PCWP, but without the systemic vasoconstriction encountered with dopamine. It too has been shown to be helpful following cardiac surgery,[7] and may be more beneficial than dopamine by causing less of an increase in peripheral vascular resistance and greater augmentation of myocardial blood flow.[5,8] Additionally, combinations of low-dose dopamine with dobutamine are occasionally useful to obtain both renal vasodilation as well as inotropic effects.

Amrinone lactate (0.75 mg/kg bolus, then 5 to 10 μg/kg per minute), a non-sympathomimetic agent that has both inotropic and vasodilatory effects, is less commonly used. Its mechanism of action is through phosphodiesterase inhibition, with a resultant increase in intracellular cyclic adenosine monophosphate (cAMP) levels.[9] Clinically, it can be useful after cardiac surgery for both mild congestive failure and for refractory left ventricular dysfunction, and it can be used in conjunction with the adrenergic agents or the intra-aortic balloon pump (IABP).[10] Its

Table 14–2. Intravenous Vasodilators after Cardiac
Surgery

Agent	Approximate Dose Range	Vascular Effect
Nitroglycerin	1–5 μg/kg per minute	Venous $\gg$ arterial
Sodium nitroprusside	0.5–10 μg/kg per minute	Arterial and venous

Source: Adapted from Elefteriades and Geha[56] 1985, p 92.

dual actions of inotropic support and vasodilation resemble that of a β-agonist in combination with a vasodilator. Significant side effects of amrinone may include hypotension, thrombocytopenia, and possibly an increase in ventricular ectopic activity.[9]

Finally, in addition to the aforementioned primarily inotropic agents, vasodilator therapy for left ventricular dysfunction can be considered (Table 14–2). In the presence of an elevated PCWP and adequate systemic arterial pressure, these agents can be helpful. They also are used frequently in the treatment of congestive heart failure in combination with an inotropic agent, which allows their systemic hypotensive effect to be better tolerated. The goals of vasodilator therapy include a decrease in preload or afterload, allowing improvement in myocardial oxygen demand and in pump performance. In general, these agents exert their effects primarily on either the venous system or the arterial system. Intravenous nitroglycerin (1 to 5 μg/kg per minute) is primarily a venodilator, resulting in preload reduction through vasodilation of venous capacitance vessels. It also exerts a modest effect on systemic arterial vessels with some decrease in afterload. Another agent, intravenous sodium nitroprusside (0.5 to 10 μg/kg per minute), causes both arterial and venous dilation, and acts to reduce both preload and afterload.[11] It is a potent agent used postoperatively for treatment of either systemic hypertension or left ventricular dysfunction with congestive heart failure. It is particularly useful in this setting in combination with dopamine.[12,13] Sodium nitroprusside also promotes forward flow in patients with acute MR or ventricular septal defect, through a reduction in afterload. One important toxicity of nitroprusside is the accumulation of cyanide and thiocyanate because of drug metabolism. Blood thiocyanate levels require monitoring, and treatment should be stopped if levels are > 10 mg/dl.[11] Following initial use of intravenous vasodilators postoperatively, the patient may be continued on long-term oral vasodilators if needed. These may include oral nitrates or hydralazine, a direct-acting arterial dilator.

Mechanical Support

Left ventricular dysfunction after open heart surgery can generally be treated with a combination of inotropic and vasodilating agents but may necessitate transient mechanical support. Initially if there is difficulty in maintaining cardiac output and systemic blood pressure after cardiopulmonary bypass, the patient may be returned to bypass for a short time to allow the myocardium to become nonischemic and to recover function. If function remains impaired, an IABP may be used to decrease afterload and improve coronary blood flow.[14] This technique has become a mainstay in management of patients with poor left ventricular function preoperatively or in the immediate postoperative period and may be required in 4% to 6% of patients undergoing cardiac surgery.[15] One early study using the IABP for patients who could not be withdrawn from cardiopulmonary bypass showed an 88% success rate in weaning from bypass.[14] Thus, in patients with severe ventricular dysfunction postoperatively, an IABP should be considered early in the course. It also may be useful in patients undergoing repair or replacement for severe MR, in which the left ventricle has lost its low-pressure outlet into the left atrium and faces a sudden increased afterload. Most patients can be successfully weaned from IABP support in 48 to 72 hours.

Complications secondary to IABP placement may include infection or embolic events, but the major complication is vascular insufficiency related to the insertion site, which occurs in about 10% of patients.[15] One representative study of 100 consecutive percutaneous insertion attempts had a 12% complication rate and suggested a difference between experienced and less experienced operators.[16]

More severe postoperative left ventricular dysfunction, generally secondary to perioperative infarction or to cardiogenic shock at the time of operation, can occasionally be treated using a left ventricular assist device.[17,18] Although it is uncommon to require such support after valvular surgery, postcardiotomy cardiogenic shock does occur and carries with it a very high mortality. Several groups have reported on short-term survival of patients treated with left ventricular assist devices and indicate that up to half of the patients can subsequently be weaned from mechanical support after short periods of stabilization.[19,20] One recent report noted long-term survival in a small number of patients after cardiac surgery who had required left ventricular assist, including four patients who had undergone valve replacement surgery.[21] Thus a ventricular assist device can be a useful adjunct in the severely ill patient, by allowing time for ventricular function to recover.

MANAGEMENT AFTER MITRAL VALVE SURGERY

Mitral Regurgitation

The aforementioned principles of cardiovascular support apply to management after correction of either MR or mitral stenosis (MS). However, specific differences in hemodynamics and left ventricular function may be encountered. In patients with significant MR, the aim is repair or replacement of the mitral valve before significant left ventricular dysfunction occurs. Even in relatively early operative repair, the left ventricle will face a significant increase in impedance to ejection postoperatively. This occurs as the left ventricle loses its low impedance outlet into the left atrium and now ejects its entire volume into the relatively high impedance aorta.[22] If MR with associated ventricular dilation and impairment of systolic function has progressed before operation, then mitral valve replacement may actually result in a drop in left ventricular ejection fraction with worsening of symptoms.[23] These patients will require specific attention to preload and afterload conditions and may benefit from early use of vasodilators, in conjunction with inotropic agents, to reduce afterload in the immediate postoperative period. Preservation of the papillary muscles and mitral apparatus may lead to improved ventricular performance postoperatively.[24-26] This is generally accomplished during mitral repair but may also be done with mitral replacement.

Mitral Stenosis

Patients with MS generally have well-preserved left ventricular function, because the ventricle has not been subjected to either volume or pressure overload. Interestingly, several groups have noted abnormalities in left ventricular wall motion or left ventricular performance in patients with MS,[27-29] although the effects on postoperative outcome are probably limited. Therefore, unless patients have had combined MS and MR, concomitant coronary artery disease, or suffered perioperative ischemia, the postoperative management should not require significant left ventricular support. In patients with longstanding MS, moderate-to-severe elevations in pulmonary artery pressures may have developed, but usually right ventricular performance remains normal.[30] Furthermore, pulmonary pressures will fall after mitral valve replacement and often remain lowered,[31,32] so that valve replacement is still generally indicated. Management of these patients should include determination of pulmonary artery pressures before valve replacement. Nitroglycerin may have a modest effect in treating pulmonary hypertension that persists postoperatively in these patients.[33] Rarely, severe pulmonary hypertension may lead to right ventricular dysfunction, and some authors have considered temporary right ventricular assist devices in this situation.[20] Another finding in patients with chronic MS is left atrial dilation with resultant atrial fibrillation. With relief of stenosis, the left atrial pressure overload and dilation may improve and allow successful cardioversion to sinus rhythm.

MANAGEMENT AFTER AORTIC VALVE SURGERY

Aortic Regurgitation

As with MR, the goal of medical management in AR is to replace the aortic valve before the development of significant left ventricular dysfunction.[34,35] This concept was supported by a series of studies by Henry and colleagues[36,37] using M-mode echocardiography in patients with AR. They found a poorer outcome after valve replacement in both symptomatic and asymptomatic patients with chronic AR who have extreme ventricular dilation preoperatively. Patients with a preoperative left ventricular end-systolic dimension of >55 mm or a fractional shortening of <25% did worse after surgery. Also associated with a poor outcome was a left ventricular end-diastolic dimension of >70 mm. Furthermore, this group found that even with improved operative technique in more recent years, preoperative left ventricular function and size were still the best predictors of outcome after surgery.[38] Impaired ejection fraction at peak exercise using radionuclide studies also has been correlated with a worse postoperative outcome.[39] Although these data indicate that early operative replacement is warranted in AR with signs of ventricular enlargement, more recent evidence also suggests that even with relatively poor preoperative function, many patients will show improvement after valve surgery.[40] Furthermore, even late after valve replacement left ventricular volumes and mass may continue to regress.[41] Nevertheless, valve replacement should be undertaken before extreme left ventricular enlargement occurs and before left ventricular function deteriorates. After surgery one should obtain a new assessment of ventricular dimension and function to help guide long-term management. The immediate care after aortic valve replacement will be similar to that for patients after mitral valve surgery. Pharmacologic support will likely be required following cardiopulmonary bypass, and recovery of ventricular function may require time.

Aortic Stenosis

Although patients with AS requiring valve replacement may or may not have progressed to left ventricular dysfunction with congestive heart failure, their surgical outcome will generally be favorable even with impaired preoperative function.[42] Along with the improvement in the aortic valve pressure gradient, there may be a postoperative decline in left ventricular filling pressure, volume index, and hypertrophy, along with an increase in ejection fraction and functional class.[42,43] The increase in ejection fraction observed even with significant preoperative ventricular dysfunction suggests that mechanical overload on the heart rather than irreversible myocardial damage was responsible for the initially depressed contractility.[22] The postoperative management will reflect this pathophysiology, in that congestive failure may be less frequent than with some of the other valvular lesions, and cardiac function may rapidly improve with the relief of the fixed afterload on the heart. However, because of the marked left ventricular hypertrophy that can occur with AS, myocardial preservation during operation may be difficult, and the possibility of intraoperative ischemia exists. Also, marked systemic hypertension following valve replacement for AS tends to occur frequently, especially when left ventricular systolic function is normal. This can be treated initially with nitroglycerin and vasodilators and may also respond well to beta-receptor blockers such as propranolol.

PERIOPERATIVE ISCHEMIA AND INFARCTION

Perioperative myocardial infarction carries with it a significant increase in operative morbidity and mortality and therefore must be considered in all patients after cardiac surgery. In general, myocardial damage may result either from significant obstructive coronary artery disease that has not been adequately revascularized or from inadequate myocardial protection during cardiopulmonary bypass. Additionally, hemodynamic instability either preoperatively or postoperatively, especially in a patient with coronary artery disease, may result in myocardial damage.[44]

Patients with valvular heart disease frequently have associated coronary artery disease, and if not surgically treated at the time of valve surgery, these patients have a worse outcome.[45] Therefore current recommendations are that men ≥ 35 years of age, women who are postmenopausal, and any patient with symptoms suggestive of coronary artery disease undergo preoperative coronary angiography.[46,47] Patients with significant coronary disease should then undergo combined valvular and coronary revascularization.

Myocardial damage because of inadequate protection during cardiopulmonary bypass has declined in frequency as better methods of cardioplegia have become standard. Surgeons may now use a variety of cardioplegic solutions, temperatures, and infusion strategies to optimize protection for the heart.[44]

Evaluation for myocardial damage postoperatively should be routine, and the diagnosis will depend primarily on changes in the electrocardiogram (ECG) and on the release of creatine kinase-MB (CK-MB) fraction.[48] Occasionally, a technetium-99m pyrophosphate myocardial scan to identify a recent infarct or a change in the lactate dehydrogenase isoenzyme ratio will also be helpful. The ECG after infarction will typically show appearance of new Q waves, new marked T-wave changes, or a new bundle-branch block, and serial ECGs may be useful. Creatine kinase may rise routinely after surgery, but with myocardial infarction, the cardiac-specific MB fraction should exceed 5% of the total serum creatine kinase or be >50 IU/L.[49] Because small elevations in CK-MB may frequently occur, some investigators recommend that at least two different tests (CK-MB, ECG, or myocardial scan) show positive results before diagnosing perioperative infarction.[48]

Evaluation after perioperative infarction should follow the same principles as after any completed infarction and should include appropriate risk stratification.[50] Left ventricular function remains the most important predictor of outcome after myocardial infarction, and therefore ejection fraction should be determined using radionuclide ventriculography or echocardiography. Recurrent ischemia is a second important predictor for adverse outcome, and this can be assessed with exercise testing performed either predischarge or at 3 to 6 weeks. For the patient with an abnormal baseline ECG, this test should be performed with a thallium-201 scan as well. Patients with either recurrent ischemia or a positive exercise test may need to be considered for coronary angiography to determine the extent of nonrevascularized disease. If the critical lesion is identified, one option in the postsurgical patient may be coronary angioplasty to dilate the culprit vessel. Finally, significant ventricular ectopy after infarction is associated with a higher mortality, and Holter monitoring should be performed in most postinfarction patients before discharge to identify patients at high risk of sudden death.

Pharmacologic treatment of the patient with perioperative infarction also should be similar to that for routine myocardial infarction. Patients with depressed ejection fractions may benefit from afterload reducing agents such as angiotensin-converting enzyme inhibitors. Aspirin (160 to 325 mg daily) should be started in any patient who will not be treated with anticoagulants. In the patient with preserved left ventricular function, β-blockers also may be considered for postinfarction prophylaxis.

POSTOPERATIVE ARRHYTHMIAS

Arrhythmias are a common complication after cardiac surgery. They are present not only because of the underlying cardiac abnormalities, but also because of the effects of surgery itself on the heart, and because of metabolic changes such as electrolyte disturbances and hypoxemia. Their management is similar to that in the nonpostoperative setting but also should take into account the disturbances frequently present after surgery. Supraventricular arrhythmias are the most frequent, particularly after mitral valve surgery, and this section will emphasize the more common rhythm disturbances seen.

Supraventricular arrhythmias occur in about 30% of postoperative patients[51] and are often related to mild pericarditis or to electrolyte abnormalities. Although a number of studies have addressed prophylactic treatment with digitalis or other agents preoperatively, most patients are only treated empirically if they have a history of supraventricular arrhythmias. If isolated atrial premature beats occur, they do not require treatment. Atrial flutter is one of the more common perioperative arrhythmias and is typically recognized because of its regular rhythm, often with a classic "sawtooth" pattern on ECG. In the postoperative patient, one can use the atrial epicardial pacing wires to record an atrial ECG and confirm the rhythm. Treatment of atrial flutter, after correction of electrolyte disturbances, can be accomplished in one of several ways. It is usually very sensitive to DC cardioversion, so that a low-energy shock (25 to 50 joules) will often restore sinus rhythm.

Alternatively, if the patient does have an atrial pacing wire in place, overdrive pacing at about 125% of the atrial rate for a few seconds is very effective.[51,52] Or, the patient may instead be treated with either verapamil or digoxin to slow AV conduction, followed by a type-1A antiarrhythmic agent such as procainamide or quinidine (Table 14–3). This last method may take somewhat longer and therefore be less useful. Finally, once the patient has returned to sinus rhythm, treatment with digoxin and a type-1A agent is usually initiated or continued and then maintained for several months postoperatively. Because the type-1A drugs are vagolytic and may speed AV conduction, their use should always be preceded by treatment with a drug to block the AV node and achieve a controlled ventricular rate in order to prevent rapid 1:1 conduction of atrial flutter.[53]

Atrial fibrillation also is quite common and may be treated with electrical cardioversion if the patient is hemodynamically compromised. If the patient is tolerating the rhythm, a usual first choice for treatment is digoxin, which may be given intravenously (see Table 14–3). Alternatively, intravenous verapamil is quite effective at slowing AV conduction and may be tried, although it can produce hypotension.[54] Once rate control is achieved, a type-1A drug should be started. The combination of digoxin and a type-1A agent often restore sinus rhythm. If atrial fibrillation persists with appropriate levels of both drugs, DC cardioversion can then be used. If a patient has a history of longstanding atrial fibrillation or has a large left atrium secondary to mitral valve disease, sinus rhythm may not be easily restored. In this case, the goal should be appropriate rate control using oral agents. Digoxin alone may be insufficient, and either propranolol or the calcium blockers verapamil or diltiazem may be added.

A less common atrial rhythm is multifocal atrial tachycardia, with its characteristic multiform P waves observed on the ECG. This is usually encountered in the setting of underlying pulmonary disease, often with hypoxemia present. It does not respond well to digoxin. Verapamil has been reported to be of some use,[55] although its effectiveness appears to be variable. Reversal of hypoxemia or electrolyte abnormalities is often necessary to restore a normal rhythm.

Ventricular arrhythmias are somewhat less common and tend to be related to an underlying cause such as hypokalemia, hypoxemia, or the effects of pressor

Table 14–3. Agents for the Treatment of Supraventricular Arrhythmias

Agent	Dosage Regimen	Comments
Digoxin	Load: IV: 0.75–1.25 mg/24 h (in 0.25-mg increments) Maintenance: IV or oral: 0.125–0.5 mg/d	Cardiac glycoside slows atrioventricular (AV) conduction
Verapamil	Bolus IV: 5–10 mg (in 5-mg increments) Maintenance: Oral: 120–480 mg/d	Calcium channel blocker slows AV conduction
Propranolol	Bolus IV: 0.1–0.15 mg/kg (in 1-mg increments) Maintenance: Oral: 40–320 mg/d	β-adrenergic blocker slows AV conduction
Procainamide	Load: IV: 10–15 mg/kg (at 20–50 mg/min) Maintenance: IV: 2–6 mg/min Maintenance: Oral: 2–8 g/d	Type-IA antiarrhythmic
Quinidine	Oral: 1200–1400 mg/d	Type-IA antiarrhythmic

Source: Adapted from Batsford,[51] 1991, p 1839.

agents. They may also occur because of myocardial ischemia or infarction. Premature ventricular beats do not require specific therapy. Nonsustained ventricular tachycardia should be treated initially with intravenous lidocaine (75 mg bolus, repeated once after 15 minutes, then 2 to 3 mg/min infusion). A second choice is procainamide. The patient can then be switched to an oral type-1A agent if further therapy is warranted. Brief episodes of nonsustained ventricular tachycardia in the immediate postoperative period, especially if associated with a correctable abnormality such as hypokalemia, usually do not require prolonged therapy. Sustained ventricular tachycardia with hemodynamic compromise or ventricular fibrillation is treated with DC cardioversion at high energy levels (300 joules). This is followed by intravenous lidocaine or procainamide until the cause of the ventricular dysrhythmia is determined and corrected. If no cause is readily apparent, these patients may need to be considered for full electrophysiologic studies.

POSTOPERATIVE BLEEDING

In the immediate postoperative period, a small degree of mediastinal bleeding and drainage is normal and reflects both the hematologic abnormalities secondary to cardiopulmonary bypass, as well as bleeding from suture lines and surgical sites. In general this should be <250 ml/hr in the first few hours, then decreased to <100 ml/hr.[56] Several hematologic factors play a role in postoperative bleeding.[57] First, large doses of heparin have been given during cardiopulmonary bypass, and the heparin effect may still be present. Protamine is administrated routinely to reverse this, and additional protamine can be given if the activated clotting time remains prolonged. Second, platelet function is impaired because of cardiopulmonary bypass, and in the event of continuing oozing despite apparently normal hematologic values, platelets (6 to 12 U) should be administered. Third, clotting factors may be depleted as reflected by a prolonged prothrombin time (PT) and partial thromboplastin time (PTT). Active bleeding associated with a prolonged PT and PTT may be corrected by administration of fresh frozen plasma. More recently, some centers have used epsilon aminocaproic acid for treatment of bleeding.[58] This is a synthetic antifibrinolytic agent that inhibits plasmin activity and the conversion of plasminogen to plasmin.

Bleeding also may contribute to a pericardial effusion postoperatively. Although early reports showed postoperative tamponade in up to 6% of cases, more recent series have identified tamponade in only 1% to 3% of postoperative patients.[59,60] These investigators also found that postoperative pericardial effusion was very common but only rarely progressed to actual tamponade. Therefore, a pericardial effusion suspected on the basis of chest x-ray or physical examination may be evaluated echocardiographically but does not require intervention unless hemodynamic evidence of tamponade is present. Occasionally, cardiac tamponade may occur due to localized hematoma formation resulting in right atrial compression, and a recent report described the detection of this syndrome by transesophageal echocardiography.[61] In these patients, there was systemic hypotension and the right atrial pressures were elevated, but standard transthoracic echocardiography did not identify a large effusion. However, the more sensitive transesophageal echocardiography did identify right atrial compression by organized thrombus or fluid. Therefore, in the patient with hemodynamic evidence of tamponade without large pericardial effusion by transthoracic echocardiogram, a transesophageal echocardiogram may be diagnostic.

ANTICOAGULATION

Initiation and maintenance of the appropriate anticoagulation regimen is an important aspect of care after valvular surgery. The goal of anticoagulation is to prevent accumulation of thrombus on the artificial valve surface and the subsequent occurrence of thromboembolic events. Two types of artificial valves are primarily used with somewhat different requirements for anticoagulation. The first group are the mechanical valves, either the caged-ball design, such as the Starr-Edwards valve, or the tilting-disc design, such as the Björk-Shiley or the St. Jude bileaflet valve. The second group are the bioprosthetic or tissue valves, typically constructed as glutaraldehyde-fixed porcine heterografts.

Because of a high incidence of thromboembolism, mechanical valves in either the aortic or mitral position all require full long-term anticoagulation.[62,63] Warfarin (Coumadin) is begun 2 days postoperatively and continued indefinitely, with the goal being prolongation of the PT to 1.5 to 2 times normal. In this range, the risk of thromboembolism is reduced without a dramatic increase in the risk of hemorrhagic complications. The addition of aspirin to this regimen has been shown to increase the risk of bleeding.[64] However, the addition of dipyridamole (Persantine) does not markedly increase the bleeding risk, and in the case of thromboembolic events while on appropriate warfarin therapy, dipyridamole should be added to the regimen.[62]

Bioprosthetic valves have the advantage of lower rates of thromboembolism and are therefore chosen specifically in patients who may be poor candidates for long-term anticoagulation because of hematologic problems, risk of trauma, childbearing potential, or comorbid disease. Their disadvantage, however, is a decrease in durability compared to mechanical valves. Postoperatively, all patients with bioprosthetic valves should be started on warfarin for 3 months until the sewing ring of the valve becomes endothelialized.[63] Patients with bioprostheses in the aortic position do not need to be continued on long-term anticoagulation. Patients with bioprostheses in the mitral position who are in sinus rhythm and have a normal size left atrium also do not require long-term anticoagulation. However, in patients with mitral bioprostheses who have atrial fibrillation or a history of systemic embolism or who are noted to have left atrial thrombus present, long-term anticoagulation is required.[62] Some authors believe that long-term anticoagulation for bioprosthetic valves may be acceptable at a somewhat lower level, with a PT of only 1.3 to 1.5 times normal.[62]

Increasingly, patients with mitral valve disease are able to undergo reconstructive surgery rather than valve replacement. In general, these patients will not require long-term anticoagulation but are usually treated with warfarin for the first 3 postoperative months because of the presence of a mitral anular sewing ring that is used in the repair.

ENDOCARDITIS PROPHYLAXIS

Patients who have received either type of prosthetic valve are at risk for the development of endocarditis, and it is of particular concern because prosthetic valve endocarditis carries with it a high mortality.[65] Typically, prosthetic valve endocarditis is divided into early onset (<60 days from surgery) and late onset (>60 days), with distinct differences in the type of infecting organism and probably in the mode of acquisition.[65,66] A number of studies have demonstrated that early prosthetic valve endocarditis is frequently caused by staphylococci, particularly *Staphylococcus epidermidis*.[67,68] Most of these infections are likely acquired at or near the time of surgery, frequently from intraoperative contamination and postoperative wound contamination. Furthermore, most of these *S. epidermidis* isolates are methicillin-resistant, indicating their origin as inhospital contaminants.[67] Antibiotic treatment of such infections usually requires a combination of agents.

In contrast, late prosthetic valve endocarditis more tyically resembles native valve endocarditis, with streptococcal infections becoming more common well after surgery. The etiology for late infection is generally transient bacteremia, often associated with medical procedures. All patients who have prosthetic valves in place must be aware of their relatively high-risk status and should be counseled as to appropriate prophylactic antibiotic use before dental, surgical, gastrointestinal, and genitourinary procedures.[69] These patients are considered at special risk and therefore in the past have been advised to receive parenteral, rather than oral, antibiotics before these procedures. However, the most recent recommendations of the American Heart Association indicate that for dental, oral, or upper respiratory tract procedures, even these patients may receive the standard oral prophylactic regimen that is given to lower-risk patients; for genitourinary or gastrointestinal procedures, parenteral antibiotics are still advised.[70] Some physicians may still wish to prescribe parenteral antibiotics in all cases for these high-risk patients. The standard oral regimen for dental, oral, or upper respiratory tract procedures is amoxicillin 3 g 1 hour before and 1.5 g 6 hours after the procedure. Penicillin-allergic patients may take erythromycin ethylsuccinate 800 mg 1 hour before and 400 mg 6 hours after the procedure. The standard regimen for genitourinary or gastrointestinal procedures is intravenous or intramuscular ampicillin 2 g, plus gentamicin 1.5 mg/kg 30 minutes before the procedure; this is followed by either oral amoxicillin 1.5 g 6 hours after the procedure or a repeat of the initial parenteral regimen 8 hours after the procedure. Alternative regimens including parenteral regimens for penicillin-allergic patients also are available, and published recommendations for their administration should be followed.[70,71]

SUMMARY

The management of the patient after valvular surgery is influenced by the preoperative left ventricular function and by the specific type of valvular lesion that has been corrected. The hemodynamics of the patient immediately after surgery must be evaluated carefully, and the patient can be supported with a variety of pharmacologic and mechanical measures as ventricular function recovers. Perioperative ischemia, arrhythmias, and bleeding may occur and should be specifically treated. Initiation of anticoagulation and adjustment of warfarin doses is an important aspect of postoperative care. Finally, the patient needs to be counseled that the presence of a prosthetic valve carries a risk for infective endocarditis and instructed on appropriate regimens for antibiotic prophylaxis.

REFERENCES

1. Kirklin, JW, Blackstone, EH, and Kirklin, JK: Cardiac surgery. In Braunwald, E (ed): Heart Disease: A Textbook of Cardiovascular Medicine, ed 3. WB Saunders, Philadelphia, 1988, p 1663.
2. Elefteriades, JA and Geha, AS: House Officer Guide to ICU Care. The Cardiothoracic Surgical Patient. Aspen Systems Corporation, Rockville, Md., 1985, p 85.

3. Weiner, N: Norepinephrine, epinephrine, and the sympathomimetic amines. In Gilman, AG, Goodman, LS, and Gilman, A (eds): Goodman and Gilman's The Pharmacologic Basis of Therapeutics, ed 6. Macmillan, New York, 1980, p 145.

4. LeJemtel, TH and Sonnenblick, EH: Nonglycosidic cardioactive agents. In Hurst, JW, Schlant, RC, Rackley, CE, et al (eds): The Heart, ed 7. McGraw-Hill, New York, 1990, p 1762.

5. Fowler, MB, Alderman, EL, Oesterle, SN, et al: Dobutamine and dopamine after cardiac surgery: Greater augmentation of myocardial blood flow with dobutamine. Circulation 70(Suppl I):I-103, 1984.

6. Sonnenblick, EH, Frishman, WH, and LeJemtel, TH: Dobutamine: A new synthetic cardioactive sympathetic amine. N Engl J Med 300:17, 1979.

7. Sakamoto, T and Yamada, T: Hemodynamic effects of dobutamine in patients following open heart surgery. Circulation 55:525, 1977.

8. VanTrigt, P, Spray, TL, Pasque, MK, et al: The comparartive effects of dopamine and dobutamine on ventricular mechanics after coronary artery bypass grafting: A pressure-dimension analysis. Circulation 70(Suppl I):I-112, 1984.

9. Mancini, D, LeJemtel, T, and Sonnenblick, E: Intravenous use of amrinone for the treatment of the failing heart. Am J Cardiol 56:8B, 1985.

10. Goenen, M, Pedemonte, O, Baele, P, et al: Amrinone in the management of low cardiac output after open heart surgery. Am J Cardiol 56:33B, 1985.

11. Cohn, NJ and Burke, LP: Nitroprusside. Ann Intern Med 91:752, 1979.

12. Stemple, DR, Kleiman, JH, and Harrison, DC: Combined nitroprusside-dopamine therapy in severe chronic congestive heart failure. Dose-related hemodynamic advantages over single drug infusions. Am J Cardiol 42:267, 1978.

13. Sturm, JT, Furhman, TM, Sterling, R, et al: Combined use of dopamine and nitroprusside therapy in conjunction with intra-aortic balloon pumping for the treatment of postcardiotomy low-output syndrome. J Thorac Cardiovasc Surg 82:13, 1981.

14. Buckley, MJ, Crave, JM, Gold, HK, et al: Intra-aortic balloon pump assist for cardiogenic shock after cardiopulmonary bypass. Circulation XLVII and XLVIII(Suppl III):III-90, 1973.

15. Sanfelippo, PM, Baker, NH, Ewy, HG, et al: Experience with intraaortic balloon counterpulsation. Ann Thorac Surg 41:36, 1986.

16. Martin, RS III, Moncure, AC, Buckley, MJ, et al: Complications of percutaneous intra-aortic balloon insertion. J Thorac Cardiovasc Surg 85:186, 1983.

17. Pae, WE Jr and Pierce, WS: Intra-aortic balloon counterpulsation, ventricular assist pumping, and the artificial heart. In Baue, AE, Geha, AS, Hammond, GL, et al (eds): Glenn's Thoracic and Cardiovascular Surgery, ed 5. Appleton and Lange, Norwalk, Conn., 1991, p 1585.

18. Pierce, WS, Parr, GVS, Myers, JL, et al: Ventricular-assist pumping in patients with cardiogenic shock after cardiac operations. N Engl J Med 305:1606, 1981.

19. Pennington, DG, McBride, LR, Swartz, MT, et al: Use of the Pierce-Donachy ventricular assist device in patients with cardiogenic shock after cardiac operations. Ann Thorac Surg 47:130, 1989.

20. Rose, DM, Connolly, M, Cunningham, JN, et al: Technique and results with a roller pump left and right heart assist device. Ann Thorac Surg 47:124, 1989.

21. Kanter, KR, Ruzevich, SA, Pennington, DG, et al: Follow-up of survivors of mechanical circulatory support. J Thorac Cardiovasc Surg 96:72, 1988.

22. Ross, JR Jr: Left ventricular function and the timing of surgical treatment in valvular heart disease. Ann Intern Med 94:498, 1981.

23. Schuler, G, Peterson, KL, Johnson, A, et al: Temporal response of left ventricular performance to mitral valve surgery. Circulation 59:1218, 1979.

24. David, TE, Uden, DE, and Strauss, HD: The importance of the mitral apparatus in left ventricular function after correction of mitral regurgitation. Circulation 68(Suppl II):II-76, 1983.

25. Wisenbaugh, T: Does normal pump function belie muscle dysfunction in patients with chronic severe mitral regurgitation? Circulation 77:515, 1988.

26. Yun, KL, Fann, JI, Rayhill, SC, et al: Importance of the mitral subvalvular apparatus for left ventricular segmental systolic mechanics. Circulation 82(Suppl IV):IV-89, 1990.

27. Hildner, FJ, Javier, RP, Cohen, LS, et al: Myocardial dysfunction associated with valvular heart disease. Am J Cardiol 30:319, 1972.

28. Curry, GC, Elliot, LP, and Ramsey, HW: Quantitative left ventricular angiocardiographic findings in mitral stenosis. Am J Cardiol 29:621, 1972.

29. Gash, AK, Carabello, BA, Cepin, D, et al: Left ventricular ejection performance and systolic muscle function in patients with mitral stenosis. Circulation 67:148, 1983.

30. Wroblewski, E, James, F, Spann, JF, et al: Right ventricular performance in mitral stenosis. Am J Cardiol 47:51, 1981.

31. Braunwald, E, Braunwald, N, Ross, J Jr, et al: Effects of mitral-valve replacement on the pulmonary vascular dynamics of patients with pulmonary hypertension. N Engl J Med 273:509, 1965.

32. Dalen, JE, Matloff, JM, Evans, GL, et al: Early reduction of pulmonary vascular resistance after mitral-valve replacement. N Engl J Med 277:387, 1967.

33. Halperin, JL, Brooks, KM, Rothlauf, EB, et al: Effect of nitroglycerin on the pulmonary venous gradient in patients after mitral valve replacement. J Am Coll Cardiol 5:34, 1985.

34. Bonow, RO, Rosing, DR, Kent, KM, et al: Timing of operation for chronic aortic regurgitation. Am J Cardiol 50:325, 1982.

35. Nishimura, RA, McGoon, MD, Schaff, HV, et al: Chronic aortic regurgitation: Indications for operation—1988. Mayo Clin Proc 63:270, 1988.

36. Henry, WL, Bonow, RO, Borer, JS, et al: Observations on the optimum time for operative intervention for aortic regurgitation. I. Evaluation of the results of aortic valve replacement in symptomatic patients. Circulation 61:471, 1980.

37. Henry, WL, Bonow, RO, Rosing, DR, et al: Observations on the optimum time for operative intervention for aortic regurgitation. II. Serial echocardiographic evaluation of asymptomatic patients. Circulation 61:484, 1980.

38. Bonow, RO, Picone, AL, McIntosh, CL, et al: Survival and functional results after valve replacement for aortic regurgitations from 1976 to 1983: Impact of preoperative left ventricular function. Circulation 72:1244, 1985.

39. Borer, JR, Rosing, DR, Kent, KM, et al: Left ventricular function at rest and during exercise after aortic valve replacement in patients with aortic regurgitation. Am J Cardiol 44:1297, 1979.

40. Carabello, BA, Usher, BW, Hendrix, GH, et al: Predictors of outcome for aortic valve replacement in patients with aortic regurgitation and left ventricular dysfunction: A change in the measuring stick. J Am Coll Cardiol 10:991, 1987.

41. Monrad, ES, Hess, OM, Murakami, T, et al: Time course of regression of left ventricular hypertrophy after aortic valve replacement. Circulation 77:1345, 1988.

42. Kennedy, JW, Doces, J, and Stewart, DK: Left ventricular function before and following aortic valve replacement. Circulation 56:944, 1977.

43. Smith, N, McAnulty, JH, and Rahimtoola, SH: Severe aortic stenosis with impaired left ventricular function and clinical heart failure: Results of valve replacement. Circulation 58:255, 1978.

44. Buckberg, GD: Myocardial protection during adult cardiac operations. In Baue, AE, Geha, AS, Hammond, GL, et al (eds): Glenn's Thoracic and Cardiovascular Surgery, ed 5. Appleton and Lange, Norwalk, Conn., 1991, p 1417.

45. Czer, LS, Gray, RJ, DeRobertis, MA, et al: Mitral valve replacement: Impact of coronary artery disease and determinants of prognosis after revascularization. Circulation 70(Suppl I):I-198, 1984.

46. Guidelines for coronary angiography: A report of the ACC/AHA Task Force on Assessment of Diagnostic and Therapeutic Cardiovascular Procedures (Subcommittee on Coronary Angiography). J Am Coll Cardiol 10:935, 1987.

47. Rahimtoola, SH: Perspective on valvular heart disease: An update. J Am Coll Cardiol 14:1, 1989.

48. Guiteras Val, P, Pelletier, LC, Hernandez, MG, et al: Diagnostic criteria and prognosis of perioperative myocardial infarction following coronary bypass. J Thorac Cardiovasc Surg 86:878, 1983.

49. Graeber, GM: Creatine kinase (CK): Its use in evaluation of perioperative myocardial infarction. Surg Clin North Am 65:539, 1985.

50. Guidelines for the early management of patients with acute myocardial infarction. A report of the ACC/AHA Task Force on Assessment of Diagnostic and Therapeutic Cardiovascular Procedures (Subcommittee to Develop Guidelines for the Early Management of Patients with Acute Myocardial Infarction). J Am Coll Cardiol 16:249, 1990.

51. Batsford, WP: Arrhythmia complications following cardiac surgery. In Baue, AE, Geha, AS, Hammond, GL, et al (eds): Glenn's Thoracic and Cardiovascular Surgery, ed 5. Appleton and Lange, Norwalk, Conn., 1991, p 1837.

52. Waldo, AL, MacLean, WAH, Karp, RB, et al: Entrainment and interruption of atrial flutter with atrial pacing. Studies in man following open heart surgery. Circulation 56:737, 1977.

53. Zipes, DP: Specific arrhythmias, diagnosis and treatment. In Braunwald, E (ed): Heart Disease: A Textbook of Cardiovascular Medicine, ed 3. WB Saunders, Philadelphia, 1988, p 658.

54. Plumb, VJ, Karp, RB, Kouchoukos, NT, et al: Verapamil therapy of atrial fibrillation and atrial flutter following cardiac operation. J Thorac Cardiovasc Surg 83:590, 1982.

55. Levine, JH, Michael, JR, and Guarnieri, T: Treatment of multifocal atrial tachycardia with verapamil. N Engl J Med 312:21, 1985.

56. Elefteriades, JA and Geha, AS: House Officer Guide to ICU Care. The Cardiothoracic Surgical Patient. Aspen Systems Corporation, Rockville, Md., 1985, p 113.

57. Sobel, M and Salzman, EW: Hemorrhagic and Thrombotic Complications of Cardiac Surgery. In Baue, AE, Geha, AS, Hammond, GL, et al (eds): Glenn's Thoracic and Cardiovascular Surgery, ed 5. Appleton and Lange, Norwalk, Conn., 1991, p 1547.

58. DelRossi, AJ, Cernaianu, AC, Botros, S, et al: Prophylactic treatment of postperfusion bleeding using EACA. Chest 96:27–30, 1989.

59. Stevenson, LW, Child, JS, Laks, H, et al: Incidence and significance of early pericardial effusions after cardiac surgery. Am J Cardiol 54:848, 1984.

60. Weitzman, LB, Tinker, WP, Kronzon, I, et al: The incidence and natural history of pericardial effusion after cardiac surgery—an echocardiographic study. Circulation 69:506, 1984.

61. Kochar, GS, Jacobs, LE, and Kotler, MN: Right atrial compression in postoperative cardiac patients: Detection by transesophageal echocardiography. J Am Coll Cardiol 16:511, 1990.

62. Stein, PD and Kantrowitz, A: Antithrombotic therapy in mechanical and biological prosthetic heart valves and saphenous vein bypass grafts. Chest 95(Suppl):107S, 1989.

63. Braunwald, E: Valvular heart disease. In Braunwald, E (ed): Heart Disease: A Textbook of Cardiovascular Medicine, ed 3. WB Saunders, Philadelphia, 1988, p 1078.

64. Chesebro, JH, Fuster, V, Elveback, LR, et al: Trial of combined warfarin plus dipyridamole or aspirin therapy in prosthetic heart valve replacement: Danger of aspirin compared with dipyridamole. Am J Cardiol 51:1537, 1983.

65. Wilson, WR, Danielson, GK, Guiliani, ER, et al: Prosthetic valve endocarditis. Mayo Clin Proc 57:155, 1982.

66. Oikawa, JH and Kaye, D: Endocarditis: Epidemiology, pathophysiology, management, and prophylaxis. In Frankl, WS and Brest, AN (eds): Valvular Heart Disease: Comprehensive Evaluation and Management. FA Davis, Philadelphia, 1986, p 335.

67. Karchmer, AW, Archer, GL, and Dismukes, WE: *Staphylococcus epidermidis* causing prosthetic valve endocarditis: microbiologic and clinical observations as guides to therapy. Ann Intern Med 98:447, 1983.

68. Ivert, TSA, Dismukes, WE, Cobbs, CG, et al: Prosthetic valve endocarditis. Circulation 69:223, 1984.

69. Weinstein, L: Infective endocarditis. In Braunwald, E (ed): Heart Disease: A Textbook of Cardiovascular Medicine, ed 3. WB Saunders, Philadelphia, 1988, p 1093.

70. Dajani, AS, Bisno, AL, Chung, KJ, et al: Prevention of bacterial endocarditis: Recommendations by the American Heart Association. J Am Med Assoc 264:2919, 1990.

71. Abramowicz, M (ed): Prevention of Bacterial Endocarditis. Med Lett Drugs Ther 31:112, 1989.

CHAPTER 15

Valvuloplasty

Zoltan G. Turi, M.D.

HISTORY OF VALVULOPLASTY

Attempts to dilate stenotic cardiac valves date to the early 1900s. A series of attempts at finger dilation and deployment of blade devices were largely unsuccessful[1] until development of closed commissurotomy for mitral stenosis in the 1940s and 1950s[2,3] led to the establishment of standard techniques still used in much of the world.

The first attempts at percutaneous commissurotomy employed urethral catheters with steel wire springs placed across stenotic pulmonic and tricuspid valves.[4] After only a small total experience, the investigators concluded precociously (in 1955) that "catheter commissurotomy should be attempted before surgical commissurotomy." The therapeutic use of balloons by Rashkind and Miller[5] (1966) for atrial septostomy and by Gruntzig and associates[6] (1977) for coronary angioplasty led to balloon valvulotomy for pulmonic stenosis (Semb and associates,[7] 1979), mitral stenosis (Inoue and coworkers,[8] 1982), and congenital pediatric and acquired adult aortic stenosis (Lababidi and colleagues,[9] 1984 and Cribier and coworkers,[10] 1986, respectively).

After a decade of work with largely prototype devices, mostly descriptive studies with short to intermediate follow-up, and few randomized comparisons, balloon valvuloplasty is now generally considered the procedure of choice in pulmonic stenosis, a reasonable alternative to surgery in many cases of mitral stenosis, and a limited option in acquired aortic stenosis. Its role in tricuspid stenosis is uncertain, and serious questions remain regarding the applicability of the procedure to bioprosthetic valve obstruction.

NOMENCLATURE

The term *valvuloplasty* may not be ideal to describe balloon dilation of stenotic valves.[11,12] Valvuloplasty has generally described reconstructive surgery to alleviate valvular regurgitation. The primary mechanism of action of balloon dilation, when it is in fact commissural splitting, is more appropriately termed a *valvulotomy* or *commissurotomy*. Thus *valvuloplasty* is potentially misleading, especially because the remodeling process suggested by the term may be the least effective mechanism of balloon dilation. Nevertheless, valvuloplasty has been adopted as the common descriptor of balloon dilation of stenotic valves and is used in this chapter.

MECHANISMS OF BALLOON VALVULOPLASTY

Three mechanisms appear to account for the results of balloon valvuloplasty: commissural splitting, stretching of the commissural orifice, and cracking of valve leaflet calcifications. The first is the typical mechanism of pulmonic valvuloplasty, of mitral and tricuspid valvuloplasty involving relatively ideal rheumatically fused valves, and of valvuloplasty for congenital and rheumatic aortic stenosis. Stretching of the orifice accounts for some of the hemodynamic improvement achieved in all valvuloplasty but may be the most short-lived. Calcification fracture improves valve leaflet compliance and mobility; it is the typical mechanism in bioprosthetic and in senile, calcific aortic valves.

MECHANISM OF AORTIC VALVULOPLASTY

Early work in postmortem valves and with intraoperative balloon dilation suggested that all three aforementioned mechanisms account for early postprocedure hemodynamic changes.[13,14] However, direct observation of stenotic aortic valves undergoing balloon dilation during heart surgery (Fig. 15–1) demonstrated only temporary dilation of the orifice, with early recoil, and minimal fracture of calcifications;[15] direct measurement of orifice size and leaflet mobility failed to show significant improvement. Similarly, a number of necropsy or intraoperative reports have claimed benefit based on fracture of valve leaflet calcifications,[16-18] but this finding has not been confirmed by others.[19] The differences between studies may have been related to balloon size, patient age, and techniques used, but the inconsistency is reflected in subsequent clinical reports. Consistent intraoperative and postmortem observations have been the more favorable anatomic results after balloon dilation of tricuspid aortic valves,[20] congenitally bicuspid or unicuspid valves (typical in the pediatric setting), and rheumatically fused aortic valves, in which the mechanism of dilation is largely due to commissural splitting.[21,22]

MECHANISMS OF MITRAL VALVULOPLASTY

X-ray analysis of 15 operatively excised valves subjected to ballooning demonstrated primarily commissural splitting,[23] whereas intraoperative study of the effect of balloon dilation demonstrated significant early benefit from commissural stretching.[24] Because fusion of commissures is the typical etiology of mitral stenosis in young patients, commissural splitting provides exceptional results.[25] In the setting of calcified leaflets (and anuli) in older patients, stretching of commissures and potential cracking of calcifications results in substantial poorer short- and long-term results.

MECHANISMS OF PULMONIC, TRICUSPID, AND BIOPROSTHETIC VALVULOPLASTY

In *pulmonic stenosis,* the primary mechanism of stenosis relief is also commissural splitting,[26] with occasional evidence of cusp tearing and avulsion;[27] anatomic examination has been reported only in young patients. *Tricuspid stenosis is*

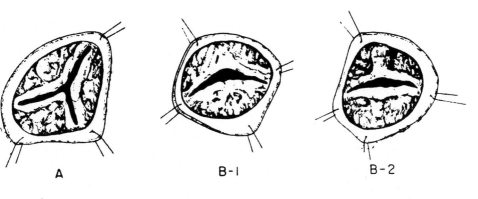

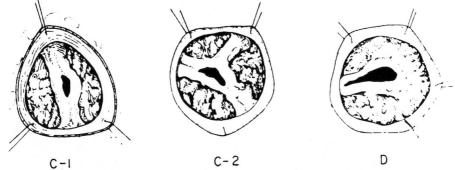

Figure 15–1. Typical anatomic features of aortic valves of patients presenting for aortic valvuloplasty. Tricuspid valve with open commissures (A); congenitally bicuspid valve with open commissures (B-1); acquired bicuspid valve with open commissures (B-2); congenitally bicuspid valve with fused commissures (C-1); acquired bicuspid valve with fused commissures (C-2); congenitally unicuspid valve (D). (From Robicsek et al.[44], with permission.)

rheumatic and similar to mitral stenosis; the differences include valve anulus size and subvalvular apparatus; the latter may predispose dilated tricuspid valves to a higher incidence of regurgitation. Inspection of eight excised *bioprosthetic valves* revealed calcified leaflets in seven; thick, rigid, and immobile leaflets in one, and commissural fusion by mounds of calcium in two. *In vitro* balloon dilation resulted in commissural splitting in two and calcification fracture in three. Debris was dislodged in three, and one valve was left with noncoapting leaflets.[28]

AORTIC VALVULOPLASTY

The typical patient undergoing aortic valvuloplasty is elderly, has rigid calcified valve leaflets, and may have associated ventricular dysfunction or systemic illness. As such, this population is at high risk for any invasive procedure, and the morbidity associated with valvuloplasty has been consistent with expectations. The disappointment has been the relatively modest gain in hemodynamics acutely and the high restenosis rate. This is not surprising, given the disappointing results with surgical commissurotomy for aortic stenosis reported 3 decades earlier.[29]

EARLY EXPERIENCE

In 1984, Lababidi and coworkers[9] reported 23 cases of aortic valvuloplasty in children. The results, a decrease in mean aortic valve gradient from 113 ± 48 to

32 ± 15 mm Hg, were apparently free of significant complications, and reflected the favorable anatomic substrate of congenital aortic stenosis for balloon valvulotomy. The first report of valvuloplasty for adult acquired aortic stenosis was by Cribier and associates[10] in 1986. Three patients (mean age = 75) underwent aortic valvuloplasty with gradient reduction $\geq 50\%$ despite use of balloons ≤ 12 mm in diameter—exceptional results given small balloons. In reporting their initial series of 92 ill elderly patients (mean age 75 ± 11 years), the same group again reported striking early results.[30] The mean gradient reduction, from 75 ± 26 to 30 ± 13 mm Hg, and increase in mean calculated valve area from 0.5 ± 0.2 to 0.9 ± 0.4 cm^2 is superior to the results reported by many groups. Representative of many others' early results were mean gradient reductions of $\leq 50\%$;[13] in a series of 32 patients (mean age = 79) McKay and colleagues[31] reported gradient reduction of 49% and valve area increase from 0.6 ± 0.2 to 0.9 ± 0.3 cm^2, using balloons as large as 23 mm in diameter.

LARGER SERIES AND FOLLOW-UP STUDIES

Even Cribier and coworkers' early data included follow-up information that raised concern about the long-term results of aortic valvuloplasty. Three-month follow-up in the original 92 patients revealed an aortic valve area no better than 0.75 ± 0.25 cm^2; although this was optimistically interpreted as sustained improvement, it also should be noted that this is still severe aortic stenosis.[32] Subsequent reports from this group have claimed generally better results, in part attributed to the use of larger balloon sizes.[33] Representative of most investigators' early experience was the 5-month follow-up data reported by Block and Palacios.[34] Of 30 patients undergoing aortic valvuloplasty, 13 were dead at 5-month follow-up, 9 had restenosed, 1 had undergone aortic valve replacement, and 7 were classified as "stable" but had not been restudied. Their initial 90 patients included 8 acute deaths, and 23 additional patients were dead by 5 months.[34] Longer follow-up in a series of 170 patients from the Beth Israel Hospital reveals no long-term improvement in valve gradient, modest improvement in valve area, and low probability of event-free survival (Fig. 15–2). Although the aortic valve areas suggest sustained improvement, patients with restenosis, aortic valve replacement, and death are excluded.

Restenosis is the second major problem in aortic valvuloplasty. The mechanism appears to be granulation, ossification, and fibrosis.[36] Restenosis has been reported as early as 3 weeks after valvuloplasty, probably related to recoil of a stretched orifice.[37] In the Beth Israel series shown in Figure 15–2, 29 of the 35 patients who returned for follow-up catheterization had restenosed at 6 months. Although a disproportionate number of those having repeat catheterization may have restenosed, an additional 25 of the 170 patients died in early follow-up and could be presumed to have restenosed as well. Further, 8 of the 14 asymptomatic patients who underwent follow-up catheterization had restenosed. Of 95 patients who underwent follow-up catheterization in the Mansfield Valvuloplasty Registry, investigators found a 73% restenosis rate at 6 months, including 62% of the patients who had symptomatically improved and 80% of those with symptoms suggesting restenosis.[38] No baseline variable predicted restenosis risk. Unfortunately, although repeat valvuloplasty can be performed, patients undergoing repeat dilations have a high early cardiac mortality.[39]

Considerable controversy has arisen regarding the overall utility of aortic val-

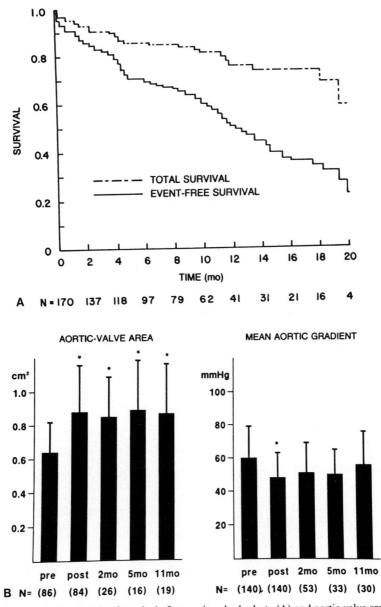

Figure 15–2. Life table analysis of survival after aortic valvuloplasty (A) and aortic valve area and gradient before and after valvuloplasty (B) in 170 patients. Note that patients with restenosis, aortic valve replacement, or who died are excluded from follow-up hemodynamic data. (From Safian et al.[35], with permission.)

vuloplasty. To many cardiologists, balloon aortic valvuloplasty has been discredited as much as surgical aortic valvuloplasty. The potential benefits, although transient, may be as a "bridging" procedure, and occasional patients have sustained improvement. The nature of the controversy has been reflected in the titles of a series of articles: "Good-bye to thoracotomy for cardiac valvulotomy,"[40] "Aortic valvuloplasty: Baby or bathwater,"[41] "Aortic valvuloplasty: Are balloon-dilated valves all they are 'cracked' up to be?,"[42] "Aortic valvuloplasty—a valid alternative?",[43] "Have balloon, will travel: Expanded indications for nonoperative intravascular balloon dilation?,"[43A] "Balloon valvuloplasty in calcified aortic stenosis: A cause for caution and alarm,"[44] and finally "Personal answer to a personal view of balloon aortic valvuloplasty."[45] The discrepancy between some groups' generally more favorable results and the mediocre results reported by many investigators may in part be explained by variations in patient age, severity of stenoses dilated, and perhaps by operator experience, although relatively experienced investigators have reported unfavorable short- and long-term results.[46]

INDICATIONS

We consider balloon valvuloplasty for severe calcific aortic stenosis to be indicated for patients who are at high or unacceptable risk for valve replacement (Table 15-1). In some patients who are poor surgical candidates owing to concurrent illness or hemodynamic decompensation, valvuloplasty can be considered a "bridge" to eventual surgery. In these patients, the short-term palliation and strong likelihood of restenosis need to be stressed so that the patient is prepared for likely subsequent surgery.

Some additional settings in which aortic valvuloplasty may be appropriate include acute treatment of aortic stenosis related cardiogenic shock[47-49] (Fig. 15-3) and as part of the preparation of patients scheduled to undergo noncardiac surgery[50] who are at increased risk of perioperative complications.[51] In some patients with low-output state, relatively low gradients, and uncertain severity of aortic stenosis, balloon aortic valvuloplasty may serve as both a diagnostic and therapeutic pro-

Table 15–1. Indications for Valvuloplasty of Severe Aortic or Mitral Stenosis

Aortic	Mitral
Indications	
Poor surgical candidate	Echo score ≤8[191]
↓ Life expectancy	
Low output state[85]	
?Advanced age[52]	
Bridging procedure	Symptomatic despite adequate heart rate lowering
Cardiogenic shock[47-49]	
Concurrent illness	
Noncardiac surgery[50]	
Congenital or rheumatic aortic stenosis[192]	Poor surgical candidate
	Pulmonary hypertension[193]
	Pregnancy[113,114]
Contraindications	
> moderate valvular regurgitation	> moderate valvular regurgitation
Clot in left ventricle	Clot in left atrium[118]
	Echo score ≥12 (relative)[146]

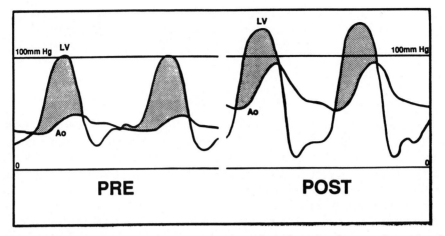

Figure 15–3. Representative pre- and post-procedure hemodynamic tracings from a patient undergoing emergency balloon aortic valvuloplasty. Note substantial improvement in systemic pressure after the procedure, without resolution of gradient; this is likely due to improved cardiac output. Ao = central aortic pressure; LV = left ventricular pressure (mm Hg).

cedure. Occasional patients in this setting will have significant hemodynamic improvement.

Should age alone be considered an indication for balloon valvuloplasty? Although this has been pronounced a "clear indicator",[52] close examination of the data may suggest otherwise. Aortic valvuloplasty in octogenarians has been reported to have inhospital mortality of 6.5% and 1-year follow-up mortality of 23%;[53] the results in octogenarians are similar to those of relatively younger patients.[54] Aortic valve replacement in elderly patients has good overall results but high early mortality (30% in 90 day follow-up) if emergency operations and a high percentage of patients with heart failure are included.[55] In more stable elderly patients, mortality appears to be lower: 12.5% mortality in those >80 years of age,[56] with no additional 3-year mortality.[57] Aortic valve replacement for aortic stenosis (especially in the setting of good left ventricular function) remains one of the best indications for open heart surgery in the elderly; as a result, aortic valve replacement may account for up to 50% of heart operations performed in octogenarians.[55] Comparison of the risk of balloon valvuloplasty vs. surgery in elderly patients is made difficult by the inclusion of inoperable candidates in balloon valvuloplasty series; the author believes that both mortality and long-term results in survivors are better with surgery. This author believes that it is a relative contraindication for balloon aortic valvuloplasty if the patient is able to present for a preliminary ambulatory visit because aortic valve replacement, which produces a gradient strikingly lower than postvalvuloplasty gradients, with a generally acceptable morbidity and mortality, is so much the superior procedure.

PREPROCEDURE EVALUATION

Patients undergoing aortic valvuloplasty should have the severity of aortic stenosis confirmed. Because the correlation between properly performed noninvasive evaluation and cardiac catheterization is strong prevalvuloplasty,[46,58,59] the indications for cardiac catheterization include coronary angiography in older patients or younger patients with risk factors for coronary artery disease. Valvuloplasty can precipitate severe myocardial ischemia; failure to take coexistent coronary disease into account can be fatal.[60,61]

Technical Approach

The current standard approach in our laboratory involves placement of a 6F sheath in the left femoral artery and 8F sheaths in the left femoral vein and right femoral artery. A 7F bipolar pacing lead-tipped pulmonary artery catheter is then used for right heart catheterization and left in place in the pulmonary artery, connected prophylactically to a temporary pacemaker generator. The use of a temporary pacemaker is justified in this setting,[62] but the catheter should be left in the pulmonary artery, inasmuch as the need to withdraw to the right ventricle to pace is rare, and the pulmonary artery pressure can provide useful hemodynamic guidance during the procedure. After 7500 units of heparin have been given intravenously and anticoagulation has been confirmed by activated clotting time, the aortic valve is crossed retrograde typically via the right femoral sheath, using standard techniques, preferably with a pigtail catheter over a 0.035 inch straight guide wire. Hemodynamics, including a Fick cardiac output, are then confirmed. An Amplatz 0.035 inch extra stiff 260 cm J guidewire (Cook, Bloomington, IN) with a "V"-shaped bend approximately 2 cm from its tip is then prepared using a metal clamp and advanced into the apex of the ventricle, withdrawing the pigtail as well as the sheath. (A 0.038 inch guidewire is preferred by some investigators for additional support.) Typically, a 9F 20-mm single foil polyethylene balloon (Mansfield, Watertown, MA) is then advanced retrograde across the aortic valve, being careful to preserve the contour of the wire in the ventricular apex (Fig. 15–4). This balloon is approved in the United States by the Food and Drug Administration for pulmonic and aortic valvuloplasty. Advancing the balloon across the aortic valve may result in a dramatic fall in systemic arterial pressure, and balloon inflation (using a diluted contrast mixture for lower viscosity and faster inflation-deflation cycles) should be initiated promptly. If the balloon has been positioned properly, a "waist" appears and then disappears as sufficient pressure is applied to overcome the resistance of the stenotic orifice. If systemic hypotension has occurred, balloon deflation should be accomplished immediately, inasmuch as wall stress is extreme, and as a consequence of both high demand and partial obstruction of coronary blood flow, the ventricle may be acutely ischemic, even in the absence of coronary artery disease.

Some investigators have routinely placed an additional catheter across the aortic valve to monitor left ventricular pressure; balloon catheters are available that allow left ventricular pressure monitoring via the distal tip. It is our practice to withdraw the balloon catheter between inflations to a point distal to the cranial vessels to minimize the chance of embolic phenomena or interference with aortic, coronary, or cranial blood flow; using standard exchange technique, one can reinsert a pigtail after several inflations to measure postinflation hemodynamics. We routinely perform a transseptal catheterization and leave a pigtail in the left ventricle across the mitral valve through a Mullins sheath (USCI, Billerica, MA) placed in the left atrium (before heparinization); thus we have continuous hemodynamic readout before, during, and after valvuloplasty, obviating any need for multiple exchanges. The hemodynamics during valvuloplasty, an example of which is presented in Figure 15–5, can be alarming to the uninitiated.

Postprocedure patient evaluation is complicated by a weaker correlation between echo-Doppler data and hemodynamics determined during catheterization. This may be explained in part by the fact that noninvasive determinations have been made 1 to 4 days after valvuloplasty; generally, a higher gradient has been found than the immediate postvalvuloplasty catheterization data.[46,58] There are two probable hemodynamic explanations: first, cardiac output may be depressed immediately after valvuloplasty[63] and improve in the first 48 hours as the myocardium recovers from the stunning effects of balloon inflation, thereby resulting in a higher gradient; second, recoil of the dilated orifice may occur early after balloon stretching. Nevertheless, postprocedure echo is helpful to assess for iatrogenically induced aortic regurgitation (AR) or mitral regurgitation (MR) (in most patients MR decreases secondary to the change in loading conditions,[59] but trauma to the mitral apparatus occasionally causes substantial insufficiency). The postprocedure evaluation of the patient also may be influenced by blood loss: this may artifactually depress the gradient, suggesting a better result than actually obtained. Some early reported "successes" were in fact due largely to blood loss.

TECHNIQUE VARIATIONS

Two prominent variations are in use: (1) an antegrade method using a transseptal approach,[64] which has particular applicability in patients with severe peripheral vascular disease precluding deployment of large catheters in the arterial tree and (2) a double-balloon technique, for which superior results have been claimed.[65–67] Because the superiority of the double-balloon technique remains unproven, and concern exists regarding possible damage to the ascending aorta, this author continues to use single balloons. Preliminary data suggest that single balloons ≤20 mm, when compared with larger single or double balloons, have lower risk of causing AR or neurologic events, with only a small sacrifice in postprocedure valve area.[68] The 20-mm balloon most commonly used in our laboratory usually suffices to adequately lower the aortic valve gradient. It can be passed through a 12F sheath, precluding the need to continuously exert pressure for hemostasis throughout the procedure; however, once it has been inflated, its withdrawal is occasionally difficult, sometimes enhanced by gentle rotation. A balloon that tapers abruptly in its distal portion can be used; this allows "predilation" of the valve with a smaller (15 mm) balloon segment. A 23-mm balloon typically requires a larger, 14F sheath. Experimental 8F polyethylene terephthelate balloons can advance through a 9F sheath.

Balloons are available in 3-cm to 5.5-cm lengths; in adults, when balloons ≤20 mm diameter are used, the longer length is preferable. Although inflation-deflation cycles are longer in the 5.5-cm length balloons, there is less tendency to abruptly slide into the apex or eject into the aorta. Bifoil, trefoil, and tapered balloon designs have been used primarily in Europe;[69] the advantage of these designs remains to be demonstrated by controlled studies,[70] although the eccentric deployment of parallel balloons in the aortic orifice may better preserve blood flow during balloon inflation.

Aortic valvuloplasty also has been performed by the brachial route[35] as well as a retrograde approach via subclavian cutdown.[71]

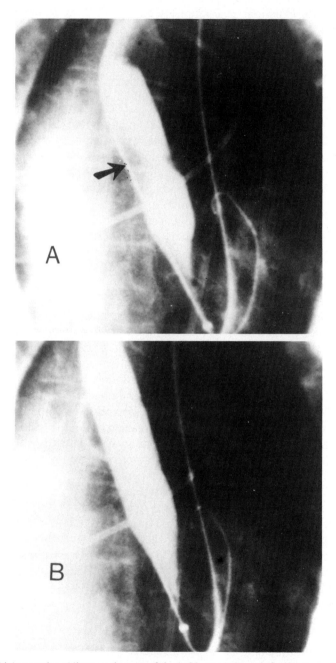

Figure 15–4. Right anterior oblique angiogram of single 20-mm balloon inflating across the aortic valve (*A*) with a waist at the level of the stenosis *(arrow);* fully inflated balloon (*B*). Note curved safety wire in the ventricular apex.

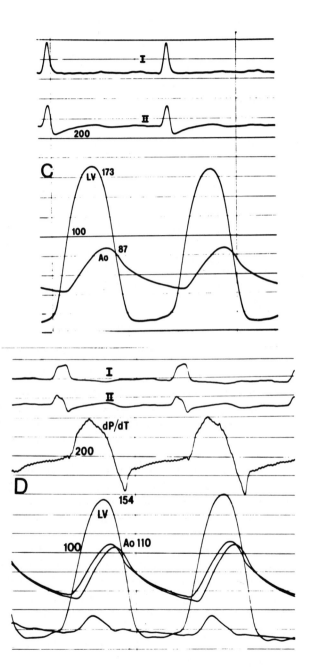

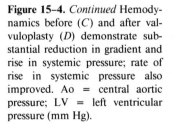

Figure 15–4. *Continued* Hemodynamics before (*C*) and after valvuloplasty (*D*) demonstrate substantial reduction in gradient and rise in systemic pressure; rate of rise in systemic pressure also improved. Ao = central aortic pressure; LV = left ventricular pressure (mm Hg).

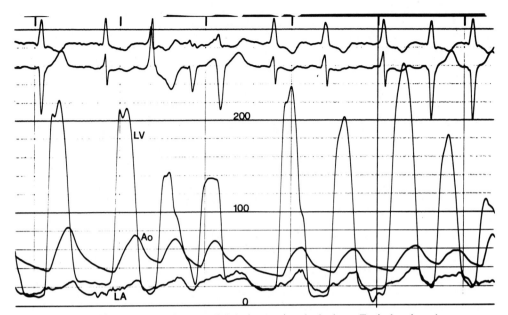

Figure 15–5. Hemodynamic tracing recorded during aortic valvuloplasty. Typical patients have severe systemic hypotension; left ventricular pressure (LV) is generally preserved, but systemic pressure (Ao) drops abruptly, and left atrial pressure (LA) may approach systemic. All pressures recorded at 200 mm Hg scale.

COMPLICATIONS OF AORTIC VALVULOPLASTY

Complications of aortic valvuloplasty can be attributed to interruption of blood flow to the cranial and coronary arteries; stunning effect on the myocardium; potential mechanical trauma to the heart, aorta, or aortic leaflets; embolization; and the effects of large catheters on peripheral vessels (Table 15–2). The potential for these complications is magnified by the advanced age of the typical adult patient.

Decreased flow to the cranial vessels may be exacerbated by the coexistence of carotid artery disease,[72] and rapid decrease in cranial blood flow velocity has been documented. In my experience, using largely single-foil balloons in elderly subjects, a decrease in systolic blood pressure to ≤60 mm Hg is common, but is rarely associated with syncope or seizure (see Fig. 15–5). Cerebral vascular events after aortic valvuloplasty are infrequent (<2%), but systemic screening for cerebral emboli suggests that subclinical embolization is relatively common.[73]

Severe aortic insufficiency, which occurs in approximately 1% of patients, can be caused by leaflet entrapment,[74] tearing,[75] disruption,[76] or possibly stretching of the anulus with failure to coapt during diastole.[77,78] Other complications include aortic-root rupture,[79,80] possibly more likely if the diameter of the balloon(s) exceeds the diameter of the aortic root (or anulus) in a calcified aorta (Fig. 15–6). Severe MR due to chordal disruption also has been reported;[81] this is due to passage of guidewire and balloon through the submitral apparatus and can also be caused by failing to keep the balloon properly positioned during antegrade aortic valvuloplasty.

Residual atrial septal defect, frequently reported in mitral valvuloplasty, also

Table 15–2. Risk and Etiology of Complications after Aortic
or Mitral Valvuloplasty in Adults

	Aortic Valvuloplasty		Mitral Valvuloplasty	
Complication	Incidence	Common Etiologies	Incidence	Common Etiologies
Death: acute follow-up	4%–9%[194] 23% (7 mo)[54]	Myocardial ischemia and stunning; trauma to heart or aorta; emboli; vascular complications. Low-output state, procedure-related complications, poor final valve area are predisposing factors.	1%[146] 3% (1 mo)	Tamponade; myocardial rupture; embolic events. High echo scores and low valve areas appear to be risk factors.
Stroke	1%[53]	Interruption cranial blood flow; calcific debris emboli.	2%[110]	Embolus from left atrial clot.
Myocardial infarction	2%[83]	↓ coronary blood flow; high wall stress; coronary embolus.	Rare	↓ coronary blood flow; coronary embolus.
Vascular injury	12%[195]	Large catheters in femoral arteries; withdrawal of balloons.	Rare	
Tamponade	2%[35]	Trauma to left ventricle from guidewire or balloon.	1%–3%[140]	Perforation during transseptal puncture; trauma from guidewire or balloons.
Severe regurgitation	1%–2%[83]	Leaflet entrapment, tearing, disruption, stretching of anulus with failure to coapt.	2%[101]	Leaflet avulsion, tearing, disruption of submitral apparatus, failure of leaflets to coapt, edema or ischemia of papillary muscles.
Atrial septal defect	Rare[82]	Torn septum during catheter passage or septal predilation; patency maintained by left atrial > right atrial pressure. Occurs only with antegrade approach.	3%[196]	Torn septum during septal dilation; withdrawal of partly inflated balloon; simultaneous withdrawal of balloons; balloon too proximal during inflation; balloons through two septostomy sites;[122] residual mitral gradient with shunt driven by left atrial > right atrial pressure.

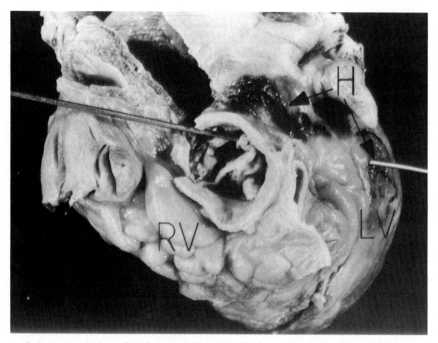

Figure 15–6. Anatomic view of aortic rupture caused by aortic valvuloplasty with an oversized balloon. The stylet is placed through the perforation; tear starts just above the aortic valve ring, follows the left main stem, and penetrates to the subepicardium. Subepicardial hemorrhage (H) can be seen. RV = right ventricle; LV = left ventricle. (From Vrolix et al.[80], with permission.)

has been reported after antegrade aortic valvuloplasty.[82] The high incidence of peripheral vascular complications reported in early series (≥10%),[35,83] including related mortality,[30] appears to have been addressed by improved technology, obviating the need for a femoral cutdown.[84] Inhospital mortality associated with aortic valvuloplasty has been reported to range from 3.5%[35] to 11.9%, the latter in a population with low cardiac output and low gradient.[85]

MITRAL VALVULOPLASTY

The typical patients undergoing percutaneous balloon mitral valvuloplasty (PBMV) are substantially younger than those undergoing aortic valvuloplasty. The relative success of PBMV, like the relatively mediocre result of aortic valvuloplasty, was predictable from the surgical literature: closed commissurotomy, performed since 1923,[86] had excellent early and long-term results,[1,2,87] but has been largely supplanted by open commissurotomy in much of the world, despite lack of evidence that open commissurotomy is superior in ideal populations.[88]

Early Experience

Inoue and colleagues[89] originally developed a "pillow-shaped" balloon constructed of rubber tubing for atrial septostomy; this balloon was adapted for mitral valvuloplasty and the results in six adult patients were reported in 1984.[8] The procedure was "successful" in five of the six, with a mean gradient reduction of 53%. In 1985, Lock and associates[90] dilated mitral valves in eight children in India using a conventional single-balloon technique; they achieved an improvement in valve area from 0.7 ± 0.3 to 1.3 ± 0.3 cm² and a mean decrease in valve gradient of 54%. Subsequently, al Zaibag and coworkers[91] introduced a double-balloon technique (see "technique variations") and also demonstrated that the procedure could be performed with relative safety with guidewires coiled in the left ventricular apex rather than advanced into the descending aorta. The latter substantially shortens the procedure. Excluding their unsuccessful cases, the author reported >100% improvement in mitral valve area and >80% reduction in gradient (final gradient 1.9 ± 1.7 mm Hg) without development of significant MR—exceptional results. In elderly patients with calcified mitral valves, gradient reduction of ≥50% and mitral valve area increases of ≥100% were reported, especially after the introduction of the double-balloon technique.[92-95]

Describing an adult population (mean age 49) of 35 patients with mitral stenosis undergoing balloon valvuloplasty, Palacios and colleagues[96] described a mean gradient decrease from 18 ± 1 mm Hg to 7 ± 1 mm Hg and mean mitral valve area increase from 0.8 ± 0.1 to 1.7 ± 0.2 cm². In this study, the initial patients underwent single-balloon dilation of the mitral valve; they then modified the technique of al Zaibag by introducing two balloons through a single septostomy site. In a subsequent analysis of 100 patients undergoing PBMV,[97] they noted postprocedure mitral valve areas 0.5 cm² greater when two balloons were used (Fig. 15–7), an increment that may result either from a larger balloon surface area (and independent of whether one large or two smaller balloons are used) or the more anatomic placement of two balloons in an elliptic opening.

Early in the PBMV experience, it became apparent that subvalvular disease, leaflet calcification, and leaflet mobility were predictors of poor outcome.[98] The

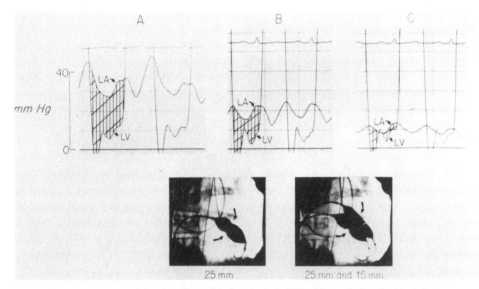

Figure 15–7. Hemodynamics at baseline (*A*), after single balloon (*B*), and after double balloon valvuloplasty (*C*). Arrows point to waist in balloon(s) during inflation. LV = left ventricular pressure; LA = left atrial pressure (mm Hg). (From Palacios et al.[96], with permission.)

Table 15–3. Echo Scoring System before Mitral
Valvuloplasty

Grade	Mobility	Subvalvular Thickening	Thickening	Calcification
1	Highly mobile valve with only leaflet tips restricted	Minimal thickening just below the mitral leaflets	Leaflets near normal in thickness (4–5 mm)	A single area of increased echo brightness
2	Leaflet mid and base portions have normal mobility	Thickening of chordal structures extending up to one third of the chordal length	Mid-leaflets normal, considerable thickening of margins (5–8 mm)	Scattered areas of brightness confined to leaflet margins
3	Valve continues to move forward in diastole, mainly from the base	Thickening extending to the distal third of the chords	Thickening extending through the entire leaflet (5–8 mm)	Brightness extending into the mid-portion of the leaflets
4	No or minimal forward movement of the leaflets in diastole	Extensive thickening and shortening of all chordal structures extending down to the papillary muscles	Considerable thickening of all leaflet tissue (>8–10 mm)	Extensive brightness throughout much of the leaflet tissue

Source: From Wilkins et al,[191] p. 300 with permission.

scoring system developed by Abascal and colleagues[99] encompasses the most commonly used noninvasive screening criteria (Table 15–3). This system assigns a maximum of 4 points to each of four parameters: leaflet mobility, subvalvular thickening, leaflet thickening, and leaflet calcification. Patients with echo scores ≤8 appear to have the best results, those with scores >12 the least favorable. The scoring system has been applied to larger series of patients, and its value confirmed,[100] although there is substantial individual variability. High echo scores do not predict occurrence of postprocedure MR;[101,102] only the surface area of the inflated balloons has shown a correlation.[103] Balloon surface area also has been shown to correlate with effectiveness of valve dilation.[100,104] There does appear to be a higher rate of restenosis when the echo score if >8;[97] in a 4-year follow-up of 320 patients, those with echo scores >8 had significantly higher mortality, need for mitral valve replacement, and had higher New York Heart Association (NYHA) classification (Figure 15–8).[105]

LARGER SERIES AND FOLLOW-UP STUDIES

Unlike the disappointing follow-up after aortic valvuloplasty, patients subjected to PBMV sustained their initial hemodynamic improvement. Restenosis appears to occur primarily in a population whose preprocedure evaluation (see above) predicts suboptimal results on the basis of leaflet or subvalvular disease anatomy. Palacios and coworkers[97] found mean valve areas of 0.9 ± 0.1 cm^2 at baseline, 1.9 ± 0.1 cm^2 immediately postvalvuloplasty, and 2.0 ± 0.1 cm^2 at 13 months average follow-up in 29 patients with echo scores ≤8. By contrast, 10 patients with echo scores >8 had valve areas of 0.9 ± 0.1, 1.8 ± 0.1, and 1.1 ± 0.1 cm^2, respectively. Reporting cardiac catheterization 8-month follow-up in 92 of 100 patients, we found sustained improvement in a young (mean age 27) popula-

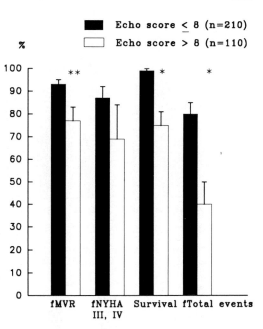

Echo score ≤ 8 (n=210)
Echo score > 8 (n=110)

Figure 15–8. Influence of echo score on follow-up (mean 20 ± 1 months) of 320 patients after mitral valvuloplasty. fMVR = freedom from mitral valve replacement. fNYHA III,IV = freedom from New York Heart Association classification III or IV. fTotal events = freedom from death, MVR, or NYHA III, IV. * = $p < 0.0001$, ** = $p < 0.002$ echo score ≤ 8 vs echo score > 8. (Adapted from Palacios et al.[105])

tion with mean echo score of 7 and no difference in early or intermediate results between balloon valvuloplasty and closed or open commissurotomy (Fig. 15–9).[106,107]

Based on the surgical closed commissurotomy experience, restenosis after PBMV can be expected to occur ≥5 years after valvuloplasty;[108] median reoperation time after open commissurotomy was 8 years.[109] Early restenosis after PBMV appears to occur primarily in patients with suboptimal initial results.[110] PBMV for restenosis after surgical commissurotomy has been reported in 90 patients; the procedure was successful (valve area >1.5 cm²) in 68. At 18 months follow-up, mean valve area was unchanged and only two patients demonstrated restenosis. However, the success rate is lower and need for mitral valve replacement higher (3 patients) than initial mitral dilations.[111]

INDICATIONS

We consider balloon valvuloplasty clearly indicated for patients with echo scores ≤8, in sinus rhythm, and without evidence of clot in the left atrium. Because the procedure is still considered experimental in the United States, we emphasize to patients that surgery is the standard alternative. For patients with echo scores ≥12, or moderate MR or AR, we prefer to recommend surgery if the patient is a reasonable risk. We have had good results with PBMV in patients with pulmonary hypertension (including pulmonary systolic pressure >100 mm Hg) who were thought to be inoperable on that basis.

Mitral stenosis is frequently first diagnosed or precipitates severe clinical symptoms during pregnancy;[112] successful PBMV has been reported by a number of groups.[113–116]

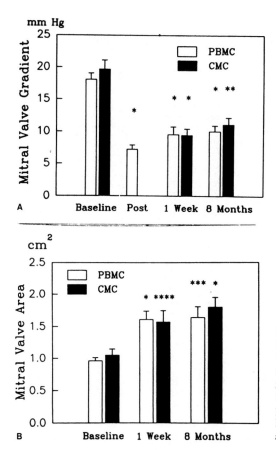

Figure 15-9. Mitral valve gradient (*A*) and mitral valve area (*B*) from cardiac catheterization data at baseline, 1 week and 8 months after balloon valvuloplasty (PBMC) and surgical closed mitral commissurotomy (CMC) in a randomized prospective trial. Immediate post-valvuloplasty gradient is shown for balloon commissurotomy only. (From Turi et al.,[106] with permission.)

PREPROCEDURE EVALUATION

The ideal patients for PBMV have no history of embolic phenomena, are in sinus rhythm, have at most moderate pulmonary hypertension, mild MR, a quiet precordium (suggesting absence of significant MR or AR), and a well-preserved first heart sound. In my experience, the latter is the single most useful physical finding to suggest absence of severe subvalvular disease.

The introduction of transesophageal echocardiography (TEE) has greatly increased the sensitivity to detect thrombus, particularly in the left atrium and the left atrial appendage.[117] Inasmuch as clot has been reported in patients with mitral stenosis in normal sinus rhythm[118] along with a high incidence of cerebral embolism,[119] I believe that all patients undergoing PBMV should have TEE if possible, although my colleagues and I have performed several hundred mitral valvuloplasties in patients with sinus rhythm without prior TEE and without known emboli. If clot is detected, the patient should have a minimum of 6 months anticoagulation and repeat TEE; serious consideration should be given to open commissurotomy as an alternative, although PBMV without complication has been performed in this setting after apparent clot resolution.[120]

As with aortic valvuloplasty, we believe that preprocedure cardiac catheterization is valuable in the patient being considered for mitral valvuloplasty. We prefer to perform diagnostic catheterization in a separate setting, particularly if angiography is performed, to allow dye to clear and the patient's cardiac and renal function to recover. Although Doppler-derived mitral valve gradients and areas are relatively accurate prevalvuloplasty,[121] coronary angiography is valuable for the safe conduct of PBMV in older patients. In young patients without other confounding issues, the hemodynamics obtained during valvuloplasty should be adequate to confirm the severity of stenosis.

TECHNICAL APPROACH

We routinely place an 8F sheath in the left femoral vein for diagnostic right heart catheterization, a 6F sheath in the left femoral artery for blood pressure monitoring, and an 8F sheath in the right femoral vein for access prior to transseptal catheterization. The initial right heart catheterization includes oxygen saturation measurement in the superior vena cava and pulmonary artery to exclude significant baseline left-to-right shunting and a determination of pulmonary wedge pressure (helpful when confirming that the transseptal needle pressure reflects left atrial pressure). The right heart catheter is also helpful as a landmark when performing transseptal puncture and provides useful hemodynamics throughout the procedure. The left femoral artery sheath provides access for a left ventricular catheter; we use this to measure transmitral gradient at the end of the procedure, avoiding having any catheters in place across the mitral valve.

After the right heart catheterization and before heparinization, we place a 0.032 inch guidewire through the right femoral vein sheath into the superior vena cava and exchange an 8F Mullins sheath (with a sidearm for pressure monitoring), then use standard technique to perform transseptal puncture. Once the sheath has been advanced into the left atrium, we administer 5000 U of intravenous heparin and place a 7F balloon flotation catheter through the sheath across the mitral valve, being careful to have the balloon inflated before advancing the catheter into the left ventricle. We feel the latter is essential protection against advancing through the submitral apparatus and causing subsequent severe MR. After a second 5000 U of heparin are given and the activating clotting time confirmed to be >300 seconds, we advance into the apex of the left ventricle a 0.035-inch Amplatz extra-stiff exchange length guidewire that has had a curve formed in the end similar to the one described for aortic valvuloplasty and a second gentle curve somewhat more proximally. The guidewire appearance needs to be identical to that seen in Figure 15–10 in order to provide adequate tracking for the valvuloplasty balloons and freedom from sustained arrhythmias. (Alternatively, the second wire can be placed through the Mullins sheath advanced into the left ventricle.) Extensive runs of ventricular tachycardia are occasionally encountered during this phase of the procedure; careful attention to maintaining the shape of the distal guidewire and occasional use of small amounts of intravenous lidocaine (≤ 50 mg) will usually suppress the arrhythmias. The Mullins sheath and balloon flotation catheter are removed at this point, leaving only the wire protruding from the femoral vein, over which a 5-mm peripheral balloon angioplasty catheter is passed and the septum dilated. A Block parallel lumen catheter (Mansfield, Watertown, MA) is advanced over the wire into the left ventricle. The second lumen is used to place a second, identical Amplatz wire.

At this point in the procedure, we have modified our technique to reflect the experience of surgeons performing closed mitral commissurotomy, in which the

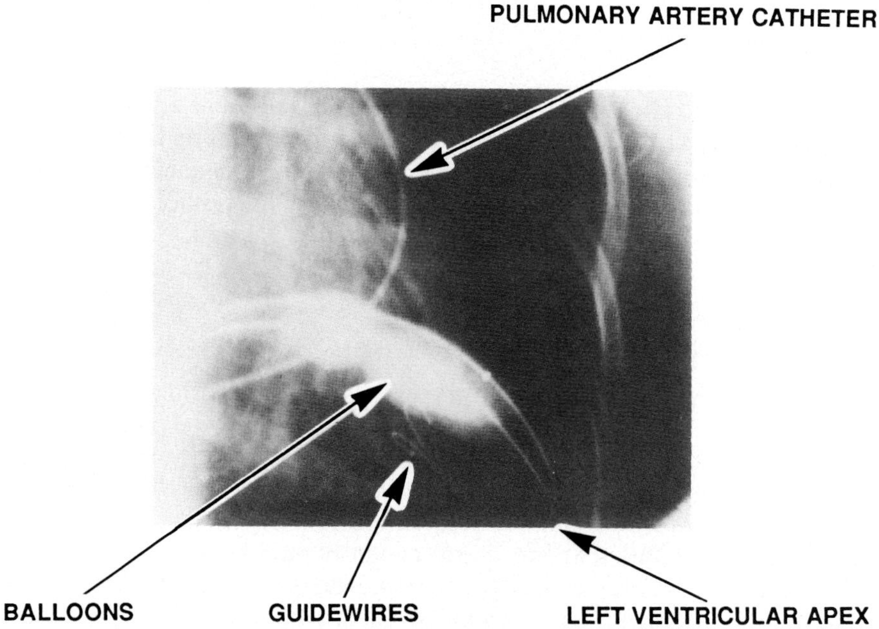

A

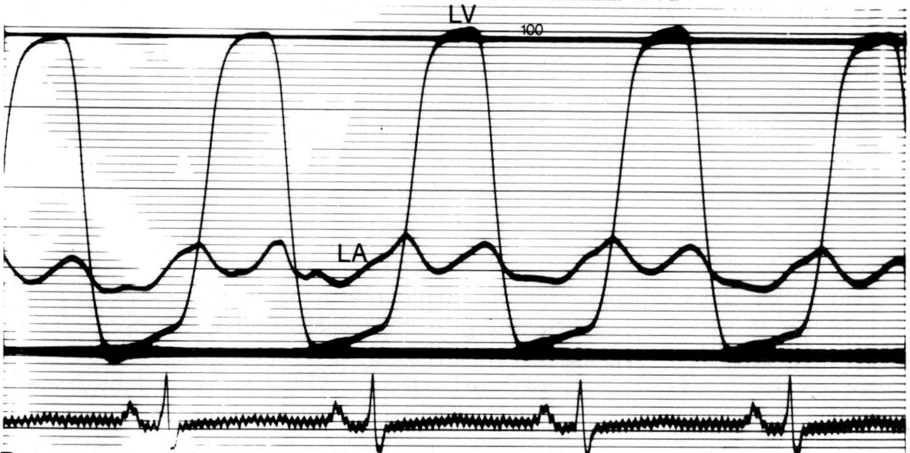

B

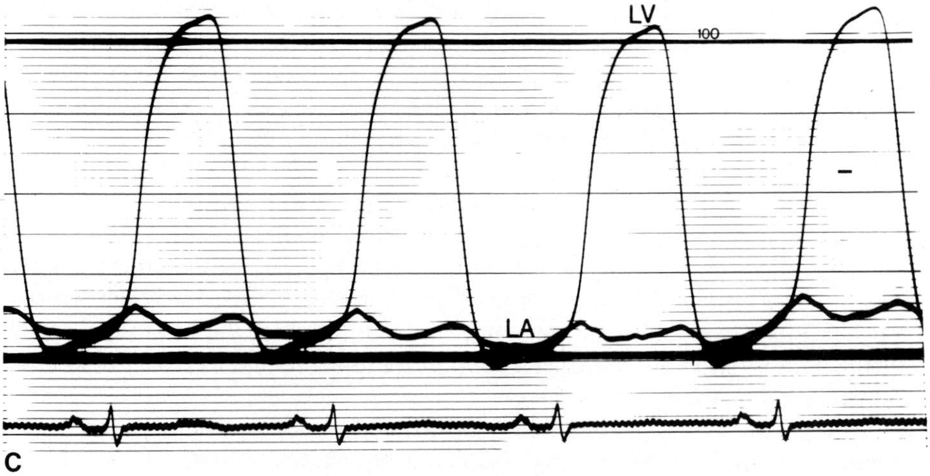

C

Figure 15–10. See legend on opposite page.

typical Tubbs dilator is stretched to a moderate position only. If no regurgitant jet is felt by the surgeon's finger in the left atrium, the dilator is stretched further, until full opening is achieved or MR becomes evident. Similarly, we typically advance one 20-mm and one 15-mm balloon across the mitral orifice of an average-sized individual; balloon inflation is performed simultaneous using a 1:8 contrast mixture to minimize viscosity and balloon inflation-deflation times. The balloons are then withdrawn in tandem (withdrawing simultaneously may predispose to residual atrial septal defects[122]), and hemodynamics are determined. If the residual gradient is ≥ 10 mm Hg and there is no hemodynamic evidence of increasing regurgitation, an 18-mm balloon is substituted for the 15 mm, and the two balloons are readvanced. We rarely go beyond the use of two 20-mm balloons.

At the end of the procedure, we withdraw one wire and both balloons completely, place a sheath over the second wire, and insert a diagnostic catheter over the remaining wire into the left atrium. A 5F pigtail is advanced retrograde into the left ventricle, and final hemodynamics are obtained. After transseptal pullback, a final oxygen saturation run is performed to assess for left-to-right shunting. In the typical patient, sheaths are withdrawn 4 or more hours after the procedure when the activating clotting time is <200 seconds; in most cases heparin is restarted, and the patient is placed on oral anticoagulation.

As with aortic valvuloplasty, postprocedure patient evaluation is complicated by the weaker correlation between echo-Doppler data and hemodynamics determined during cardiac catheterization after valvuloplasty.[98,123] However, Doppler measurements made late after PBMV correlate better with catheterization data.[124] This may be due to changes in left atrial compliance after valvuloplasty,[125] and to limitations of the Gorlin formula in the setting of MR, the latter a setting in which the pressure half-time may be particularly valuable.[126] Hemodynamics 1 week after PBMV demonstrate a trend toward slight increase in gradient and reduced valve area, also suggesting early recoil.[106] A residual atrial septal defect may decompress the left atrium, yielding a decrease in mitral valve gradient and a factitious improvement in mitral valve area; in addition, the resultant increase in pulmonary blood flow may suggest an additional increase in mitral valve area if a pulmonary catheter thermal dilution technique is used to assess cardiac output. Postprocedure echo helps exclude significant iatrogenically induced MR or atrial septal defect.

TECHNIQUE VARIATIONS

The unique balloon design developed by Inoue and associates[8] inflates distally first and has a barbell shape, securing the balloon in a relatively ideal position across the mitral valve and preventing forward or retrograde motion of the inflated balloon (Fig. 15–11). Its relative advantages are theoretical prevention of trauma to the ventricular apex or atrial septum; its potential drawbacks include the deployment of a spherical balloon in an elliptical orifice. Other balloon types used for PBMV have included a single large balloon[127] and bifoil and trefoil balloons.[128] A

Figure 15–10. Simplified double balloon technique with parallel wires in apex of ventricle in a patient undergoing mitral valvuloplasty (*A*); associated pre- (*B*) and postprocedure hemodynamics (*C*). LA = left atrial pressure; LV = left ventricular pressure (mm Hg). Hemodynamic tracings all at 100 mm Hg scale; courtesy of Dr. B. Soma Raju, Nizam's Institute of Medical Sciences, Hyderabad, India. (Angiogram from Turi,[190] with permission.)

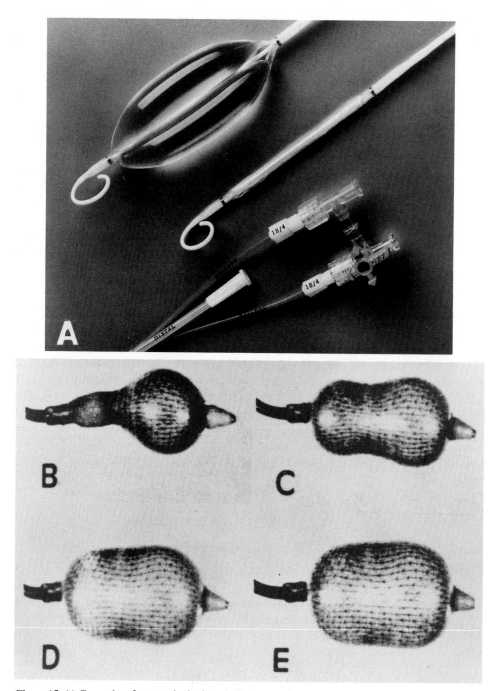

Figure 15–11. Examples of some valvuloplasty balloons used in mitral valvuloplasty: (*A*) Mansfield double balloon (Courtesy Mansfield Scientific, Watertown, MA); Inoue balloon with distal inflation first (*B*); then proximal segment (*C*); then progressive complete inflation (*D–E*). (From Inoue et al.,[8] with permission.)

comparison of balloon types revealed no difference in valve areas,[129,130] but bifoil balloons were associated with lower success rate than double balloons and a higher incidence of postprocedure MR and atrial septal defect than Inoue balloons. Another variation is the placement of two balloons via two transseptal punctures;[91] the potential drawback of this technique, besides the addition of a second transseptal puncture, is the apparent greater incidence of iatrogenically induced atrial septal defect.[122] A technique involving passage of balloons retrograde across the mitral valve, via a wire originally positioned transseptally from the femoral vein into the descending aorta, has the potential advantage of avoiding the placement of catheter shafts or balloons across the interatrial septum; the technique has several drawbacks, including potential trauma to two femoral arteries, and the need to perform a more complex procedure.[94] Finally, PBMV via a retrograde approach without transseptal puncture has been reported.[131,132]

Intraprocedural TEE has been suggested to facilitate transseptal puncture[133] and to guide the positioning of balloons.[134,135] I believe that neither indication outweighs the small risks and discomfort of TEE if PBMV is performed by experienced cardiologists.

COMPLICATIONS

Mitral valvuloplasty is associated with a significant complication rate. This is in part due to the technical complexity of the procedure; the biggest single source of misadventure is the transseptal puncture. Transseptal catheterization is rarely performed in most adult cardiovascular laboratories; this procedure requires training and regular performance to maintain skills and prevent serious morbidity.[136] The complications of transseptal catheterization during PBMV include a pericardial tamponade (see general considerations at the end of this chapter), residual atrial septal defect, cerebral embolization, iatrogenically induced aortic–right atrial fistula, and death. Transseptal puncture in mitral stenosis is made somewhat more difficult by distorted left atrial anatomy, frequently including a stretched foramen and a thickened interatrial septum.[137] Left-to-right shunting secondary to an iatrogenic atrial septal defect is detected in the majority of patients[138] if sensitive techniques are used. Most shunts resolve within weeks or months, and need for surgical repair is rare; however, right heart failure has been reported.[139]

Tamponade occurs in ≤3% of patients undergoing PBMV but much more frequently with relatively inexperienced operators;[140] in larger series ≤1% can be expected. The most common etiologies are inadvertent entry into the pericardium, injudicious advancement of the transseptal apparatus after entering the left atrium, tear of the base of the septum during balloon dilation (more likely to occur if the septal puncture is low), and "harpooning" of a balloon or guidewire through the ventricular apex during valvuloplasty. The likelihood of the latter is decreased when two balloons, the Inoue balloon, or a trefoil/regular balloon combination is used.[141] Vigorous anticoagulation during the procedure and manipulation of the septum and heart during balloon inflation predispose to pericardial hemorrhage; it can occur at any time during and in the early period after PBMV.[142–144]

Mitral regurgitation after balloon valvuloplasty has several possible etiologies: disruption of the submitral apparatus, avulsion of the mitral leaflets, failure of the leaflets to coapt early after valvuloplasty, or edema or ischemia of the papillary muscles. Myocardial ischemia is induced during balloon valvuloplasty by hypotension and concurrent decrease in coronary blood flow, and occasionally by coronary artery embolism.[145] Stroke or death occurs in 1% to 2% of mitral valvuloplasty patients;[140] operator experience and clinical status of the patient contribute significantly. The National Heart, Lung, and Blood Institute Registry of 737 patients includes 1% catheterization lab mortality, with a high echo score and severely stenosed valves as predictors.[146]

VALVULOPLASTY OF PULMONIC, TRICUSPID, AND BIOPROSTHETIC VALVES

PULMONIC VALVES

Pulmonic stenosis, when caused by congenital commissural fusion rather than dysplasia, is particularly amenable to balloon valvuloplasty. Deployment of devices is technically easy, fused commissures are the primary pathology in young patients, secondary regurgitation is typically well tolerated, and there is a background of excellent results after surgical commissurotomy with rare restenosis.[147]

Credit for the first balloon valvuloplasty goes to Semb and coworkers[7] although the technique is radically different from subsequent approaches; a balloon catheter was withdrawn from the pulmonary artery to the right ventricle to "rupture" the pulmonic valve. Kan and coworkers[148] used a more conventional balloon technique, straddling the pulmonary valve during dilation. The modern technique initially involved single balloons matched in size to the valve anulus;[149] subsequent introduction of oversized balloons (20% to 30% larger than the anulus) appears to have increased gradient reduction and decreased restenosis rate[150] without increasing complications.[151] In adolescents and adults, single balloons generally are too small; the double-balloon technique allows larger effective balloon size[152] as well as theoretically allowing forward blood flow between the inflated balloons and diminishing systemic hypotension.[153,154]

Results of balloon pulmonary valvuloplasty in 784 patients[155] included reduction of pulmonary outflow systolic gradients from 71 ± 33 to 28 ± 21 mm Hg, mortality of 0.2%, and total major complication rate of only 0.6%. Balloon valvotomy of calcified pulmonic valves in adults appears to be equally effective,[153,156] although pulmonic valvuloplasty in the elderly has been reported only sporadically.[157] In general, complication rates of pulmonic valvuloplasty may be lower than for surgery (surgical mortality has been reported as approximately 3%,)[158] although this is not a matched population, and restenosis appears to be uncommon. Thus, balloon valvuloplasty has become the procedure of choice and is indicated in patients with gradients ≥ 50 mm Hg; the major contraindication appears to be a hypoplastic valve anulus.

TRICUSPID VALVES

The physiology of the obstructed tricuspid valve, like the mitral valve, is typically secondary to rheumatic heart disease, and involves fused leaflets. Using a double-balloon technique,[159] several case reports have presented excellent hemodynamic improvement,[160,161] although there appears to be less benefit in patients with moderate tricuspid regurgitation.[162] Because the surgical experience with tricuspid commissurotomy has been associated with good relief of obstruction but significant tricuspid regurgitation, caution is advised until more experience is reported.

BIOPROSTHETIC VALVES

Bioprosthetic valve stenosis is typically the result of calcific deposition and secondary leaflet noncompliance.[163] Balloon valvuloplasties of bioprostheses in the tricuspid, pulmonic, mitral, and aortic position as well as valves in extracardiac conduits have been reported.

Initial results dilating tricuspid bioprostheses[164,165] have been promising, but the only follow-up report to date[166] demonstrated early recurrence; examination of the valve revealed rigid calcification, no leaflet fusion, and no anatomic evidence of the valvuloplasty—results similar to restenosed calcified native aortic valves. Successful tricuspid valvuloplasty in a patient with fungal endocarditis[167] and double-balloon dilation has been reported.[168] Similar results were noted in three reports of mitral bioprosthesis dilation.[169-171] One-year follow-up showed sustained improvement.[172] Balloon dilation of stenotic bioprosthetic aortic,[173] pulmonary,[174] and conduit valves[175] has been reported as successful, although high failure rate and high restenosis rate also have been reported in the latter.[176]

McKay and colleagues[177] reported two unsuccessful aortic valve bioprosthesis dilations, one resulting in valve replacement and one in death. Pathologic examination revealed cuspal tears and perforations and broken and friable calcium deposits. Because of concern regarding embolization, a mitral prosthetic valvuloplasty has been reported in which a debris-catching device was deployed.[178]

MULTIVALVE DILATION

Combined valvuloplasty of both stenotic mitral and aortic valves was reported by Kritzer and associates,[179] and subsequently by Berman and coworkers.[180] Two series totaling 16 patients[180,181] were generally successful. Combined dilation of rheumatic mitral and tricuspid stenosis,[182,183] apparent pulmonary and tricuspid stenosis,[184] and aortic, mitral, and tricuspid stenosis[185] also have been described. In general, dilation of a valve proximal to a second stenosis can result in proximal volume overload and heart failure (e.g., dilation of a stenosed mitral valve before relieving aortic outflow obstruction). Hence, I prefer to dilate the most distal valve first, typically the aortic and then the mitral valve. Occasionally, a patient may not tolerate lying flat until mitral stenosis is relieved[180] and valvuloplasty of a mitral valve before aortic valve dilation has been performed without incident.[179]

GENERAL CONSIDERATIONS

Oral anticoagulation is discontinued several days before the procedure; we prefer prothrombin times to be ≤25% elevated preprocedure. Heparin is discontinued at least 4 hours in advance and transseptal puncture is performed only if the activating clotting time is <170 seconds. We prescribe antiplatelet drugs (aspirin and dipyridamole) before valvuloplasty. Except for mitral valvuloplasty or in patients with atrial fibrillation, heparin and antiplatelet drugs are not continued postprocedure.

A cardiac surgeon, operating room, and perfusion team are on standby for every case, although in our experience emergency surgery is rarely necessary. Because tamponade is a potential complication of *every* valvuloplasty, a pericardiocentesis kit should be readily available, and any bout of hypotension or bradycardia should raise a suspicion of tamponade; continuous monitoring of left atrial or pulmonary artery pressure along with systemic pressure and fluoroscopy of the left heart border (looking for a characteristic absence of left heart border motion) should allow prompt diagnosis. Tamponade during valvuloplasty occurs very quickly and, except for myocardial rupture caused by a valvuloplasty balloon, is usually readily treated by pericardiocentesis.

Patients after valvuloplasty may have transiently decreased cardiac output due to ischemia or valvular regurgitation and may have fluctuations in vascular loading conditions and renal blood flow due to blood loss, changes in levels of atrial natriuretic peptides, vasopressin,[186,187] and activation of the renin angiotensin system.[188] Some patients will demonstrate dramatic diuresis postvalvuloplasty; this should be anticipated, and careful attention needs to be paid to fluid management in the first 24 hours.

COST COMPARISON

My colleagues and I compared the cost of percutaneous balloon mitral valvuloplasty and closed mitral commissurotomy.[106] In the United States, the cost of

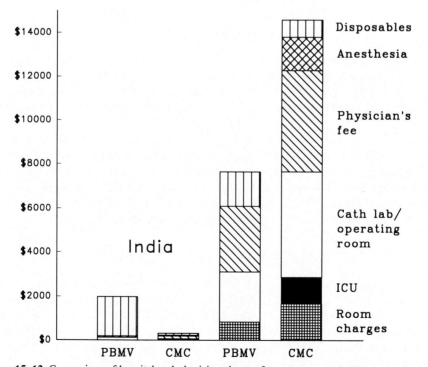

Figure 15–12. Comparison of hospital and physician charges for percutaneous balloon mitral valvuloplasty (PBMV) and surgical closed mitral commissurotomy (CMC) in India and the United States. (Adapted from Turi et al.[106])

balloon valvuloplasty was half that of commissurotomy, primarily because of the shorter hospital stay and lower physician and hospital fees. These costs were compared with charges in a representative institution in India. The cost of valvuloplasty was six times greater than for surgery (Fig. 15–12). The difference is explained by the disproportionately lower cost of hospital stay and physician's fees in India and the relatively high cost of disposables in developing countries.

Thus, despite initially optimistic pronouncements[40] that balloon valvuloplasty will significantly improve care for rheumatic valve disease in developing countries, the low cost and excellent results of closed commissurotomy continue to make it the procedure of choice in many parts of the world where valvular heart disease is prevalent.[189] Development of cheaper and possibly reusable technology is needed.

ACKNOWLEDGMENT

I wish to thank Luis Tami, M.D. for providing translation from Spanish[4] and Dr. Suryadavera Rao for obtaining references.

REFERENCES

1. Bailey, CP: The surgical treatment of mitral stenosis (mitral commissurotomy). Dis Chest 15:377, 1949.
2. Harken, DE: The surgical treatment of mitral stenosis. N Engl J Med 239:801, 1948.
3. Baker, C, Brock, RC, and Campbell, M: Valvulotomy for mitral stenosis. Br Med J 1283, 1950.
4. Rubio-Alvarez, V and Limon-Lason, R: Comisurotomia tricuspidea por medio de un cateter modificado. Archivos del Instituto de Cardiologia de Mexico 25:57, 1955.
5. Rashkind, WJ and Miller, WW: Creation of an atrial septal defect without thoracotomy. J Am Med Assoc 196:991, 1966.
6. Gruntzig, AR, Senning, A, and Siegenthaler, WE: Nonoperative dilatation of coronary-artery stenosis: Percutaneous transluminal coronary angioplasty. N Engl J Med 301:61, 1979.
7. Semb, BK, Tjonneland, S, Stake, G, et al: "Balloon valvulotomy" of congenital pulmonary valve stenosis with tricuspid valve insufficiency. Cardiovasc Radiol 2:239, 1979.
8. Inoue, K, Owaki, T, Nakamura, T, et al: Clinical application of transvenous mitral commissurotomy by a new balloon catheter. J Thorac Cardiovasc Surg 87:394, 1984.
9. Lababidi, Z, Wu, JR, and Walls, JT. Percutaneous balloon aortic valvuloplasty: Results in 23 patients. Am J Cardiol 53:194, 1984.
10. Cribier, A Savin, T, Saoudi, N, et al: Percutaneous transluminal valvuloplasty of acquired aortic stenosis in elderly patients: An alternative to valve replacement. Lancet 1:63, 1986.
11. Ribeiro, PA, al Zaibag, M, and Sawyer, W: Nomenclature for the use of balloon catheters (letter). Am J Cardiol 63:262, 1989.
12. Smucker, ML: Percutaneous mitral balloon valvulotomy or balloon valvuloplasty? It's not just semantics anymore (comment). Circulation 82:643, 1990.
13. McKay, RG, Safian, RD, Lock, JE, et al: Balloon dilatation of calcific aortic stenosis in elderly patients: Postmortem, intraoperative, and percutaneous valvuloplasty studies. Circulation 74:119, 1986.
14. Safian, RD, Mandell, VS, Thurer, RE, et al: Postmortem and intraoperative balloon valvuloplasty of calcific aortic stenosis in elderly patients: Mechanisms of successful dilation. J Am Coll Cardiol 9:655, 1987.
15. Robicsek, F and Harbold, NB, Jr: Limited value of balloon dilatation in calcified aortic stenosis in adults: Direct observations during open heart surgery. Am J Cardiol 60:857, 1987.
16. Isner, JM, Samuels, DA, Slovenkai, GA, et al: Mechanism of aortic balloon valvuloplasty: Fracture of valvular calcific deposits. Ann Intern Med 108:377, 1988.
17. Letac, B, Gerber, LI, and Koning, R. Insights on the mechanism of balloon valvuloplasty in aortic stenosis. Am J Cardiol 62:1241, 1988.

18. Kalan, JM, Mann, JM, Leon, MB, et al: Morphologic findings in stenotic aortic valves that have had "successful" percutaneous balloon valvuloplasty. Am J Cardiol 62:152, 1988.

19. Commeau, P, Grollier, G, Lamy, E, et al: Percutaneous balloon dilatation of calcific aortic valve stenosis: Anatomical and haemodynamic evaluation. Br Heart J 59:227, 1988.

20. Kennedy, KD, Hauck, AJ, Edwards, WD, et al: Mechanism of reduction of aortic valvular stenosis by percutaneous transluminal balloon valvuloplasty: Report of five cases and review of literature. Mayo Clin Proc 63:769, 1988.

21. Ribeiro, PA, al Zaibag, M, and Rajendran, V: Double balloon aortic valvotomy for rheumatic aortic stenosis: In vivo studies. Eur Heart J 10:417, 1989.

22. Perry, SB, Zeevi, B, Keane, JF, et al: Interventional catheterization of left heart lesions, including aortic and mitral valve stenosis and coarctation of the aorta. Cardiol Clin 7:341, 1989.

23. Kaplan, JD, Isner, JM, Karas, RH, et al: In vitro analysis of mechanisms of balloon valvuloplasty of stenotic mitral valves. Am J Cardiol 59:318, 1987.

24. Nabel, E, Bergin, PJ, and Kirsh, MM: Morphological analysis of balloon mitral valvuloplasty: Intra-operative results (abstract). J Am Coll Cardiol 15:97A, 1990.

25. Benedetti, M, Biagini, A, Anastasio, G, et al: Evaluation of in vivo morphological results of balloon mitral valvotomy. Eur J Cardiothorac Surg 4:337, 1990.

26. Ettedgui, JA, Ho, SY, Tynan, M, et al: The pathology of balloon pulmonary valvoplasty. Int J Cardiol 16:285, 1987.

27. Walls, JT, Lababidi, Z, and Curtis, JJ: Morphologic effects of percutaneous balloon pulmonary valvuloplasty. South Med J 80:475, 1987.

28. Ledesma Velasco, M, Verdin Vazquez, R, Acosta Valdez, JL, et al: Valvuloplasty with balloon catheter in biologic prosthesis. Reality or illusion. Arch Inst Cardiol Mex 59:69, 1989.

29. Harken, DE, Black, H, and Taylor, WJ: The surgical correction of calcific aortic stenosis in adults. Results in the first 100 consecutive transaortic valvuloplasties. J Thorac Surg 36:759, 1958.

30. Cribier, A, Savin, T, Berland, J, et al: Percutaneous transluminal balloon valvuloplasty of adult aortic stenosis: Report of 92 cases. J Am Coll Cardiol 9:381, 1987.

31. McKay, RG, Safian, RD, Lock, JE, et al: Assessment of left ventricular and aortic valve function after aortic balloon valvuloplasty in adult patients with critical aortic stenosis. Circulation 75:192, 1987.

32. Grossman, W and Baim, DS: Cardiac Catheterization, Angiography, and Intervention, ed. 4. Lea & Febiger, Philadelphia, 1991, p 504.

33. Cribier, A and Letac, B: Two years' experience of percutaneous balloon valvuloplasty in aortic stenosis. Herz 13:110, 1988.

34. Block, PC and Palacios, IF: Clinical and hemodynamic follow-up after percutaneous aortic valvuloplasty in the elderly. Am J Cardiol 62:760, 1988.

35. Safian, RD, Berman, AD, Diver, DJ, et al: Balloon aortic valvuloplasty in 170 consecutive patients. N Engl J Med 319:125, 1988.

36. Feldman, T, Glagov, S, Chiu, YC, et al: Second dilatation for restenosis following successful balloon aortic valvuloplasty (abstract). J Am Coll Cardiol 13:17A, 1989.

37. Gambino, A, Zeldis, SM, Goodman, M, et al: Early aortic valve restenosis after successful balloon valvuloplasty. Am Heart J 116:207, 1988.

38. Bashore, TM and Davidson, CJ: Follow-up recatheterization after balloon aortic valvuloplasty. Mansfield Scientific Aortic Valvuloplasty Registry Investigators. J Am Coll Cardiol 17:1188, 1991.

39. Davidson, CJ, Harrison, JK, Leithe, ME, et al: Left ventricular performance and clinical outcome after repeat balloon aortic valvuloplasty. Ann Intern Med 113:250, 1990.

40. Roberts, WC: Good-bye to thoracotomy for cardiac valvulotomy. Am J Cardiol 59:198, 1987.

41. Smucker, ML: Aortic valvuloplasty: Baby or bathwater. Cathet Cardiovasc Diagn 16:113, 1989.

42. Isner, JM: Aortic valvuloplasty: Are balloon-dilated valves all they are "cracked" up to be? Mayo Clin Proc 63:830, 1988.

43. Block, PC: Aortic valvuloplasty—A valid alternative? (editorial) N Engl J Med 319:169, 1988.

43a. Dash, H: Have balloon will travel: expanded indications for nonoperative intravascular balloon dilation? J Am Coll Cardiol 9:387, 1987.

44. Robicsek, F, Harbold, NB, Jr, Daugherty, HK, et al: Balloon valvuloplasty in calcified aortic stenosis: A cause for caution and alarm. Ann Thorac Surg 45:515, 1988.

45. Letac, B and Cribier, A: Personal answer to a personal view on balloon aortic valvuloplasty (letter). Eur Heart J 9:195, 1988.

46. Bernard, Y, Bassand, JP, Anguenot, T, et al: Aortic valve area evolution after percutaneous aortic

valvuloplasty: A prospective trial using a combined Doppler echocardiographic and haemodynamic method. Eur Heart J 11:98, 1990.

47. Losordo, DW, Ramaswamy, K, Rosenfield, K, et al: Use of emergency balloon dilation to reverse acute hemodynamic decompensation developing during diagnostic catheterization for aortic stenosis (bailout valvuloplasty). Am J Cardiol 63:388, 1989.

48. Friedman, HZ, Cragg, DR, and O'Neill, WW: Cardiac resuscitation using emergency aortic balloon valvuloplasty. Am J Cardiol 63:387, 1989.

49. Desnoyers, MR, Salem, DN, Rosenfield, K, et al: Treatment of cardiogenic shock by emergency aortic balloon valvuloplasty. Ann Intern Med 108:833, 1988.

50. Levine, MJ, Berman, AD, Safian, RD, et al: Palliation of valvular aortic stenosis by balloon valvuloplasty as preoperative preparation for noncardiac surgery. Am J Cardiol 62:1309, 1988.

51. Goldman, L, Caldera, DL, Nussbaum, SR, et al: Multifactorial index of cardiac risk in noncardiac surgical procedures. N Engl J Med 297:845, 1977.

52. Cheitlin, MD: Severe aortic stenosis in the sick octogenarian. A clear indicator for balloon valvuloplasty as the initial procedure [comment]. Circulation 80:1906, 1989.

53. Letac, B, Cribier, A, Koning, R, et al: Aortic stenosis in elderly patients aged 80 or older. Treatment by percutaneous balloon valvuloplasty in a series of 92 cases [see comments]. Circulation 80:1514, 1989.

54. Reeder, GS, Nishimura, RA, and Holmes, DR, Jr: Patient age and results of balloon aortic valvuloplasty: The Mansfield Scientific Registry experience. The Mansfield Scientific Aortic Valvuloplasty Registry Investigators. J Am Coll Cardiol 17:909, 1991.

55. Edmunds, LH, Jr, Stephenson, LW, Edie, RN, et al: Open-heart surgery in octogenarians. N Engl J Med 319:131, 1988.

56. Craver, JM, Weintraub, WS, Jones, EL, et al: Predictors of mortality, complications, and length of stay in aortic valve replacement for aortic stenosis. Circulation 78:I85, 1988.

57. Culliford, AT, Galloway, AC, Colvin, SB, et al: Aortic valve replacement for aortic stenosis in persons aged 80 years and over. Am J Cardiol 67:1256, 1991.

58. Litvack, F, Jakubowski, AT, Buchbinder, NA, et al: Lack of sustained clinical improvement in an elderly population after percutaneous aortic valvuloplasty. Am J Cardiol 62:270, 1988.

59. Come, PC, Riley, MF, Safian, RD, et al: Usefulness of noninvasive assessment of aortic stenosis before and after percutaneous aortic valvuloplasty. Am J Cardiol 61:1300, 1988.

60. Romanello, PP, Moses, JW, Wilentz, JR, et al: Acute myocardial infarction complicating percutaneous aortic valvuloplasty successfully treated by percutaneous coronary angioplasty. Am Heart J 119:953, 1990.

61. Deligonul, U, Kern, MJ, Bell, ST, et al: Acute myocardial infarction during percutaneous aortic balloon valvuloplasty. Cathet Cardiovasc Diagn 15:164, 1988.

62. Harvey, JR, Wyman, RM, McKay, RG, et al: Use of balloon flotation pacing catheters for prophylactic temporary pacing during diagnostic and therapeutic catheterization procedures. Am J Cardiol 62:941, 1988.

63. Egeblad, H and Wennevold, A: Left ventricular function during balloon dilatation of the aortic valve in elderly patients: A blind study of echocardiograms. Br Heart J 63:32, 1990.

64. Block, PC and Palacios, IF: Comparison of hemodynamic results of anterograde versus retrograde percutaneous balloon aortic valvuloplasty. Am J Cardiol 60:659, 1987.

65. Dorros, G, Lewin, RF, King, JF, et al: Percutaneous transluminal valvuloplasty in calcific aortic stenosis: The double balloon technique. Cathet Cardiovasc Diagn 13:151, 1987.

66. Ribeiro, PA, al Zaibag, M, Halim, M, et al: Percutaneous single- and double-balloon aortic valvotomy in adolescents and young adults with congenital aortic stenosis. Eur Heart J 9:866, 1988.

67. Midei, MG, Brennan, M, Walford, GD, et al: Double vs single balloon technique for aortic balloon valvuloplasty. Chest 94:245, 1988.

68. Brinker, JA, Powers, E, Slater, J, et al: Influence of procedure variables on the acute hemodynamic results of balloon aortic valvuloplasty: A report of the NHLBI valvuloplasty registry (abstract). Circulation 82:III-78, 1990.

69. Meier, B, Friedli, B, and von Segesser, L: Valvuloplasty with trefoil and bifoil balloons and the long sheath technique. Herz 13:1, 1988.

70. Voudris, V, Drobinski, G, L'Epine, Y, et al: Results of percutaneous valvuloplasty for calcific aortic stenosis with different balloon catheters. Cathet Cardiovasc Diagn 17:80, 1989.

71. Heyndrickx, GR, Vanermen, H, Wellens, F, et al: Dilatation of stenotic aortic valves through a temporary vascular prosthesis on the subclavian artery. Am J Cardiol 60:1193, 1987.

72. Karnik, R, Valentin, A, Bonner, G, et al: Transcranial Doppler monitoring during percutaneous transluminal aortic valvuloplasty. Angiology 41:106, 1990.

73. Davidson, CJ, Skelton, TN, Kisslo, KB, et al: The risk for systemic embolization associated with percutaneous balloon valvuloplasty in adults. A prospective comprehensive evaluation. Ann Intern Med 108:557, 1988.

74. Treasure, CB, Schoen, FJ, Treseler, PA, et al: Leaflet entrapment causing acute severe aortic insufficiency during balloon aortic valvuloplasty. Clin Cardiol 12:405, 1989.

75. Lewin, RF, Dorros, G, King, JF, et al: Aortic annular tear after valvuloplasty: the role of aortic annulus echocardiographic measurement. Cathet Cardiovasc Diagn 16:123, 1989.

76. Seifert, PE and Auer, JE: Surgical repair of annular disruption following percutaneous balloon aortic valvuloplasty. Ann Thorac Surg 46:242, 1988.

77. Sadaniantz, A, Malhotra, R, and Korr, KS: Transient acute severe aortic regurgitation complicating balloon aortic valvuloplasty. Cathet Cardiovasc Diagn 17:186, 1989.

78. Dean, LS, Chandler, JW, Saenz, CB, et al: Severe aortic regurgitation complicating percutaneous aortic valve valvuloplasty. Cathet Cardiovasc Diagn 16:130, 1989.

79. Lembo, NJ, King, SB III, Roubin, GS, et al: Fatal aortic rupture during percutaneous balloon valvuloplasty for valvular aortic stenosis. Am J Cardiol 60:733, 1987.

80. Vrolix, M, Piessens, J, Moerman, P, et al: Fatal aortic rupture: An unusual complication of percutaneous balloon valvuloplasty for acquired valvular aortic stenosis. Cathet Cardiovasc Diagn 16:119, 1989.

81. de Ubago, JL, Vazquez de Prada, JA, Moujir, F, et al: Mitral valve rupture during percutaneous dilation of aortic valve stenosis. Cathet Cardiovasc Diagn 16:115, 1989.

82. Lemmer, JH, Jr, Winniford, MD, and Ferguson, DW: Surgical implications of atrial septal defect complicating aortic balloon valvuloplasty. Ann Thorac Surg 48:295, 1989.

83. Lewin, RF, Dorros, G, King, JF, et al: Percutaneous transluminal aortic valvuloplasty: acute outcome and follow-up of 125 patients. J Am Coll Cardiol 14:1210, 1989.

84. Isner, JM, Salem, DN, Desnoyers, MR, et al: Treatment of calcific aortic stenosis by balloon valvuloplasty. Am J Cardiol 59:313, 1987.

85. Nishimura, RA, Holmes, DR, Jr, and Michela, MA: Follow-up of patients with low output, low gradient hemodynamics after percutaneous balloon aortic valvuloplasty: The Mansfield Scientific Aortic Valvuloplasty Registry. J Am Coll Cardiol 17:828, 1991.

86. Cutler, EC and Levine, SA: Cardiotomy and valvulotomy for mitral stenosis. Boston Med Surg J 188:1023, 1923.

87. John, S, Bashi, VV, Jairaj, PS, et al: Closed mitral valvotomy: Early results and long-term follow-up of 3724 consecutive patients. Circulation 68:891, 1983.

88. Hickey, MS, Blackstone, EH, Kirklin, JW, et al: Outcome probabilities and life history after surgical mitral commissurotomy: Implications for balloon commissurotomy. J Am Coll Cardiol 17:29, 1991.

89. Inoue, K, Kitamura, F, Chikusa, H, et al: Atrial septostomy by a new balloon catheter. Jpn Circ J 45:730, 1981.

90. Lock, JE, Khalilullah, M, Shrivastava, S, et al: Percutaneous catheter commissurotomy in rheumatic mitral stenosis. N Engl J Med 313:1515, 1985.

91. al Zaibag, M, Ribeiro, PA, Al Kasab, S, et al: Percutaneous double-balloon mitral valvotomy for rheumatic mitral-valve stenosis. Lancet 1:757, 1986.

92. McKay, RG, Lock, JE, Keane, JF, et al: Percutaneous mitral valvuloplasty in an adult patient with calcific rheumatic mitral stenosis. J Am Coll Cardiol 7:1410, 1986.

93. Palacios, IF, Lock, JE, Keane, JF, et al: Percutaneous transvenous balloon valvotomy in a patient with severe calcific mitral stenosis. J Am Coll Cardiol 7:1416, 1986.

94. Babic, UU, Pejcic, P, Djurisic, Z, et al: Transarterial balloon mitral valvuloplasty. Z Kardiol 76:111, 1987.

95. McKay, CR, Kawanishi, DT, and Rahimtoola, SH: Catheter balloon valvuloplasty of the mitral valve in adults using a double-balloon technique. Early hemodynamic results. J Am Med Assoc 257:1753, 1987.

96. Palacios, I, Block, PC, Brandi, S, et al: Percutaneous balloon valvotomy for patients with severe mitral stenosis. Circulation 75:778, 1987.

97. Palacios, IF, Block, PC, Wilkins, GT, et al: Follow-up of patients undergoing percutaneous mitral balloon valvotomy. Analysis of factors determining restenosis. Circulation 79:573, 1989.

98. Reid, CL, McKay, CR, Chandraratna, PA, et al: Mechanisms of increase in mitral valve area and influence of anatomic features in double-balloon, catheter balloon valvuloplasty in adults with

rheumatic mitral stenosis: A Doppler and two-dimensional echocardiographic study. Circulation 76:628, 1987.

99. Abascal, VM, Wilkins, GT, Choong, CY, et al: Echocardiographic evaluation of mitral valve structure and function in patients followed for at least 6 months after percutaneous balloon mitral valvuloplasty. J Am Coll Cardiol 12:606, 1988.

100. Abascal, VM, Wilkins, GT, O'Shea, JP, et al: Prediction of successful outcome in 130 patients undergoing percutaneous balloon mitral valvotomy (comments). Circulation 82:448, 1990.

101. Pan, JP, Lin, SL, Go, JU, et al: Frequency and severity of mitral regurgitation one year after balloon mitral valvuloplasty. Am J Cardiol 67:264, 1991.

102. Abascal, VM, Wilkins, GT, Choong, CY, et al: Mitral regurgitation after percutaneous balloon mitral valvuloplasty in adults: Evaluation by pulsed Doppler echocardiography. J Am Coll Cardiol 11:257, 1988.

103. Roth, RB, Block, PC, and Palacios, IF: Predictors of increased mitral regurgitation after percutaneous mitral balloon valvotomy. Cathet Cardiovasc Diagn 20:17, 1990.

104. Reid, CL, Chandraratna, PA, Kawanishi, DT, et al: Influence of mitral valve morphology on double-balloon catheter balloon valvuloplasty in patients with mitral stenosis. Analysis of factors predicting immediate and 3-month results. Circulation 80:515, 1989.

105. Palacios, IF, Tuzcu, EM, Newell, JB, et al: Four year clinical follow-up of patients undergoing percutaneous mitral balloon valvotomy (abstract). Circulation 82:III-545, 1990.

106. Turi, ZG, Reyes, VP, Raju, BS, et al: Percutaneous balloon versus surgical closed commissurotomy for mitral stenosis. A prospective, randomized trial (comments). Circulation 83:1179, 1991.

107. Reyes, VP, Raju, BS, Turi, ZG, et al: Percutaneous balloon vs open surgical commissurotomy for mitral stenosis: A randomized trial (abstract). Circulation 82:III-545, 1990.

108. John, S, Perianayagam, WJ, Abraham, KA, et al: Restenosis of the mitral valve: Surgical considerations and results of operation. Ann Thorac Surg 25:316, 1978.

109. Housman, LB, Bonchek, L, Lamberg, L, et al: Prognosis of patients after open mitral commissurotomy. Actuarial analysis of late results in 100 patients. J Thorac Cardiovasc Surg 73:742, 1977.

110. Vahanian, A, Michel, PL, Cormier, B, et al: Results of percutaneous mitral commissurotomy in 200 patients. Am J Cardiol 63:847, 1989.

111. Vahanian, A, Michel, PL, Cormier, B, et al: Mid-term results of mitral balloon valvotomy for restenosis after surgical commissurotomy (abstract). Circulation 82:III-80, 1990.

112. Ueland, K: Pregnancy and cardiovascular disease. Med Clin North Am 61:17, 1977.

113. Palacios, IF, Block, PC, Wilkins, GT, et al: Percutaneous mitral balloon valvotomy during pregnancy in a patient with severe mitral stenosis. Cathet Cardiovasc Diagn 15:109, 1988.

114. Safian, RD, Berman, AD, Sachs, B, et al: Percutaneous balloon mitral valvuloplasty in a pregnant woman with mitral stenosis. Cathet Cardiovasc Diagn 15:103, 1988.

115. Mangione, JA, Zuliani, MF, Del Castillo, JM, et al: Percutaneous double balloon mitral valvuloplasty in pregnant women. Am J Cardiol 64:99, 1989.

116. Smith, R, Brender, D, and McCredie, M: Percutaneous transluminal balloon dilatation of the mitral valve in pregnancy. Br Heart J 61:551, 1989.

117. Casale, PN, Whitlow, P, Currie, PJ, et al: Transesophageal echocardiography in percutaneous balloon valvuloplasty for mitral stenosis. Cleve Clin J Med 56:597, 1989.

118. Kronzon, I, Tunick, PA, Glassman, E, et al: Transesophageal echocardiography to detect atrial clots in candidates for percutaneous transseptal mitral balloon valvuloplasty. J Am Coll Cardiol 16:1320, 1990.

119. Rao, VD, Cherian, G, Krishnaswami, S, et al: Systemic embolism in rheumatic mitral valve disease. J Assoc Physicians India 27:299, 1979.

120. Hung, JS, Lin, FC, and Chiang, CW: Successful percutaneous transvenous catheter balloon mitral commissurotomy after warfarin therapy and resolution of left atrial thrombus. Am J Cardiol 64:126, 1989.

121. Smith, MD, Wisenbaugh, T, Grayburn, PA, et al: Value and limitations of Doppler pressure half-time in quantifying mitral stenosis: A comparison with micromanometer catheter recordings. Am Heart J 121:480, 1991.

122. Fields, CD, Slovenkai, GA, and Isner, JM: Atrial septal defect resulting from mitral balloon valvuloplasty: Relation of defect morphology to transseptal balloon catheter delivery. Am Heart J 119:568, 1990.

123. Dev, V, Singh, LS, Radhakrishnan, S, et al: Doppler echocardiographic assessment of transmitral

gradients and mitral valve area before and after mitral valve balloon dilatation. Clin Cardiol 12:629, 1989.

124. Come, PC, Riley, MF, Diver, DJ, et al: Noninvasive assessment of mitral stenosis before and after percutaneous balloon mitral valvuloplasty. Am J Cardiol 61:817, 1988.

125. Thomas, JD, Wilkins, GT, Choong, CY, et al: Inaccuracy of mitral pressure half-time immediately after percutaneous mitral valvotomy. Dependence on transmitral gradient and left atrial and ventricular compliance. Circulation 78:980, 1988.

126. Wisenbaugh, T, Berk, M, Essop, R, et al: Effect of mitral regurgitation and volume loading on pressure half-time before and after balloon valvotomy in mitral stenosis. Am J Cardiol 67:162, 1991.

127. Herrmann, HC, Kussmaul, WG, and Hirshfeld, JW, Jr: Single large-balloon percutaneous mitral valvuloplasty. Cathet Cardiovasc Diagn 17:59, 1989.

128. Patel, J, Vythilingum, S, and Mitha, AS: Balloon dilatation of the mitral valve by a single bifoil (2 × 19 mm) or trefoil (3 × 15 mm) catheter. Br Heart J 64:342, 1990.

129. Shim, WH, Jang, YS, Cho, SY, et al: Comparison of outcome among double, bifoil, and Inoue balloon techniques for percutaneous mitral valvuloplasty in severe mitral stenosis (abstract). Circulation 82:III-498, 1990.

130. Bassand, JP, Schiele, F, Bernard, Y, et al: The double balloon technique or the Inoue's technique in percutaneous mitral valvuloplasty: Comparative results in a consecutive series of 200 patients (abstract). Circulation 82:III-80, 1990.

131. Orme, EC, Wray, RB, and Mason, JW: Balloon mitral valvuloplasty via retrograde left atrial catheterization. Am Heart J 117:680, 1989.

132. Buchler, JR, Armelin, E, and Pimentel, WA: Isolated transarterial percutaneous mitral valvuloplasty: The double balloon technique. Int J Cardiol 28:253, 1990.

133. Ballal, RS, Mahan, EF, Nanda, NC, et al: Utility of transesophageal echocardiography in interatrial septal puncture during percutaneous mitral balloon commissurotomy. Am J Cardiol 66:230, 1990.

134. Orihashi, K, Matsuura, Y, Ishihara, H, et al: Transvenous mitral commissurotomy examined with transesophageal echocardiography. Heart Vessels 3:209, 1987.

135. Kronzon, I, Tunick, PA, Schwinger, ME, et al: Transesophageal echocardiography during percutaneous mitral valvuloplasty. J Am Soc Echocardiogr 2:380, 1989.

136. Schoonmaker, FW, Vijay, NK, and Jantz, RD: Left atrial and ventricular transseptal catheterization review: Losing skills. Cathet Cardiovasc Diagn 13:233, 1987.

137. Sheikh, KH, Davidson, CJ, Skelton, TN, et al: Interatrial septal thickening preventing percutaneous mitral valve balloon valvuloplasty. Am Heart J 117:206, 1989.

138. Yoshida, K, Yoshikawa, J, Akasaka, T, et al: Assessment of left-to-right atrial shunting after percutaneous mitral valvuloplasty by transesophageal color Doppler flow-mapping. Circulation 80:1521, 1989.

139. L'Epine, Y, Drobinski, G, Sotirov, Y, et al: Right heart failure due to an inter-atrial shunt after percutaneous mitral balloon dilatation. Eur Heart J 10:285, 1989.

140. Block, PC and Palacios, IF: Aortic and mitral balloon valvuloplasty: The United States experience. In Topol, E (ed): Textbook of Interventional Cardiology. WB Saunders, Philadelphia, 1990, p 845.

141. Vahanian, A, Michel, PL, Cormier, B, et al: Mitral valvuloplasty: The French experience. In Topol, EJ (ed): Textbook of Interventional Cardiology. WB Saunders, Philadelphia, 1990, p 876.

142. Butany, J, D'Amati, G, Charlesworth, D, et al: Fatal left ventricular perforation following balloon mitral valvuloplasty. Can J Cardiol 6:343, 1990.

143. Shawl, FA, Domanski, MJ, Yackee, JM, et al: Left ventricular rupture complicating percutaneous mitral commissurotomy: Salvage using percutaneous cardiopulmonary bypass support. Cathet Cardiovasc Diagn 21:26, 1990.

144. Berland, J, Gerber, L, Gamra, H, et al: Percutaneous balloon valvuloplasty for mitral stenosis complicated by fetal pericardial tamponade in a patient with extreme pulmonary hypertension. Cathet Cardiovasc Diagn 17:109, 1989.

145. Wiegand, V, Tebbe, U, Helmchen, U, et al: Coronary arterial embolism due to valvular debris after percutaneous valvuloplasty of calcific mitral stenosis. Clin Cardiol 11:793, 1988.

146. Dean, LS, Davis, K, Feit, F, et al: Complications and mortality of percutaneous balloon mitral commissurotomy (abstract). Circulation 82:III-545, 1990.

147. Kopecky, SL, Gersh, BJ, McGoon, MD, et al: Long-term outcome of patients undergoing surgical repair of isolated pulmonary valve stenosis. Follow-up at 20–30 years. Circulation 78:1150, 1988.

148. Kan, JS, White, RI, Jr, Mitchell, SE, et al: Percutaneous balloon valvuloplasty: A new method for treating congenital pulmonary-valve stenosis. N Engl J Med 307:540, 1982.

149. Lababidi, Z and Wu, JR: Percutaneous balloon pulmonary valvuloplasty. Am J Cardiol 52:560, 1983.

150. Rao, PS, Thapar, MK, and Kutayli, F: Causes of restenosis after balloon valvuloplasty for valvular pulmonary stenosis. Am J Cardiol 62:979, 1988.

151. Radtke, W, Keane, JF, Fellows, KE, et al: Percutaneous balloon valvotomy of congenital pulmonary stenosis using oversized balloons. J Am Coll Cardiol 8:909, 1986.

152. Nishimura, RA, Holmes, DR, Jr, Reeder, GS, et al: Doppler evaluation of results of percutaneous aortic balloon valvuloplasty in calcific aortic stenosis. Circulation 78:791, 1988.

153. Al Kasab, S, Ribeiro, P, and al Zaibag, M: Use of a double balloon technique for percutaneous balloon pulmonary valvotomy in adults. Br Heart J 58:136, 1987.

154. Mullins, CE, Nihill, MR, Vick, GW III, et al: Double balloon technique for dilatation of valvular or vessel stenosis in congenital and acquired heart disease. J Am Coll Cardiol 10:107, 1987.

155. Stanger, P, Cassidy, SC, Girod, DA, et al: Balloon pulmonary valvuloplasty: Results of the Valvuloplasty and Angioplasty of Congenital Anomalies Registry. Am J Cardiol 65:775, 1990.

156. Pepine, CJ, Gessner, IH, and Feldman, RL: Percutaneous balloon valvuloplasty for pulmonic valve stenosis in the adult. Am J Cardiol 50:1442, 1982.

157. Goudevenos, J, Wren, C, and Adams, PC: Balloon valvotomy of calcified pulmonary valve stenosis. Cardiology 77:55, 1990.

158. Nugent, EW, Freedom, RM, Nora, JJ, et al: Clinical course of pulmonic stenosis. Circulation 56:I-18, 1977.

159. al Zaibag, M, Ribeiro, P, and Al Kasab, S: Percutaneous balloon valvotomy in tricuspid stenosis. Br Heart J 57:51, 1987.

160. Khalilullah, M, Tyagi, S, Yadav, BS, et al: Double-balloon valvuloplasty of tricuspid stenosis. Am Heart J 114:1232, 1987.

161. Goldenberg, IF, Pedersen, W, Olson, J, et al: Percutaneous double balloon valvuloplasty for severe tricuspid stenosis. Am Heart J 118:417, 1989.

162. Ribeiro, PA, al Zaibag, M, Al Kasab, S, et al: Percutaneous double balloon valvotomy for rheumatic tricuspid stenosis. Am J Cardiol 61:660, 1988.

163. Ribeiro, PA, al Zaibag, M, and Sawyer, W: The value and extent of valve area increase by balloon dilatation of the stenosed bioprosthesis: In vitro studies. Rev Port Cardiol 8:515, 1989.

164. Feit, F, Stecy, PJ, and Nachamie, MS: Percutaneous balloon valvuloplasty for stenosis of a porcine bioprosthesis in the tricuspid valve position. Am J Cardiol 58:363, 1986.

165. Chow, WH, Cheung, KL, Tai, YT, et al: Successful percutaneous balloon valvuloplasty of a stenotic tricuspid bioprosthesis. Am Heart J 119:666, 1990.

166. Wren, C and Hunter, S: Balloon dilatation of a stenosed bioprosthesis in the tricuspid valve position. Br Heart J 61:65, 1989.

167. Benedick, BA, Davis, SF, and Alderman, E: Balloon valvuloplasty for fungal endocarditis induced stenosis of a bioprosthetic tricuspid valve. Cathet Cardiovasc Diagn 21:248, 1990.

168. Attubato, MJ, Stroh, JA, Bach, RG, et al: Percutaneous double-balloon valvuloplasty of porcine bioprosthetic valves in the tricuspid position. Cathet Cardiovasc Diagn 20:202, 1990.

169. Arie, S, Arato Goncalves, MT, Rati, MA, et al: Balloon dilatation of a stenotic dura mater mitral bioprothesis. Am Heart J 117:201, 1989.

170. Calvo, OL, Sobrino, N, Gamallo, C, et al: Balloon percutaneous valvuloplasty for stenotic bioprosthetic valves in the mitral position. Am J Cardiol 60:736, 1987.

171. Fernandez, JJ, DeSando, CJ, Leff, RA, et al: Percutaneous balloon valvuloplasty of a stenosed mitral bioprosthesis. Cathet Cardiovasc Diagn 19:39, 1990.

172. Cox, DA, Friedman, PL, Selwyn, AP, et al: Improved quality of life after successful balloon valvuloplasty of a stenosed mitral bioprosthesis. Am Heart J 118:839, 1989.

173. Ramondo, A, Gemelli, M, and Chioin, R: Balloon dilatation of a porcine bioprosthetic valve in aortic position. Int J Cardiol 24:105, 1989.

174. Waldman, JD, Schoen, FJ, Kirkpatrick, SE, et al: Balloon dilatation of porcine bioprosthetic valves in the pulmonary position. Circulation 76:109, 1987.

175. Ensing, GJ, Hagler, DJ, Seward, JB, et al: Caveats of balloon dilation of conduits and conduit valves. J Am Coll Cardiol 14:397, 1989.

176. Zeevi, B, Keane, JF, Perry, SB, et al: Balloon dilation of postoperative right ventricular outflow obstructions. J Am Coll Cardiol 14:401, 1989.

177. McKay, CR, Waller, BF, Hong, R, et al: Problems encountered with catheter balloon valvuloplasty of bioprosthetic aortic valves. Am Heart J 115:463, 1988.

178. Babic, UU, Grujicic, S, and Vucinic, M: Balloon valvoplasty of mitral bioprosthesis. Int J Cardiol 30:230, 1991.
179. Kritzer, GL, Block, PC, and Palacios, I: Simultaneous percutaneous mitral and aortic balloon valvotomies in an elderly patient. Am Heart J 114:420, 1987.
180. Berman, AD, Weinstein, JS, Safian, RD, et al: Combined aortic and mitral balloon valvuloplasty in patients with critical aortic and mitral valve stenosis: Results in six cases. J Am Coll Cardiol 11:1213, 1988.
181. Medina, A, Bethencourt, A, Coello, I, et al: Combined percutaneous mitral and aortic balloon valvuloplasty. Am J Cardiol 64:620, 1989.
182. Shrivastava, S, Radhakrishnan, S, and Dev, V: Concurrent balloon dilatation of tricuspid and calcific mitral valve in a patient of rheumatic heart disease. Int J Cardiol 20:133, 1988.
183. Bethencourt, A, Medina, A, Hernandez, E, et al: Combined percutaneous balloon valvuloplasty of mitral and tricuspid valves. Am Heart J 119:416, 1990.
184. Chen, CR, Lo, ZX, Huang, ZD, et al: Concurrent percutaneous balloon valvuloplasty for combined tricuspid and pulmonic stenoses. Cathet Cardiovasc Diagn 15:55, 1988.
185. Konugres, GS, Lau, FY, and Ruiz, CE: Successive percutaneous double-balloon mitral, aortic, and tricuspid valvotomy in rheumatic trivalvular stenoses. Am Heart J 119:663, 1990.
186. Lewin, RF, Raff, H, Findling, JW, et al: Stimulation of atrial natriuretic peptide and vasopressin during retrograde mitral valvuloplasty. Am Heart J 120:1305, 1990.
187. Waldman, HM, Palacios, IF, Block, PC, et al: Responsiveness of plasma atrial natriuretic factor to short-term changes in left atrial hemodynamics after percutaneous balloon mitral valvuloplasty. J Am Coll Cardiol 12:649, 1988.
188. Tsai, RC, Yamaji, T, Ishibashi, M, et al: Atrial natriuretic peptide and vasopressin during percutaneous transvenous mitral valvuloplasty and relation to renin-angiotensin-aldosterone system and renal function. Am J Cardiol 65:882, 1990.
189. Roberts, WC: India and Indian cardiology. Am J Cardiol 62:1326, 1988.
190. Turi, ZG: Percutaneous balloon mitral valvuloplasty. Cardiac Chronicle 4:1, 1990.
191. Wilkins, GT, Weyman, AE, Abascal, VM, et al: Percutaneous balloon dilatation of the mitral valve: An analysis of echocardiographic variables related to outcome and the mechanism of dilatation. Br Heart J 60:299, 1988.
192. Rao, PS, Thapar, MK, Wilson, AD, et al: Intermediate-term follow-up results of balloon aortic valvuloplasty in infants and children with special reference to causes of restenosis. Am J Cardiol 64:1356, 1989.
193. Dev, V and Shrivastava, S: Time course of changes in pulmonary vascular resistance and the mechanism of regression of pulmonary arterial hypertension after balloon mitral valvuloplasty. Am J Cardiol 67:439, 1991.
194. Holmes, DR, Jr., Nishimura, RA, and Reeder, GS: In-hospital mortality after balloon aortic valvuloplasty: Frequency and associated factors. J Am Coll Cardiol 17:189, 1991.
195. Cribier, A, Berland, J, Koning, R, et al: Percutaneous transluminal aortic valvuloplasty: Indications and results in adult aortic stenosis. Eur Heart J 9:149, 1988.
196. Ruiz, CE, Allen, JW, and Lau, FY: Percutaneous double balloon valvotomy for severe rheumatic mitral stenosis. Am J Cardiol 65:473, 1990.

Index